Genetics of Diabetes Mellitus

ENDOCRINE UPDATES

Shlomo Melmed, M.D., Series Editor

---

1. E.R. Levin and J.L. Nadler (eds.): Endocrinology of Cardiovascular Function. 1998. ISBN: 0-7923-8217-X
2. J.A. Fagin (ed.): Thyroid Cancer. 1998. ISBN: 0-7923-8326-5
3. J.S. Adams and B.P. Lukert (eds.): Osteoporosis: Genetics, Prevention and Treatment. 1998. ISBN: 0-7923-8366-4.
4. B.-Å. Bengtsson (ed.): Growth Hormone. 1999. ISBN: 0-7923-8478-4
5. C. Wang (ed.): Male Reproductive Function. 1999. ISBN 0-7923-8520-9
6. B. Rapoport and S.M. McLachlan (eds.): Graves' Disease: Pathogenesis and Treatment. 2000. ISBN: 0-7923-7790-7.
7. W. W. de Herder (ed.): Functional and Morphological Imaging of the Endocrine System. 2000. ISBN 0-7923-7923-9
8. H.G. Burger (ed.): Sex Hormone Replacement Therapy. 2001. ISBN 0-7923-7965-9
9. A. Giustina (ed.): Growth Hormone and the Heart. 2001. ISBN 0-7923-7212-3
10. W.L. Lowe, Jr. (ed.): Genetics of Diabetes Mellitus. 2001. ISBN 0-7923-7252-2

Genetics of Diabetes Mellitus

edited by

William L. Lowe, Jr., M.D.

Northwestern University Medical School
Chicago, Illinois, USA

KLUWER ACADEMIC PUBLISHERS
BOSTON/DORDRECHT/LONDON

Distributors for North, Central and South America:
Kluwer Academic Publishers
101 Philip Drive
Assinippi Park
Norwell, Massachusetts 02061 USA
Telephone (781) 871-6600
Fax (781) 681-9045
E-Mail <kluwer@wkap.com>

Distributors for all other countries:
Kluwer Academic Publishers Group
Distribution Centre
Post Office Box 322
3300 AH Dordrecht, THE NETHERLANDS
Telephone 31 78 6392 392
Fax 31 78 6392 254
E-Mail <services@wkap.nl>

Electronic Services <http://www.wkap.nl>

Library of Congress Cataloging-in-Publication Data

Genetics of diabetes mellitus / edited by William L. Lowe, Jr.
p. ; cm. -- (Endocrine updates ; 10)
Includes bibliographical references and index.
ISBN 0-7923-7252-2 (hardback : alk. paper)
1. Diabetes--Genetic aspects. I. Lowe, William L., 1954- II. Series.
[DNLM: 1. Diabetes Mellitus--genetics. WK 810 G3293 2001]
RC660 .G432 2001
616.4'62042--dc21

00-048767

Printed on acid-free paper.

Printed in the United States of America

The Publisher offers discounts on this book for course use and bulk purchases. For further information, send email to <barbara.murphy@wkap.com>.

TABLE OF CONTENTS

LIST OF CONTRIBUTORS

DOMENICO ACCILI, Department of Medicine, Columbia University, New York, NY 10032

JOSEPH AVRUCH, Diabetes Unit and Department of Molecular Biology, Massachusetts General Hospital, Boston, MA 02114

MATTHIAS F. BAUER, Institute of Diabetes Research of the Academic Hospital Munich-Schwabing, D-80804 Munich, GERMANY

PAMELA R. FAIN, Barbara Davis Center for Childhood Diabetes, University of Colorado Health Sciences Center, Denver, CO 80262 USA

GEORGE S. EISENBARTH, Barbara Davis Center for Childhood Diabetes, University of Colorado Health Sciences Center, Denver, CO 80262 USA

PHILIPPE FROGUEL, Queen Mary and Westfield College Genomic Center, University of London, London, UK

KLAUS-DIETER GERBITZ, Institute of Diabetes Research of the Academic Hospital Munich-Schwabing, D-80804 Munich, GERMANY

SOUMITRA GHOSH, Max McGee National Research Center for Juvenile Diabetes, Medical College of Wisconsin, Milwaukee, WI 53226

SABINE HOFMANN, Institute of Diabetes Research of the Academic Hospital Munich-Schwabing, D-80804 Munich, GERMANY

WEN-CHI HSUEH, Department of Genetics, Southwest Foundation for Biomedical Research, San Antonio, TX 78227

STEVEN E. KAHN, University of Washington and VA Puget Sound Health Care System,Seattle, WA 98108

WILLIAM L. LOWE, JR., Center for Endocrinology, Metabolism, and Molecular Medicine, Northwestern University Medical School, Chicago, IL 60611

BRAXTON D. MITCHELL, Department of Genetics, Southwest Foundation for Biomedical Research, San Antonio, TX 78227

STEPHEN H. NYE, Max McGee National Research Center for Juvenile Diabetes, Medical College of Wisconsin, Milwaukee, WI 53226

BYUNG-CHUL PARK, Department of Medicine, Columbia University, New York, NY 10032

ALBERTO PUGLIESE, Diabetes Research Institute, University of Miami School of Medicine, Florida 33136

CONSTANTIN POLYCHRONAKOS, Children's Hospital Research Institute and the Department of Pediatrics, McGill University, Quebec, CANADA H3H 1P3

ALAN R. SHULDINER, Department of Medicine, University of Maryland School of Medicine, Baltimore, MD 21201

GILBERTO VELHO, INSERM U342, Institut Cochin de Génétique Moléculaire, Paris, FRANCE

JOSEP VIDAL, University of Washington and VA Puget Sound Health Care System,Seattle, WA 98108

1
GENETICS OF COMPLEX DISEASES

Steven H. Nye, Ph.D.
Soumitra Ghosh, M.D., Ph.D.
Max McGee National Research Center for Juvenile Diabetes
Medical College of Wisconsin, Milwaukee, WI 53226 USA

INTRODUCTION

In recent years, the emphasis in the field of human disease gene mapping has shifted towards the isolation of genes involved in complex diseases. Complex diseases are characterized as those traits that run in families and are commonly found in the population, but do not exhibit a simple mode of inheritance. They are often referred to as multifactorial because evidence suggests that complex diseases are caused by more than one gene, likely in combination with environmental factors. Screening efforts to identify genes for complex diseases appear complicated when considering that the risk for developing these disorders may depend on a particular combination of susceptibility alleles in many unlinked genes, with the effect of a single locus being small. Recent reports have described efforts to identify genes for multiple sclerosis (1-4), rheumatoid arthritis (5) and obesity (6-9). Other than the insulin gene for type 1 diabetes (10-13) and apolipoprotein E for late-onset Alzheimer's disease (14-16), few genes have been confirmed to have a functional role in the etiology of complex human disease. However, newer developments in molecular methodologies make the prospects of finding complex disease genes more likely.

In this review, we update the progress being made, and describe the tools employed in genetic studies of type 1 and type 2 diabetes. We also describe gene and protein expression profiling technologies that will advance our understanding of the genetic basis of complex human diseases. The Human Genome Project will soon provide complete genome sequence overlaid with a highly dense marker set of single nucleotide polymorphisms (SNPs). This will enable placement of all genes and markers in regions of linkage on the human genetic map providing additional power for candidate gene and allelic association studies.

BOTH GENES AND ENVIRONMENTAL FACTORS CONTRIBUTE TO COMPLEX DISEASE

Measurements of familial aggregation for a trait must take into account the genetic relationship between individuals, the number of family members, the disease frequency in the population, and the genetic model for the disease. However, families may share predisposing environments as well as genes acting either alone or in concert together. Therefore, by itself familial aggregation is insufficient evidence to assume that its etiology is entirely genetic (17).

Evidence for Genetic Components in Complex Diseases

Concordance rate for a trait is defined as the proportion of affected twins that have affected co-twins. By estimating and comparing the phenotypic concordance amongst monozygotic (MZ) and dizygotic (DZ) twins, one can measure the relative importance of genes versus the environment. It has been noted that studies for autism (18), attention deficit hyperactivity disorder (19) and multiple sclerosis (20) suggest major roles for genetic factors (17). Yet, twin studies require careful interpretation because sample size is often limited and they are subject to inaccurate assumptions and ascertainment bias (21). In addition, twins typically share the same family environment early in life, confounding the contributions of environmental and genetic influences. Therefore, studying twins reared apart is important for distinguishing genetic effects from those due to a common environment (22). While adoption studies may be biased by selective placement of individuals, a role for genetic factors in the etiology of alcoholism (23) and obesity (24) has been supported by these studies. At best though, twin studies merely provide evidence for the extent of genetic determination, but do not prove genetic susceptibility (25).

Twin studies have contributed to defining the genetic component for both type 1 and type 2 diabetes. The proband concordance rate (defined as 2C/(2C+D) where C is the number of pairs with both twins affected and D is the number of pairs with one twin affected) measured in a type 1 diabetes study was 53% for MZ twin pairs compared to 11% for DZ twin pairs, indicating that a significant genetic component exists (26). For type 2 diabetes, the MZ proband concordance rate (58%) has also been reported to be significantly higher than the DZ rate (17%) (27). One exception has been the recent, population-based study of Danish twin pairs where the probandwise concordance estimate for MZ twins was higher (~50%), but not significantly different from the DZ estimate (~37%) (28). However, when impaired glucose tolerance was studied and those with diabetes included, the difference reached statistical significance (~63% vrs. ~43%; $p<0.01$).

Since concordance rates are not easy to establish and require careful epidemiologic studies, a related approach to verify that the disease has a familial component is to estimate the risk-to-relative ratio for a relative of type R, termed λ_R (29). This ratio is defined as the risk to relative of a proband divided by the population prevalence and it is a measure of the extent of familiality for a discrete trait. Again, one has to be cautious because biases can be introduced (30). For type 1 diabetes, the population prevalence is 0.4%, but the risk to siblings of affected individuals is 6%, resulting in λ_S of 15.0 (31). The λ_S value for type 2 diabetes (approximately 3.5) is dependent on the population under study (32). It is also possible to quantify the size of a specific gene effect by assigning a locus-specific λ (31). Locus-specific risk ratios may be obtained from allele-sharing data observed at a given marker locus, which is assumed tightly linked with a disease locus (22).

Evidence for environmental components in complex diseases

Multiple environmental factors are often cited as possible triggers in a complex disease, thereby making it difficult to prove which one(s) is the primary causative agent(s). For example, important components considered in the pathogenesis of asthma are breast-feeding, diet, viral respiratory infections in early childhood, exposure to allergens and parental smoking (33, 34). Environmental factors can also confuse efforts to map disease genes by creating phenocopies. Phenocopies are those individuals who are affected, but not due to genetic predisposition. Rather, they develop a disease because of some unspecified environmental factor(s) or the phenotype is due to genes at other locations (22). Proper identification of phenocopies is key to mapping disease genes because misclassification of the disease state will reduce evidence for linkage.

For type 1 diabetes, a variety of factors that may accelerate the pathogenic process (such as climate, stress and infections) have been proposed (35). Recently, two prospective reports showed the role that viruses may play in initiating the disease in children. One group analyzed serum of high-risk individuals collected periodically after birth, and found association between the incidence of rotavirus infection (a common cause of childhood gastroenteritis) and levels of type 1 autoantibodies (36). A second study of Finnish children followed the development of both type 1 autoantibodies and enteroviral specific antibodies every 3-12 months following birth (37). Prior to the appearance of type 1 autoantibodies, more at-risk children were found to have enteroviral infections compared to controls, suggesting that a temporal relationship exists between viral infection and the induction of autoimmunity. However, due to the high prevalence of common viral infections found in the population, it may be difficult to prove whether a virus is a true causative agent in complex disease. A long-standing debate still resides over the effect of cow's milk for developing type 1 diabetes in humans. Lack of passively-transferred maternal immunity, molecular mimicry with GAD65 epitopes and impaired mucosal immunity have been suggested as a plausible mechanism for this autoimmunity along with the association of HLA type (38). However, these risk factors alone do not explain the vast majority of type 1 diabetes cases.

Environmental factors also influence the incidence of type 2 diabetes. Rapid changes in lifestyle (such as moving from a rural to an urban environment) that may significantly alter diet or physical activity have been studied in migrant populations. Increases in disease prevalence with Westernization have been found in diverse populations including Japanese immigrants to the United States and some Native American populations (39). Changes in prevalence for type 2 diabetes have also been studied within a population. For example, a 40% increase in the age-adjusted prevalence rate was measured within the Pima Indians for a 10-year period. Interestingly, 30 years earlier the prevalence of diabetes in the Pima Indian population was similar to that of the general population (40). The large increase in disease occurrence in this short period further exemplifies the role that environmental factors can play in complex disease. Some studies suggest that the intrauterine environment has a long-range effect on the likelihood of developing type 2 diabetes at an early age (41). But similar to type 1 diabetes, it is difficult to convincingly prove the relative contribution of any single environmental factor in the etiology of type 2 diabetes.

One the most important advances in complex disease genetics in the next few years will be the study of gene-environmental interactions. Recent developments in statistical methodology now make this possible (42-44).

LINKAGE ANALYSIS PRINCIPLES FOR POSITIONAL CLONING

Positional cloning methods try to establish whether a specific marker is linked to a gene underlying the disease of interest. This is a powerful strategy to localize a gene responsible for a trait because it assumes no prior knowledge of the pathways involved in a disease process, but merely tries to identify the genes that are responsible. Using tools like linkage analysis, linkage disequilibrium, physical mapping, sequence analysis and mutation detection, genes for over 100 monogenic diseases have been isolated. Examples include genes for cystic fibrosis, Huntington's disease and Duchenne muscular dystrophy (45).

Linkage Analysis of Monogenic Diseases

Finding the causative gene for a monogenic disease is easier since these are rare, highly penetrant disorders that follow a Mendelian inheritance pattern. Linkage analysis methods for monogenic diseases first require specifying a model. In the model, the mode of inheritance (e.g., dominant, recessive, sex-linked), allele frequency (for both disease and marker), recombination fraction and penetrance (probability of disease, given a genotype) are all considered. Next, co-segregation of markers with the disease gene is measured. In principle, if a marker locus is linked to the disease gene, then a particular allele at the marker locus is likely to segregate with the disease within a family. In an unrelated family, a different allele from the same marker may segregate with the disease gene. The marker loci chosen are ideally polymorphic thereby enabling the inheritance of the four grandparental chromosomes (in informative meioses) to be tracked. The most commonly used markers are microsatellites, which are short, tandemly repeated sequences that are easily amplified by PCR and found widely dispersed throughout the genome. For multiple linkage analysis, information is gathered from multiple linked markers thereby increasing power and reducing the false-positive rate (46).

The extent of linkage is measured by formulating a LOD score (47), which is the logarithm (base 10) of the likelihood (or probability) ratio comparing the hypothesis of linkage with the hypothesis of free recombination. The recombination fraction (θ) refers to the probability that a gamete produced by a parent is a recombinant between two loci (in this case, the marker locus and the disease gene). The closer the marker is to the disease gene, the greater the extent of co-segregation (smaller θ) and the bigger the LOD score. A LOD score of 3 (1,000:1 odds for linkage) is the conventional cutoff point above which the significance of a linkage is declared. Genetic distance is measured in centiMorgans (cM), where 1 cM is the distance between two loci that on average shows 1% recombination during meiosis. This translates to approximately 1,000,000 base pairs of DNA across the genome. Maps with an average resolution of approximately 1 cM are available and genotyping of these markers has become routine (48, 49).

Physical mapping begins after a candidate region for a gene is located. The traditional path has been to utilize yeast artificial chromosomes (YACs), P1 artificial clones (PACs), bacterial artificial chromosomes (BACs) and radiation hybrid mapping to integrate genetic and physical maps by use of STSs (sequence tagged sites). The accurate assembly of clones into an ordered contig usually requires significant depth of clone coverage (6-10 fold recommended) and restriction-digest fingerprinting (to verify extent of overlap and to detect deletions/rearrangements) (50). Chromosome walking (used to isolate sequentially overlapping genomic clones) is undertaken to close any gaps in the physical map. For this purpose, end sequencing of large clones has now become extremely efficient (51). Genomic sequence sampling is then carried out to develop a high-resolution sequence-based physical map, generate more STSs and polymorphic markers, and to identify genes (52, 53). The method relies on first-pass sequencing of ends of clones (resulting in approximately 30-50% of complete DNA sequencing of the contig) and provides a bridge towards the eventual isolation of a disease gene.

However, the Human Genome Project will soon make many of these methods unnecessary. Rather, positional cloning, by fully sequencing a region under investigation and using computational tools to find functional sites that encode elements responsible for gene structure, regulation and transcription, is rapidly becoming the method of choice. As a final step in identifying a disease gene, it is necessary to demonstrate that a mutation appears only in affected individuals and not in unrelated controls. In a monogenic disorder, the presence of the mutation typically correlates with the disease making functional studies initially less critical. However, this is not so for complex disorders, where functional studies are often essential in the accurate identification of the disease variant.

Positional cloning is easier in forms of common disease that show evidence for major gene segregation. Thus, the genetic study of a simpler, single-gene trait that resembles a multifactorial disorder may offer valuable insight into distinct parts of the whole disease. One example is maturity onset diabetes of the young (MODY). MODY is a rare, monogenic form of the disease that accounts for approximately 1-5% of diabetic cases, depending on the population. MODY has an autosomal dominant mode of inheritance and an earlier age-of-onset compared with common type 2 diabetes. This makes it is possible to collect large multigenerational MODY pedigrees, a feature of this subtype (54). At least six different genes (MODY 1-6), located on chromosomes 20 (hepatocyte nuclear factor-4α or *HNF-4α*), 7 (glucokinase), 12 (*HNF-1α*), 13 (insulin promoter factor-1 or *IPF-1*), 17 (*HNF-1β*) and 2 (NeuroD1) independently cause MODY within single pedigrees (55-60). At present, it appears that MODY genes play a minor role in common type 2 diabetes (61).

Linkage Analysis of Multifactorial Diseases

While positional cloning efforts have isolated genes responsible for monogenic diseases, the same is not true for complex traits like hypertension, multiple sclerosis and type 1 and type 2 diabetes. This is primarily because the inheritance patterns for complex diseases do not fit any simple genetic model, making it far more difficult to map underlying loci. Thus far, most complex disease studies have been candidate gene analyses, where linkage information is not taken into account. Functional candidate gene approaches require that some basic information is known about the biochemical defect of the trait. The goal is to identify a candidate molecule in order to study the association between sequence variants and the phenotype of interest. However, one could create a long list of plausible candidate genes for many complex diseases, making it too impractical to carry out a thorough molecular genetic analysis for each gene.

Because of this and limited understanding of the exact pathogenesis for complex diseases, many investigators have turned to genome-wide analysis. In a genome-wide scan, microsatellite markers covering the entire genome are used to detect areas of linkage. Current genotyping and analysis methods are robust and have been successfully used to isolate genes for monogenic disorders. However, it may not be possible to evaluate the effects of each and every locus determining a complex disease with this technology (62). In addition, while a genome-wide scan for a monogenic disease gene is essentially completed when linkage is found, data from the entire genome must be considered in order to assess the relative significance of a candidate region for multifactorial diseases.

Statistical tools for gene mapping involving complex traits should make minimal assumptions and model-independent (nonparametric) approaches are of primary importance in the analysis of a complex disease. However, standard linkage analysis can be relatively robust to model misspecification in certain situations (63) and in applicable cases, is more powerful than a model-independent method. Therefore, it is advisable to consider both approaches in any one study. The most common model-independent approach makes use of affected relatives and assesses sharing of genes using identity-by-descent (IBD) information. In affected relative-pair analysis, no logistical problems arise because of incomplete penetrance or absent environmental triggers since only affected individuals are studied. Parental genotype information is required in IBD-based methods for affected sib pairs (ASP). In the absence of parents, pedigree-based allele frequency estimates may be used to infer IBD probabilistically (64-67). The ultimate aim is to look for skewing in the distribution of allele sharing from the expected proportions of 0.25:0.50:0.25 for affected sib pairs sharing 0, 1 or 2 genes IBD. A significant distortion from this ratio with a decrease in sibs sharing zero alleles IBD (and an increase in sibs sharing two alleles IBD) suggests that the marker is linked to a disease locus. A LOD score can also be formulated comparing the most likely estimates for allele sharing, given nuclear family structure, with the null hypothesis expected under Mendelian segregation ratios (64, 65).

Theoretical calculations show that to detect a single locus that has a λ_s of 1.6 with 90% power would require 300 affected sib pairs provided that heterozygosity of the marker is 1 (perfect information) and the map consists of markers every cM (64, 65). If markers are spaced every 5 cM the power drops to 70%. Therefore, more than 300 sib pairs are required to detect linkage to type 2 diabetes with adequate power, where a single locus may have, at best, a locus-specific λ_s value of 1.6. The markers are less than 100% informative and density of maps used for a genome scan rarely have an average resolution of less than 10 cM. Where multiple genes are thought to be acting, it is reasonable to perform linkage analysis on multiple unlinked loci simultaneously. Thus, regions from the initial linkage scan with interesting signals could be analyzed together as a second tier approach. There are several methods of statistical modeling in the presence of multiple unlinked disease loci and both model-based approaches and those that make fewer assumptions have been explored. In nearly all cases, multi-trait-locus linkage analysis has been shown to be more powerful than single-trait-locus analysis (68-71).

PHENOTYPES

In this discussion we use the term trait and phenotype interchangeably. The phenotype for a study must be clearly and accurately defined, since misclassification will reduce power in any genetic analysis. Clinical end points for disease (e.g. diabetes, high blood pressure) are not necessarily always the best genetic traits to analyze. In fact, there may be a more homogenous subgroup of individuals in whom a genetic mechanism is clearly apparent. For example, in a sample with a younger age-of-onset for a specific disease, the λ_R may be increased, as compared to the whole group. Ideally, the stratification will define a trait, which is influenced by fewer loci, each with a bigger individual effect. Thus, if the underlying cause for increased λ_R is genetic, the power to detect a locus per family unit will be increased. This process of stratification requires close collaboration between clinical and genetics experts along with an element of luck as it is difficult a priori to think of an appropriate stratification variable.

A chronic disease process often has many stages with intermediate phenotypes. For example, impaired glucose tolerance and fasting hyperglycemia are clearly defined states prior to diabetes (72). In addition, there are several clinical measurements that are purely quantitative in nature, such as blood pressure or cholesterol levels. Very high levels of these traits are associated with clinical complications. All of these phenotypes can be analyzed by quantitative trait locus (QTL) linkage analysis, if the underlying variation has a strong genetic component. In QTL analysis, investigators look for an inverse relationship between the IBD status at a locus of two related individuals and their difference in quantitative trait values. For example, if two sibs are sharing a chromosomal region (high sharing) and both have either high or low trait values (meaning a small overall trait difference), then this contributes to the evidence for linkage (46, 73). As in all genetic analyses, where the relationship between genetic variation and a phenotype is being sought, it is important to eliminate other confounding influences and to get a measure of a more homogenous, informative trait. Thus, simple analysis of insulin levels (affected also by antibody assay and liver metabolism) and glucose levels (affected also by levels of food intake, medication, and numerous metabolic pathways) could be complemented by better measures of beta cell function and insulin resistance, under stricter control of external influences (74, 75). Considering loss of information through categorizing of discrete trait data and the impact of diabetes on both insulin resistance and beta-cell function (76), several groups have endeavored to study at-risk unaffected individuals for other heritable, predictive quantitative traits such as insulin resistance (77-82).

In the future, better ways to classify type 2 diabetes phenotypes will become available when more discriminatory molecules for disease detection are discovered.

RESULTS OF GENOME-WIDE STUDIES FOR COMPLEX DISEASE

Type1 diabetes was the first complex disorder to be studied by genome-wide screening of affected sib-pair families with initial studies suggesting approximately 20 regions with evidence for linkage (83-85). These findings were followed up by a study including an additional 263 multiplex families (total of 356 ASP families using 348 microsatellite markers) (86). Four regions outside of the major locus *IDDM1*/MHC (multipoint maximum LOD score (MLS) =34, $p<1x10^{-6}$) were not excluded at λ_s =3 and LOD=-2, including *IDDM10* (10p13-q11; MLS=4.7, $p=3x10^{-6}$) and a novel region at markers D16S515-D16S520 (16q22-24; MLS=3.4, $p=6.5x10^{-5}$). Fourteen other regions outside of *IDDM1* and *IDDM2*/INS (MLS=2.8, $p=2.7x10^{-4}$) had MLS greater than or equal to 1.5. A different group performed a second-generation screen with 467 ASPs on all 22 autosomes using 438 markers (87). A region located on chromosome 1q at marker D1S1617 was found to have a significant LOD score (MLS=3.31), in addition to the well-characterized *IDDM1* (MLS=32.5). The second study generally did not replicate the first screen results illustrating a common phenomenon in many genome-wide scan studies (88).

Many groups have now completed genome scans for type 2 diabetes. Genome-wide significance was reported on chromosome 2q37 with a combined data set of 440 Mexican-American ASP families (MLS for the locus known as NIDDM1 is 4.10; $p<10^{-4}$) (89). A second genome scan in a different Mexican-American population and scans in several Caucasian populations failed to detect significant evidence for linkage on 2q37 (90-94). However, a special form of a two-locus approach was used to increase the power to detect a disease locus and to narrow down the confidence interval thought to contain the susceptibility gene, NIDDM1 (95). This method makes few prior assumptions and is based on the correlation between linkage results at two unlinked loci in sets of independent families. By looking only at families who have a significant correlation (in their case, a positive correlation signifying epistasis between chromosomes 2 and 15), they were able to increase a single locus MLS from 4 to 7 and considerably narrow down the confidence interval containing the susceptibility locus (95).

In a sample from Botnia, Western Finland, six selected pedigrees with the lowest quartile for mean 30 minute insulin levels following oral glucose tolerance tests (OGTT) showed significant evidence for linkage to type 2 diabetes on chromosome 12q (locus known as NIDDM2 with MLS=3.65, p=2x10^{-5}), near the MODY3 locus (96). The overall data set of 26 families showed no strong evidence for linkage. More recently, evidence for linkage was obtained on chromosome 11q for both age-adjusted diabetes (MLS=1.7, p=0.003) and body mass index (MLS=3.6, p=2.6 x 10^{-5}) in 264 Pima Indian families (97). Bivariate analysis (analysis of both diabetes and body mass index) gave a MLS of 5.0 (two-tailed p value=1.8x10^{-6}). Genetic correlation analysis confirmed that the same locus seemed to affect both diabetes and BMI. An additional strong signal was seen on chromosome 1q (multipoint LOD score 4.10, p< 10^{-6}) in affected sib pairs (n=55) with age of onset less than 25 years.

In the Genetics of NIDDM (GENNID) study, 1,783 individuals from four distinct ethnic groups (white, Mexican American, black and Japanese) were ascertained, diagnosed and genotyped for type 2 diabetes (98). Individuals were sampled from outbred populations at multiple centers throughout the United States with linkage limited to two phenotypes, either diabetes or "impaired glucose homeostasis". Multipoint, nonparametric linkage analysis found five significant regions (p<.001) ranging from LOD scores of 1.38 to 3.91.

The Finland-US Investigation of NIDDM (FUSION) study has completed a genome scan at an average resolution of 8 cM for type 2 diabetes susceptibility genes in 719 affected sib pairs. The best evidence for linkage to diabetes is on chromosome 20 with potentially separable peaks located on both the long and short arms. The weighted MLSs were 2.15 at 69.5 cM from pter and secondary MLS peaks of 2.04 at 56.5 cM and 1.99 at 17.5 cM. At least three other groups had previously reported similar results on 20q for type 2 diabetes in Caucasians of European descent (99-101). This level of replication is reassuring and is quite rare in studies of complex disease. All groups are now fine mapping the regions for eventual positional cloning and the MODY 1 gene (present in this region) has been excluded. Other regions of interest in the FUSION scan include a MLS of 1.75 for diabetes at 84 cM on chromosome 11 (Ghosh et al., ms submitted). Quantitative trait analysis has also revealed MLSs of 3.11 at 21 cM on chromosome 10 for acute insulin response and 3.20 at 9 cM on chromosome 17 for fasting insulin/fasting glucose. These were in unaffected individuals in families with type 2 diabetes (Watanabe et al., ms submitted).

In conclusion, genome-wide scanning studies have pointed towards many interesting regions of linkage for type 1 and type 2 diabetes. But, only a few of these regions have been confirmed by replication studies.

FINE MAPPING USING LINKAGE DISEQUILIBRIUM AND SNPs

Linkage equilibrium is said to exist when the haplotype frequency equals the product of individual population allele frequencies for adjacent loci. Disequilibrium exists when this is not so. This definition can be extended to a disease locus and a nearby marker. If linkage disequilibrium exists, specific alleles at markers are said to be in association with the disease gene at the population level. Linkage disequilibrium mapping seeks to enhance the resolution that is gained by linkage analysis and has proved to be helpful in the positional cloning of a number of disease genes (102-106). Information from meiotic events throughout many generations is evaluated under the assumption that the disease mutation occurred in one individual as a founder effect. One method of detecting population association is to study two groups of people, cases and controls. Some investigators have used intrafamily methods of association to reduce the chances of spurious associations, due for example to ethnic differences between the affected (case) population and the control population. For example, the transmission disequilibrium test (TDT) seeks to detect association in the presence of linkage and measures the extent of the segregation distortion of specific allele transmission from heterozygous parents to affected offspring (107).

Since linkage disequilibrium is often not a monotonic function of physical distance, it is necessary to understand the factors that influence the relationship. Besides recombination over many generations and differences in allele frequencies at marker and disease loci, admixture (defined as the proportion of genes that have ancestry from the high-risk population), selection, mutation (both at the disease and marker locus) and drift (fixation or loss of an allele due to stochastic behavior in small populations) all affect this relationship. Something may be known about these factors beforehand (e.g. admixture in the sample and mutation rates for markers), but others are, at best, somewhat unpredictable.

An approach that is gaining popularity is to conduct whole genome association studies (108-111). Association analysis has been suggested to be more powerful than linkage analysis in detecting genes with moderate to weak effect (111, 112). However, there are many preconditions before this can be considered to be true, the principal being that there should exist one (through a founder effect), or at most, a limited number of disease variants at the given locus. In order for whole-genome linkage disequilibrium analysis to be successful there needs to be significant disequilibrium over distances which can be adequately covered by SNPs. Recent studies have looked at the density of SNPs in and around disease genes and across disease populations (113-115). The lipoprotein lipase gene was sequenced across 9700 base pairs in over 20 individuals from three ethnic groups. 88 SNPs were identified and in 34 sites, variation was found in only one population. There were 88 haplotypes in this region and these could be clustered into two ancient ancestral groups. In addition, for 64% of adjacently paired SNPs, all four gametes were present reflecting a rich history of past recombination. Pairwise disequilibrium between SNPs was also present, but very often its extent was not related to physical distance (113, 115). If these findings are typical of most genes, then a large number of SNPs will need to be typed in order to capture the information present in the genome when using common populations.

To address this issue, a population simulation study determined that an average distance of roughly 3kb on either side of a locus will be useful for linkage equilibrium, corresponding to about 500,00 SNPs required for whole-genome association studies in samples from large outbred populations (116). This study has generated intense debate mainly because the simulations were performed assuming a continuously expanding population (117). A different study calculated extent of disequilibrium based on autosomal haplotype data collected from the literature and found allelic association such that 1 SNP per 100kb would be adequate for most studies (118, 119). Thus, the ability to measure significant disequilibrium at much greater distances than those predicted by the simulation study, means that the required number of SNPs chosen for genome-wide screening may be as small as 30,000.

In conclusion, more sophisticated and specific linkage analysis methods along with association analyses must be used to map a disease susceptibility gene. The strengths of each method will obviously depend on the underlying genetic model and population structure. In addition, standard methods for positional cloning must also be employed. However, in all cases a functional assessment will ultimately give credence to whether a candidate variant is the disease allele.

FUNCTIONAL GENOMICS

Sophisticated, high-throughput molecular technologies are now in place for analysis of cellular processes that identify global gene and protein expression profile differences (EPDs) between normal and disease states. "Functional genomics" has been coined to describe the study of the complete set of gene expression events taking place within a given cell type in response to external stimuli or following some underlying pathological process. With a DNA microarray, one uses thousands of immobilized "probe" sequences to simultaneously interrogate complex cellular mRNA "targets" (120). For example, DNA microarrays were used to analyze the response of human fibroblasts in culture to serum. It was found that certain genes involved in cellular proliferation responded in a coordinated manner, while genes eliciting the immune and repair response were also induced (121). Other studies include detecting EPDs in cancer (122, 123), inflammation (124) and those that result from specific mutations in key components of the transcription machinery in yeast (125). Solution-based hybridization technologies are used to isolate differentially expressed genes without the need to separate or characterize the probe population. These include subtractive hybridization methods based on representational difference analysis (126), suppressive PCR (127) and FACs-based microbead capture (128). Relevant to diabetes, a PCR-based subtractive hybridization procedure was used to clone 80 mRNAs specific for pancreatic beta-cells (129), while a suppressive version found genes that are expressed when pancreas-specific gene transcription is either initiated or transiently expressed during early stages of pancreas development (130).

Alone, global gene expression profiles may present a misleading view of the true molecular differences found in normal and disease states. With current microarray technology, small mRNA differences between two samples (less than 2-fold) and differentially spliced mRNAs (unless all exon specific probes are generated on the array) are difficult to detect. In addition, coding region changes that may give rise to disease will go undetected because the level of gene expression remains constant. The protein component of the cell cannot be ignored because: 1) the rates of degradation of mRNAs and proteins differ, 2) differential mRNA splicing events may result in different protein forms, and 3) many proteins are post-translationally modified. As a consequence, "functional proteomics" has emerged as a technology that complements gene expression studies to generate a better pattern of cellular EPDs.

Proteomics refers to the study of the complete set of proteins that is expressed and modified following expression by the entire genome in the lifetime of a cell (131). The field still relies on 2-D polyacrylamide gel electrophoresis, as a first step in whole cell protein analysis, although on-line separation technologies such as liquid chromatography combined with refined sub-cellular fractionation procedures and more sensitive, high-throughput detection methods like tandem mass spectrometry will help in the characterization of protein expression profiles. For type 1 diabetes studies, a 2-D "catalog" of IL-1 beta changes in rat islets has been reported (132). More advanced high-throughput analytical methods such as protein chips and differential whole-cell protein labeling methods with isotope-coded affinity tags (ICAT) (133) are now emerging. A new structural genomics initiative for high-throughput X-ray crystallography aimed at developing a comprehensive mechanistic understanding of normal and abnormal human and microbial physiology at the molecular level has been reported (134).

Screening for EPDs provides a fast way to generate a great amount of data for further study. Experimental designs must include appropriate controls and careful sample handling issues must be addressed to ensure that a true representation of cellular expression is captured. After the data is collected, a major effort will be undertaken to decipher differences between the normal and disease expression patterns and to create a list of potential candidate genes for further study. With this strategy, it is hoped that expression profile differences will lead to the causative disease genes. However, inter-individual differences or genes that are the consequence of the disease may be isolated as well. It may turn out that a gene identified this way either maps to a region previously found by linkage analysis studies or is homologous to a known molecule isolated from a different organism. This would provide some level of confidence for downstream discovery of a functional variant(s).

IMPORTANCE OF ANIMAL MODELS

For several reasons, animals will help to define the functional role of genes in complex human diseases. First, once a human gene is isolated, the homologous rodent molecule can be studied. The ability to knockin or knockout genes has made the mouse a popular system for understanding gene function and a wealth of knowledge can be found in the literature regarding transgenic animal experiments. Importantly, the framework for comparative mapping between the mouse, rat and human genomes is being constructed. Second, the clinical heterogeneity found in human patients has redirected researchers to use inbred animal models because measurement of a trait can be conducted with animals having genetically identical backgrounds and under environmentally controlled conditions. Third, rodent models are readily available in large numbers, enabling the first whole genome screens to be completed in rodents several years before the first human genome screens (135-138). Fourth, the genotype of inbred animals can be experimentally manipulated to test a small region of the genome. For example, congenic non-obese diabetic (NOD) mouse strains have been created to study the role of MHC in type 1 diabetes (139) and for fine mapping *Idd3* to a 780-kb region of mouse chromosome 3, where the gene for interleukin 2 maps (140).

Traditionally, inbred animal models have been used to study complex disease because physiologic investigations can be conducted to relate genetic factors with specific phenotypes. For example, physiological characterization and linkage analysis in the Goto-Kakizaki rat was used to identify three different loci involved in type 2 diabetes that influence glucose tolerance, insulin secretion, and fat distribution (141, 142). While diseases in rodent strains are not equivalent to their human disease counterpart, it is easier to predict the timing of pathogenic events. For type 1 diabetes, the NOD mouse and BioBreeding rat spontaneously develop diabetes during which most individuals proceed through the same stages (insulitis, T cell infiltration, beta cell death) at similar times in development. In one study, protracted peri-insulitis involving minimal T cell contribution in the non-obese diabetes-resistant (NOR) mouse was compared to insulitis normally seen in the NOD mouse. NOD and NOR share the diabetogenic MHC haplotype but differ at 5 of the remaining 18 *Idd* loci. Insulitis severity was scored as an intermediate phenotype (but not as a quantitative trait) and linkage analysis was performed in (NODxNOR)F2 progeny to locate a subset of essential genes. Progression from peri- to invasive insulitis was found to be controlled by an interaction between *Idd5* and *Idd13*. Orthologous regions in rat and human were identified for *Idd5* and *Idd13* and a mechanism was suggested by which these alleles drive insulitis progression via T cell recruitment to, or retention in, islet lesions (143).

Together, the use of inbred animal strains along with high-throughput expression profiling and mapping methods are likely to identify new candidate genes. In this regard, generating a gene list based on EPDs may point us towards particular pathways where disease-related biological events may be taking place. As an example, the Cd36 gene (which encodes fatty acid translocase) was identified in the insulin resistant, spontaneously hypertensive rat (SHR) using a combination of cDNA microarrays, congenic mapping and radiation hybrid mapping (144).

CONCLUSIONS

Geneticists are now armed with better tools to dissect the genetic components of type 1 and type 2 diabetes. Rapid advances in high-throughput molecular technologies have continued a trend towards hypothesis-limited studies of diabetes and other complex diseases. While few complex disease genes have been cloned from genome-wide scans, it is likely that expression profile differences will be found at key stages in diabetes progression leading to a new set of candidate genes. Insights learned from the discovery of these new molecules plus more detailed descriptions of intra- and extra-cellular pathways will add power to the next series of genome analysis studies. Global screening efforts will, thus, be an aid to time-consuming classical mapping strategies, ultimately leading to the detection of the responsible disease variant(s). New advances in statistical methodologies for gene-environment interactions should also greatly enhance efforts to identify genes for complex diseases. Unexpected surprises may be waiting as networks of detailed metabolic pathways unfold, especially if broader roles are discovered for known molecules.

ACKNOWLEDGEMENTS

The authors are grateful to Dr. Ake Lernmark for providing valuable references. S.H.N. is indebted to members of the McGee Center for valuable scientific discussions and to Dr. S.L. Nye for continued support throughout writing this chapter. S.H.N. dedicates his efforts to Mr. Julius Gollup in memory of his battle with diabetes.

REFERENCES

1. Ebers GC, Kukay K, Bulman DE, Sadovnick AD, Rice G and others. 1996. A full genome search in multiple sclerosis. *Nat Genet* 13:472-476.
2. Sawcer S, Jones HB, Feakes R, Gray J, Smaldon N and others. 1996. A genome screen in multiple sclerosis reveals susceptibility loci on chromosome 6p21 and 17q22. *Nat Genet* 13:464-468.
3. Haines JL, Ter-Minassian M, Bazyk A, Gusella JF, Kim DJ and others. 1996. A complete genomic screen for multiple sclerosis underscores a role for the major histocompatability complex. The Multiple Sclerosis Genetics Group. *Nat Genet* 13:469-471.
4. Kuokkanen S, Gschwend M, Rioux JD, Daly MJ, Terwilliger JD and others. 1997. Genomewide scan of multiple sclerosis in Finnish multiplex families. *Am J Hum Genet* 61:1379-1387.
5. Cornelis F, Faure S, Martinez M, Prud'homme JF, Fritz P and others. 1998. New susceptibility locus for rheumatoid arthritis suggested by a genome-wide linkage study. *Proc Natl Acad Sci U S A* 95:10746-10750.
6. Comuzzie AG, Hixson JE, Almasy L, Mitchell BD, Mahaney MC and others. 1997. A major quantitative trait locus determining serum leptin levels and fat mass is located on human chromosome 2. *Nat Genet* 15:273-276.
7. Hager J, Dina C, Francke S, Dubois S, Houari M and others. 1998. A genome-wide scan for human obesity genes reveals a major susceptibility locus on chromosome 10. *Nat Genet* 20:304-308.
8. Norman RA, Thompson DB, Foroud T, Garvey WT, Bennett PH and others. 1997. Genomewide search for genes influencing percent body fat in Pima Indians: suggestive linkage at chromosome 11q21-q22. Pima Diabetes Gene Group. *Am J Hum Genet* 60:166-173.
9. Norman RA, Tataranni PA, Pratley R, Thompson DB, Hanson RL and others. 1998. Autosomal genomic scan for loci linked to obesity and energy metabolism in Pima Indians. *Am J Hum Genet* 62:659-668.
10. Bell GI, Horita S, Karam JH. 1984. A polymorphic locus near the human insulin gene is associated with insulin-dependent diabetes mellitus. *Diabetes* 33:176-183.
11. Julier C, Lucassen A, Villedieu P, Delepine M, Levy-Marchal C and others. 1994. Multiple DNA variant association analysis: application to the insulin gene region in type I diabetes. *Am J Hum Genet* 55:1247-1254.
12. Owerbach D, Gabbay K. 1993. Localization of a type 1 diabetes susceptibility locus to the variable tandem repeat region flanking the insulin gene. *Diabetes* 42:1708-1714.
13. Bennett ST, Lucassen AM, Gough SC, Powell EE, Undlien DE and others. 1995. Susceptibility to human type 1 diabetes at IDDM2 is determined by tandem repeat variation at the insulin gene minisatellite locus. *Nat Genet* 9:284-292.
14. Corder EH, Saunders AM, Strittmatter WJ, Schmechel DE, Gaskell PC and others. 1993. Gene dose of apolipoprotein E type 4 allele and the risk of Alzheimer's disease in late onset families. *Science* 261:921-923.
15. Saunders AM, Schmader K, Breitner JC, Benson MD, Brown WT and others. 1993. Apolipoprotein E epsilon 4 allele distributions in late-onset Alzheimer's disease and in other amyloid-forming diseases. *Lancet* 342:710-711.
16. Strittmatter WJ, Saunders AM, Schmechel D, Pericak-Vance M, Enghild J and others. 1993. Apolipoprotein E: high-avidity binding to beta-amyloid and increased

frequency of type 4 allele in late-onset familial Alzheimer disease. *Proc Natl Acad Sci U S A* 90:1977-1981.
17. Martin N, Boomsma D, Machin G. 1997. A twin-pronged attack on complex traits. *Nat Genet* 17:387-392.
18. Folstein S, Rutter M. 1977. Infantile autism: a genetic study of 21 twin pairs. *J Child Psychol Psychiatry* 18:297-321.
19. Stevenson J. 1992. Evidence for a genetic etiology in hyperactivity in children. *Behav Genet* 22:337-344.
20. Ebers GC, Bulman DE, Sadovnick AD, Paty DW, Warren S and others. 1986. A population-based study of multiple sclerosis in twins. *N Engl J Med* 315:1638-1642.
21. Rowe RE, Leslie RD. 1995. Twin studies in insulin dependent diabetes and other autoimmune diseases. *Diabetes Metab Rev* 11:121-135.
22. Ott J. 1991. Analysis of Human Genetic Linkage. 1st revised ed. John Hopkins University Press, Baltimore.
23. Goodwin DW, Schulsinger F, Moller N, Hermansen L, Winokur G and others. 1974. Drinking problems in adopted and nonadopted sons of alcoholics. *Arch Gen Psychiatry* 31:164-169.
24. Stunkard AJ, Sorensen TI, Hanis C, Teasdale TW, Chakraborty R and others. 1986. An adoption study of human obesity. *N Engl J Med* 314:193-198.
25. Hopper J. 1996. Commentary: genes for osteoarthritis: interpreting twin data. *BMJ* 312:943-944.
26. Kyvik KO, Green A, Beck-Nielsen H. 1995. Concordance rates of insulin dependent diabetes mellitus: a population based study of young Danish twins. *BMJ* 311:913-917.
27. Newman B, Selby JV, King MC, Slemenda C, Fabsitz R and others. 1987. Concordance for type 2 (non-insulin-dependent) diabetes mellitus in male twins. *Diabetologia* 30:763-768.
28. Poulsen P, Kyvik KO, Vaag A, Beck-Nielsen H. 1999. Heritability of type 2 (non-insulin-dependent) diabetes mellitus and abnormal glucose tolerance-a population-based twin study. *Diabetologia* 42:139-145.
29. Risch N. 1990. Linkage strategies for genetically complex traits. I. Multilocus models. *Am J Hum Genet* 46:222-228.
30. Guo SW. 1998. Inflation of sibling recurrence-risk ratio, due to ascertainment bias and/or overreporting. *Am J Hum Genet* 63:252-258.
31. Risch N. 1987. Assessing the role of HLA-linked and unlinked determinants of disease. *Am J Hum Genet* 40:1-14.
32. Rich SS. 1990. Mapping genes in diabetes. Genetic epidemiological perspective. *Diabetes* 39:1315-1319.
33. Arshad SH, Hide DW. 1992. Effect of environmental factors on the development of allergic disorders in infancy. *J Allergy Clin Immunol* 90:235-241.
34. Bleecker ER. 1998. Mapping susceptibility genes for asthma and allergy. *Clin Exp Allergy* 28 Suppl 5:6-12; discussion 26-18.
35. Dahlquist G. 1998. The aetiology of type 1 diabetes: an epidemiological perspective. *Acta Paediatr Suppl* 425:5-10.
36. Honeyman MC, Coulson BS, Stone NL, Gellert SA, Goldwater PN and others. 2000. Association between rotavirus infection and pancreatic islet autoimmunity in children at risk of developing type 1 diabetes. *Diabetes* 49:1319-1324.
37. Lonnrot M, Korpela K, Knip M, Ilonen J, Simell O and others. 2000. Enterovirus infection as a risk factor for beta-cell autoimmunity in a prospectively observed birth cohort: the Finnish Diabetes Prediction and Prevention Study. *Diabetes* 49:1314-1318.
38. Harrison LC, Honeyman MC. 1999. Cow's milk and type 1 diabetes: the real debate is about mucosal immune function. *Diabetes* 48:1501-1507.

39. Raffel LJ, Scheuner MT, Rotter JI. 1997. Genetics of Diabetes. In: Porte D, Jr., Sherwin RS (eds) *Diabetes Mellitus* 5th ed. Elsevier Science. Stamford, Connecticut:401-454.
40. Bennett PH. 1996. Epidemiology of non-insulin-dependent diabetes. In: LeRoith D, Taylor SI, Olefsky JM (eds) *Diabetes Mellitus: A Fundamental and Clinical Text*. Lippincott-Raven. Philadelphia:455-458.
41. Bennett PH, Rewers MJ, Knowler WC. 1997. Epidemiology of Diabetes Mellitus. In: Porte D, Jr., Sherwin RS (eds) *Diabetes Mellitus* 5th ed. Elsevier Science. Stamford, Connecticut:373-400.
42. Guo S. 2000. Gene-environment interactions and the affected-sib-pair designs. *Hum Hered* 50:271-285.
43. Guo S. 2000. Gene-environment interaction and the mapping of complex traits: some statistical models and their implications. *Hum Hered* 50:286-303.
44. Schaid DJ. 1999. Case-parents design for gene-environment interaction. *Genet Epidemiol* 16:261-273.
45. Collins FS. 1995. Positional cloning moves from perditional to traditional. *Nat Genet* 9:347-350.
46. Almasy L, Blangero J. 1998. Multipoint quantitative-trait linkage analysis in general pedigrees. *Am J Hum Genet* 62:1198-1211.
47. Morton NE. 1955. Sequential tests for the detection of linkage. *Am J Hum Genet* 7:277-318.
48. Dib C, Faure S, Fizames C, Samson D, Drouot N and others. 1996. A comprehensive genetic map of the human genome based on 5,264 microsatellites. *Nature* 380:152-154.
49. Ghosh S, Karanjawala ZE, Hauser ER, Ally D, Knapp JI and others. 1997. Methods for precise sizing, automated binning of alleles, and reduction of error rates in large-scale genotyping using fluorescently labeled dinucleotide markers. FUSION (Finland-U.S. Investigation of NIDDM Genetics) Study Group. *Genome Res* 7:165-178.
50. Marra MA, Kucaba TA, Dietrich NL, Green ED, Brownstein B and others. 1997. High throughput fingerprint analysis of large-insert clones. *Genome Res* 7:1072-1084.
51. Marra M, Weinstock LA, Mardis ER. 1996. End sequence determination from large insert clones using energy transfer fluorescent primers. *Genome Res* 6:1118-1122.
52. Kupfer K, Smith MW, Quackenbush J, Evans GA. 1995. Physical mapping of complex genomes by sampled sequencing: a theoretical analysis. *Genomics* 27:90-100.
53. Smith MW, Holmsen AL, Wei YH, Peterson M, Evans GA. 1994. Genomic sequence sampling: a strategy for high resolution sequence-based physical mapping of complex genomes. *Nat Genet* 7:40-47.
54. Fajans SS, Bell GI, Bowden DW, Halter JB, Polonsky KS. 1996. Maturity onset diabetes of the young (MODY). *Diabet Med* 13:S90-95.
55. Yamagata K, Furuta H, Oda N, Kaisaski P, Menzel S and others. 1996. Mutations in the hepatocyte nuclear factor-4α gene in maturity-onset diabetes of the young (MODY1). *Nature* 384:458-460.
56. Yamagata K, Oda N, Kaisaki PJ, Menzel S, Furuta H and others. 1996. Mutations in the hepatocyte nuclear factor-1α gene in maturity-onset diabetes of the young (MODY 3). *Nature* 384:455-458.
57. Vionnet N, Stoffel M, Takeda J, Yasuda K, Bell GI and others. 1992. Nonsense mutation in the glucokinase gene causes early-onset non-insulin-dependent diabetes mellitus. *Nature* 356:721-722.
58. Stoffers DA, Ferrer J, Clarke WL, Habener JF. 1997. Early-onset type-II diabetes mellitus (MODY4) linked to IPF1. *Nat Genet* 17:138-139.

59. Horikawa Y, Iwasaki N, Hara M, Furuta H, Hinokio Y and others. 1997. Mutation in hepatocyte nuclear factor-1 beta gene (TCF2) associated with MODY. *Nat Genet* 17:384-385.
60. Malecki MT, Jhala US, Antonellis A, Fields L, Doria A and others. 1999. Mutations in NEUROD1 are associated with the development of type 2 diabetes mellitus. *Nat Genet* 23:323-328.
61. Shuldiner AR, Silver KD. 1996. Candidate genes for non-insulin-dependent diabetes mellitus. In: LeRoith D, Taylor S, Olefsky JM (eds) *Diabetes Mellitus*. Lippincott-Raven. Philadelphia:565-574.
62. Suarez BK, Hampe CL, Van Eerdewegh P. 1994. Genetic Approaches to Mental Disorders. In: Gershon ES, Cloninger CR (eds). American Psychiatric Press. Washington, D.C.:23.
63. Clerget-Darpoux F, Bonaiti-Pellie C, Hochez J. 1986. Effects of misspecifying genetic parameters in Lod score analysis. *Biometrics* 42:393-399.
64. Risch N. 1990. Linkage strategies for genetically complex traits. II. The power of affected relative pairs. *Am J Hum Genet* 46:229-241.
65. Risch N. 1990. Linkage strategies for genetically complex traits. III. The effect of marker polymorphism on analysis of affected relative pairs. *Am J Hum Genet* 46:242-253.
66. Hauser ER, Boehnke M. 1998. Genetic linkage analysis of complex genetic traits by using affected sibling pairs. *Biometrics* 54:1238-1246.
67. Boehnke M. 1991. Allele frequency estimation from data on relatives. *Am J Hum Genet* 48:22-25.
68. Schork NJ, Boehnke M, Terwilliger JD, Ott J. 1993. Two-trait-locus linkage analysis: a powerful strategy for mapping complex genetic traits. *Am J Hum Genet* 53:1127-1136.
69. Dupuis J, Brown PO, Siegmund D. 1995. Statistical methods for linkage analysis of complex traits from high- resolution maps of identity by descent. *Genetics* 140:843-856.
70. Cordell HJ, Todd JA, Bennett ST, Kawaguchi Y, Farrall M. 1995. Two-locus maximum lod score analysis of a multifactorial trait: joint consideration of IDDM2 and IDDM4 with IDDM1 in type 1 diabetes. *Am J Hum Genet* 57:920-934.
71. Knapp M, Seuchter SA, Baur MP. 1994. Two-locus disease models with two marker loci: the power of affected- sib-pair tests. *Am J Hum Genet* 55:1030-1041.
72. Gavin JR, Alberti KGMM, Davidson MB, DeFronzo RA, Drash A and others. 1998. Report of the Expert Committee on the Diagnosis and Classification of Diabetes Mellitus. *Diabetes Care* 21, supplement 1:S5-S19.
73. Haseman JK, Elston RC. 1972. The investigation of linkage between a quantitative trait and a marker locus. *Behavior Genetics* 2:3-19.
74. Bergman R. 1989. Toward physiological understanding of glucose tolerance: minimal-model approach. *Diabetes* 38:1512-1527.
75. DeFronzo RA, Beckles AD. 1979. Glucose intolerance following chronic metabolic acidosis in man. *Am J Physiol* 236:E328-334.
76. Taylor SI, Accili D, Imai Y. 1994. Insulin resistance or insulin deficiency. Which is the primary cause of NIDDM? *Diabetes* 43:735-740.
77. Valle T, Tuomilehto J, Bergman RN, Ghosh S, Hauser ER and others. 1998. Mapping genes for NIDDM. Design of the Finland-United States Investigation of NIDDM genetics (FUSION) study. *Diabetes Care* 21:949-958.
78. Ghosh S, Schork NJ. 1996. Genetic analysis of NIDDM. The study of quantitative traits. *Diabetes* 45:1-14.
79. Martin BC, Warram JC, Krolewski AS, Bergman RN, Soeldner JS and others. 1992. Role of glucose and insulin resistance in the development of type 2 diabetes mellitus: results of a 25-year follow-up study. *Lancet* 340:925-929.

80. McCance DR, Pettitt DJ, Hanson RL, Jacobsson LT, Bennett PH and others. 1994. Glucose, insulin concentrations and obesity in childhood and adolescence as predictors of NIDDM. *Diabetologia* 37:617-623.
81. Lillioja S, Mott DM, Spraul M, Ferraro R, Foley JE and others. 1993. Insulin resistance and insulin secretory dysfunction as precursors of non-insulin-dependent diabetes mellitus. Prospective studies of Pima Indians. *N Engl J Med* 329:1988-1992.
82. Pratley RE, Thompson DB, Prochazka M, Baier L, Mott D and others. 1998. An autosomal genomic scan for loci linked to prediabetic phenotypes in Pima Indians. *J Clin Invest* 101:1757-1764.
83. Davies JL, Kawaguchi Y, Bennett ST, Copemen JB, Cordell HJ and others. 1994. A genome-wide search for human type 1 diabetes susceptibility genes. *Nature* 371:130-136.
84. Hashimoto L, habita C, Beressi JP, Delephine M, Besse C and others. 1994. Genetic mapping of a susceptibility locus for insulin-dependent diabetes mellitus on chromosome 11q. *Nature* 371:161-164.
85. Todd JA, Farrall M. 1996. Panning for gold: genome-wide scanning for linkage in type 1 diabetes. *Hum Mol Genet* 5:1443-1448.
86. Mein CA, Esposito L, Dunn MG, Johnson GC, Timms AE and others. 1998. A search for type 1 diabetes susceptibility genes in families from the United Kingdom. *Nat Genet* 19:297-300.
87. Concannon P, Gogolin-Ewens KJ, Hinds DA, Wapelhorst B, Morrison VA and others. 1998. A second-generation screen of the human genome for susceptibility to insulin-dependent diabetes mellitus. *Nat Genet* 19:292-296.
88. Todd JA. 1999. Interpretation of results from genetic studies of multifactorial diseases. *Lancet* 354 Suppl 1:SI15-16.
89. Hanis CL, Boerwinkle E, Chakraborty R, Ellsworth DL, Concannon P and others. 1996. A genome-wide search for human non-insulin-dependent (type 2) diabetes genes reveals a major susceptibility locus on chromosome 2. *Nat Genet* 13:161-166.
90. McCarthy M, Cassell P, Saker P, Armstrong M, Turner R and others. 1997. No excess allele-sharing on chromosome 2q (region of NIDDM1) in a large European sibship collection. *Diabetes* 46:abstract 0201.
91. Hani EH, Suaud L, Boutin P, Chevre JC, Durand E and others. 1998. A missense mutation in hepatocyte nuclear factor-4 alpha, resulting in a reduced transactivation activity, in human late-onset non-insulin- dependent diabetes mellitus. *J Clin Invest* 101:521-526.
92. Ghosh S, Hauser ER, Magnuson VL, Valle T, Ally DS and others. 1998. A large sample of finnish diabetic sib-pairs reveals no evidence for a non-insulin-dependent diabetes mellitus susceptibility locus at 2qter. *J Clin Invest* 102:704-709.
93. Duggirala R, Blangero J, Almasy L, Dyer TD, Williams KL and others. 1999. Linkage of type 2 diabetes mellitus and of age at onset to a genetic location on chromosome 10q in Mexican Americans. *Am J Hum Genet* 64:1127-1140.
94. Ciccarese M, Tonolo G, Delin I, Wong FK, Holm P and others. 1997. Preliminary data on a genome search in NIDDM siblings: the NIDDM1 locus on chromosome 2 is not linked to NIDDM in the Sardinian population. Study Group for the Genetics of Diabetes in Sardinia. *Diabetologia* 40:1366-1367.
95. Cox NJ, Frigge M, Nicolae DL, Concannon P, Hanis CL and others. 1999. Loci on chromosomes 2 (NIDDM1) and 15 interact to increase susceptibility to diabetes in Mexican Americans. *Nat Genet* 21:213-215.
96. Mahtani MM, Widen E, Lehto M, Thomas J, McCarthy M and others. 1996. Mapping of a gene for type 2 diabetes associated with an insulin secretion defect by a genome scan in Finnish families. *Nat Genet* 14:90-94.
97. Hanson RL, Ehm MG, Pettitt DJ, Prochazka M, Thompson DB and others. 1998. An autosomal genomic scan for loci linked to type II diabetes mellitus and body-mass index in Pima Indians. *Am J Hum Genet* 63:1130-1138.

98. Ehm MG, Karnoub MC, Sakul H, Gottschalk K, Holt DC and others. 2000. Genomewide Search for Type 2 Diabetes Susceptibility Genes in Four American Populations. *Am J Hum Genet* 66:1871-1881.

99. Bowden DW, Sale M, Howard TD, Qadri A, Spray BJ and others. 1997. Linkage of genetic markers on human chromosomes 20 and 12 to NIDDM in Caucasian sib pairs with a history of diabetic nephropathy. *Diabetes* 46:882-886.

100. Ji L, Malecki M, Warram JH, Yang Y, Rich SS and others. 1997. New susceptibility locus for NIDDM is localized to human chromosome 20q. *Diabetes* 46:876-881.

101. Zouali H, Hani EH, Philippi A, Vionnet N, Beckmann JS and others. 1997. A susceptibility locus for early-onset non-insulin dependent (type 2) diabetes mellitus maps to chromosome 20q, proximal to the phosphoenolpyruvate carboxykinase gene. *Hum Mol Genet* 6:1401-1408.

102. Hastbacka J, de la Chapelle A, Kaitila I, Sistonen P, Weaver A and others. 1992. Linkage disequilibrium mapping in isolated founder populations: diastrophic dysplasia in Finland. *Nat Genet* 2:204-211.

103. Yu C-Y, Oshima J, Fu Y-H, Wijsman E, Hisama F and others. 1996. Positional cloning of the Werner's syndrome gene. *Science* 272:258-262.

104. Roy N, Mahadevan MS, McLean M, Shutler G, Yaraghi Z and others. 1995. The gene for neural apoptosis inhibitory protein is partially deleted in individuals with spinal muscular atrophy. *Cell* 80:167-178.

105. Petrukhin K, Fischer SG, Pirastu M, Tanzi RE, Chernov I and others. 1993. Mapping, cloning and genetic characterization of the region containing the Wilson disease gene. *Nat Genet* 5:338-343.

106. Stone EM, Fingert JH, Alward WLM, Nguyen TD, Polansky JR and others. 1997. Identification of a gene that causes primary open angle glaucoma. *Science* 275:668-670.

107. Spielman RS, McGinnis RE, Ewens WJ. 1993. Transmission test for linkage disequilibrium: the insulin gene region and insulin-dependent diabetes mellitus (IDDM). *Am J Hum Genet* 52:506-516.

108. Collins FS, Guyer MS, Charkravarti A. 1997. Variations on a theme: cataloging human DNA sequence variation. *Science* 278:1580-1581.

109. Chapman NH, Wijsman EM. 1998. Genome screens using linkage disequilibrium tests: optimal marker characteristics and feasibility. *Am J Hum Genet* 63:1872-1885.

110. Camp NJ. 1997. Genomewide transmission/disequilibrium testing--consideration of the genotypic relative risks at disease loci. *Am J Hum Genet* 61:1424-1430.

111. Risch N, Merikangas K. 1996. The future of genetic studies of complex human disease. *Science* 273:1516-1517.

112. Lander E, Schork N. 1994. Genetic analysis of complex traits. *Science* 265:2037-2048.

113. Lai E, Riley J, Purvis I, Roses A. 1998. A 4-Mb high-density single nucleotide polymorphism-based map around human APOE. *Genomics* 54:31-38.

114. Clark AG, Weiss KM, Nickerson DA, Taylor SL, Buchanan A and others. 1998. Haplotype structure and population genetic inferences from nucleotide- sequence variation in human lipoprotein lipase. *Am J Hum Genet* 63:595-612.

115. Nickerson DA, Taylor SL, Weiss KM, Clark AG, Hutchinson RG and others. 1998. DNA sequence diversity in a 9.7-kb region of the human lipoprotein lipase gene. *Nat Genet* 19:233-240.

116. Kruglyak L. 1999. Prospects for whole-genome linkage disequilibrium mapping of common disease genes. *Nat Genet* 22:139-144.

117. Ott J. 2000. Predicting the range of linkage disequilibrium. *Proc Natl Acad Sci U S A* 97:2-3.

118. Jorde LB, Watkins WS, Carlson M, Groden J, Albertsen H and others. 1994. Linkage disequilibrium predicts physical distance in the adenomatous polyposis coli region. *Am J Hum Genet* 54:884-898.

119. Collins A, Lonjou C, Morton NE. 1999. Genetic epidemiology of single-nucleotide polymorphisms. *Proc Natl Acad Sci U S A* 96:15173-15177.
120. Schena M, Shalon D, Heller R, Chai A, Brown PO and others. 1996. Parallel human genome analysis: microarray-based expression monitoring of 1000 genes. *Proc Natl Acad Sci U S A* 93:10614-10619.
121. Iyer VR, Eisen MB, Ross DT, Schuler G, Moore T and others. 1999. The transcriptional program in the response of human fibroblasts to serum. *Science* 283:83-87.
122. Alizadeh AA, Eisen MB, Davis RE, Ma C, Lossos IS and others. 2000. Distinct types of diffuse large B-cell lymphoma identified by gene expression profiling. *Nature* 403:503-511.
123. Khan J, Simon R, Bittner M, Chen Y, Leighton SB and others. 1998. Gene expression profiling of alveolar rhabdomyosarcoma with cDNA microarrays. *Cancer Res* 58:5009-5013.
124. Heller RA, Schena M, Chai A, Shalon D, Bedilion T and others. 1997. Discovery and analysis of inflammatory disease-related genes using cDNA microarrays. *Proc Natl Acad Sci U S A* 94:2150-2155.
125. Holstege FC, Jennings EG, Wyrick JJ, Lee TI, Hengartner CJ and others. 1998. Dissecting the regulatory circuitry of a eukaryotic genome. *Cell* 95:717-728.
126. Welford SM, Gregg J, Chen E, Garrison D, Sorensen PH and others. 1998. Detection of differentially expressed genes in primary tumor tissues using representational differences analysis coupled to microarray hybridization. *Nucleic Acids Res* 26:3059-3065.
127. Diatchenko L, Lau YF, Campbell AP, Chenchik A, Moqadam F and others. 1996. Suppression subtractive hybridization: a method for generating differentially regulated or tissue-specific cDNA probes and libraries. *Proc Natl Acad Sci U S A* 93:6025-6030.
128. Brenner S, Williams SR, Vermaas EH, Storck T, Moon K and others. 2000. In vitro cloning of complex mixtures of DNA on microbeads: physical separation of differentially expressed cDNAs. *Proc Natl Acad Sci U S A* 97:1665-1670.
129. Neophytou PI, Muir EM, Hutton JC. 1996. A subtractive cloning approach to the identification of mRNAs specifically expressed in pancreatic beta-cells. *Diabetes* 45:127-133.
130. Hebrok M, Kim SK, Melton DA. 1999. Screening for novel pancreatic genes expressed during embryogenesis. *Diabetes* 48:1550-1556.
131. Abbott A. 1999. A post-genomic challenge: learning to read patterns of protein synthesis. *Nature* 402:715-720.
132. Andersen HU, Fey SJ, Larsen PM, Nawrocki A, Hejnaes KR and others. 1997. Interleukin-1beta induced changes in the protein expression of rat islets: a computerized database. *Electrophoresis* 18:2091-2103.
133. Gygi SP, Rist B, Gerber SA, Turecek F, Gelb MH and others. 1999. Quantitative analysis of complex protein mixtures using isotope-coded affinity tags. *Nat Biotechnol* 17:994-999.
134. Burley SK, Almo SC, Bonanno JB, Capel M, Chance MR and others. 1999. Structural genomics: beyond the human genome project. *Nat Genet* 23:151-157.
135. Todd JA, Aitman TJ, Cornall RJ, Ghosh S, Hall JRS and others. 1991. Genetic analysis of autoimmune type 1 diabetes mellitus in mice. *Nature* 351:542-547.
136. Rise ML, Frankel WN, Coffin JM, Seyfried TN. 1991. Genes for epilepsy mapped in the mouse. *Science* 253:669-673.
137. Jacob HJ, Lindpaintner K, Lincoln SE, Kusumi K, Bunker RK and others. 1991. Genetic mapping of a gene causing hypertension in the stroke-prone spontaneously hypertensive rat. *Cell* 67:213-224.

138. Hilbert P, Lindpaintner K, Beckmann JS, Serikawa T, Soubrier F and others. 1991. Chromosomal mapping of two genetic loci associated with blood-pressure regulation in hereditary hypertensive rats. *Nature* 353:521-529.
139. Todd JA. 1999. From genome to aetiology in a multifactorial disease, type 1 diabetes. *Bioessays* 21:164-174.
140. Lyons PA, Armitage N, Argentina F, Denny P, Hill NJ and others. 2000. Congenic mapping of the type 1 diabetes locus, Idd3, to a 780-kb region of mouse chromosome 3: identification of a candidate segment of ancestral DNA by haplotype mapping. *Genome Res* 10:446-453.
141. Galli J, Li LS, Glaser A, Ostenson CG, Jiao H and others. 1996. Genetic analysis of non-insulin dependent diabetes mellitus in the GK rat. *Nat Genet* 12:31-37.
142. Gauguier D, Froguel P, Parent V, Bernard C, Bihoreau MT and others. 1996. Chromosomal mapping of genetic loci associated with non-insulin dependent diabetes in the GK rat. *Nat Genet* 12:38-43.
143. Fox CJ, Paterson AD, Mortin-Toth SM, Danska JS. 2000. Two genetic loci regulate T cell-dependent islet inflammation and drive autoimmune diabetes pathogenesis. *Am J Hum Genet* 67:67-81.
144. Aitman TJ, Glazier AM, Wallace CA, Cooper LD, Norsworthy PJ and others. 1999. Identification of Cd36 (Fat) as an insulin-resistance gene causing defective fatty acid and glucose metabolism in hypertensive rats. *Nat Genet* 21:76-83.

2
GENETIC FACTORS IN TYPE 1 DIABETES

Alberto Pugliese, M.D.
University of Miami School of Medicine, Miami, FL 33134 USA

INTRODUCTION

Insulin-dependent diabetes mellitus (IDDM), or type 1 diabetes, is a chronic and yet incurable disease characterized by autoimmune destruction of pancreatic ß-cells and complete insulin deficiency (1). The disease develops predominantly in children or adolescents, but it can develop at a much later age, and it is quite heterogeneous in its clinical expression. A large body of evidence indicates that inherited genetic factors influence both susceptibility to and resistance from the disease. During the past few years, dramatic improvements in the ability to investigate the genetics of complex diseases have been introduced. The increasing availability of polymorphic microsatellite markers, automated typing technology (2), and large collections of families with affected sib-pairs have enabled the design of large scale, genome-wide scans to map IDDM susceptibility genes. Such scans have provided evidence to link diabetes susceptibility with numerous chromosomal regions and suggested that type 1 diabetes is a polygenic disorder. Moreover, there is evidence for epistatic phenomena involving several loci, and complex parental effects appear to influence susceptibility by modifying the transmission and expression of inherited genes. It is an intriguing and yet unproven possibility that additional genetic factors or their expression may be acquired after birth, perhaps through environmental exposures. Such factors may play a key role in triggering ß-cell autoimmunity in susceptible individuals. This chapter will review the current knowledge about the genetics of type 1 diabetes.

INHERITED SUSCEPTIBILITY LOCI

Susceptibility loci for type 1 diabetes are conventionally noted using the abbreviation *IDDM* and a number, e.g. *IDDM1*, *IDDM2*, etc., with the number usually reflecting the order in which such loci were reported. Using the candidate gene approach, association studies dating now to about two decades ago provided evidence for two susceptibility loci, namely the HLA class II region (*IDDM1*), a major susceptibility locus, and the insulin gene (*INS*) locus (*IDDM2*). The observation that *IDDM1* and *IDDM2* only contribute a portion of the disease familial clustering suggested that additional loci must exist and influence the development of diabetes. Genome scans conducted by several groups confirmed linkage with *IDDM1* and *IDDM2* and provided direct evidence for the existence of at least 15 additional loci. A list of the known susceptibility loci (as of April 2000) is shown in Table 1.

Table 1. Susceptibility Loci for Type 1 Diabetes

Locus	Chromosome	Candidate Genes	Markers
IDDM1	6p21.3	*HLA DR/DQ*	-
IDDM2	11p15.5	*INS* VNTR	-
IDDM3	15q26	?	D15S107
IDDM4	11q13.3	*MDU1, ZFM1, RT6, ICE, LRP5, FADD, CD3*	FGF3, D11S1917
IDDM5	6q25	*MnSOD*	ESR, aO46Xa9
IDDM6	18q12-q21	*JK* (Kidd Locus), *ZNF236*	D18S487, D18S64
IDDM7	2q31-33	*NEUROD*	D2S152, D2S326
IDDM8	6q25-27	?	D6S281, D6S264, D6S446
IDDM9	3q21-25	?	D3S1303
IDDM10	10p11-q11	?	D10S193, D10S208
IDDM11	14q24.3-q31	*ENSA, SEL-1L*	D14S67
IDDM12	2q33	*CTLA*-4	(AT)n 3' UTR, A/G Exon 1
IDDM13	2q34	*IGFBP2, IGFBP5, NEUROD, HOXD8*	D2S137, D2S164, D2S1471
IDDM15	6q21	?	D6S283, D6S434, D6S1580
IDDM17	10q25	?	D10S1750, D10S1773

Candidate gene abbreviations are explained in the main text. The *IDDM14* and *IDDM16* denominations have not been officially assigned to any locus.

IDDM1

The major susceptibility locus lies within the HLA (Human Leukocyte Antigen) region on the short arm of chromosome 6 (3), and it provides up to 40-50% of the inheritable diabetes risk. Alleles at the HLA-DQ and DR loci appear to be mainly responsible for *IDDM1*-encoded susceptibility. The HLA-DR4, DQB1*0302 and HLA-DR3, DQB1*0201 haplotypes appear to be the strongest determinants of diabetes susceptibility, and heterozygosity for these haplotypes is associated with the highest risk of disease (4-6). In contrast, the HLA-DR2 (DRB1*1501), DQB1*0602 haplotype has been shown to mediate a dominant protective effect from the development of type 1 diabetes (7-9). However, other loci within or near the HLA complex appear to modulate diabetes risk, and add further complexity to the analysis of *IDDM1*-encoded susceptibility. The *IDDM1* locus may be involved in antigen presentation and control immune responsiveness to one or more islet cell molecules targeted as autoantigens by the autoimmune responses leading to type 1 diabetes (insulin, glutamic acid decarboxylase (GAD), tyrosine-phosphatase-like protein IA-2/ICA512) (1). Alleles, modes of inheritance and putative mechanisms of susceptibility encoded at the *IDDM1* locus are extensively discussed in Chapter 3.

IDDM2

The insulin gene (*INS*) and its flanking regions on chromosome 11p15 have long been known to affect diabetes susceptibility (10-16). All of the polymorphisms identified in this region lie outside coding sequences, suggesting that susceptibility must derive from variability in the expression of the insulin gene. Extensive studies finally mapped *IDDM2* to the VNTR (variable number of tandem repeats) minisatellite located at the 5' end of the insulin gene (13,15-17). Both diabetes-predisposing alleles (Class I VNTRs) and diabetes-protective alleles (Class III VNTRs) have been reported at this locus. However, not all class III VNTR alleles are protective, and there is evidence that parental effects (imprinting) may inhibit the function of class III VNTR alleles and cause loss of the protective effect in certain individuals. It appears that VNTR alleles may control levels of *INS* expression in the thymus and in turn influence thymic selection of T-cells recognizing insulin, a key autoantigen in type 1 diabetes (18,19). *IDDM2*-encoded susceptibility is discussed in detail in Chapter 4.

IDDM3

Linkage with the marker D15S107 on chromosome 15q26 was initially detected in 250 Caucasian families from the U.K., U.S.A., and Canada. Families lacking the typical HLA predisposition provided most of the evidence for linkage. In these families, sibling pair disease concordance or discordance was strongly related to allele sharing at D15S107 (20). Linkage was confirmed in additional studies of 104 U.S. Caucasian families

(21) and 81 Danish families (22). In the Danish data set, the D15S107*130 allele provided increased susceptibility with a relative risk of 3.55, and the D15S107 locus was found to contribute up to 16% of the familial clustering of Type 1 diabetes (22). However, linkage was not confirmed in another data set of 265 Caucasian families (23). There is no known candidate gene in the 15q26 region.

IDDM4

IDDM4 is located on chromosome 11q13 tightly linked to the FGF3 marker, as reported by several groups (21,23-27). A number of candidate genes lie near FGF3. *MDU1*, encoding a cell-surface cell protein regulating intracellular calcium, and *ZFM1*, a nuclear protein, are both expressed in the pancreas. The *RT6* gene, which also lies in this region, encodes a T-cell protein with decreased expression in the BB rat model of type 1 diabetes (25). The interleukin-converting enzyme (*ICE*) and *CD3* genes were also proposed as candidates to explain *IDDM4* susceptibility. However, the *CD3* gene has been excluded by both association and linkage analysis (28), suggesting that a previous report of an association of the *CD3* gene with IDDM could have been due to population stratification (29). The gene encoding the low-density lipoprotein receptor related protein 5 (*LRP5*) has recently been mapped within the boundaries of the *IDDM4* locus and proposed as yet another candidate (30). However, it is unclear by what mechanism this molecule could influence diabetes susceptibility. Finally, the gene coding for the Fas-associated death domain protein, *FADD/MORT1*, has been mapped to chromosome 11q13.3 (31). Both its chromosomal localization and function in apoptosis, a mechanism of cell death recently implicated in the autoimmune destruction of ß-cells (32,33), make it a plausible susceptibility gene at the *IDDM4* locus. Further efforts to fine map susceptibility within the boundaries of the *IDDM4* region should help reduce the list of potential candidate genes to be analyzed for polymorphisms relevant to diabetes. In the most recent report, researchers found evidence for decreased transmission (46.4%) to the affected offspring of a 15 Kb stretch of DNA containing two tightly linked alleles (D11S1917*03 and H0570polyA*02). In contrast, the D11S1917*03-H0570polyA*02 haplotype showed increased transmission (56.6%) to unaffected siblings. These results suggest that *IDDM4* susceptibility may derive from a gene very close to the D11S1917 marker. Moreover, similar to that discussed for *IDDM1* and *IDDM2*, these findings show that analysis of both predisposing and non-predisposing alleles may be of value when mapping genes for common polygenic diseases (34).

IDDM5

Linkage with the a046xa9 and ESR markers on chromosome 6q25 has been shown by a number of studies (23,24,27,35,36). The Mn-superoxide dismutase (*MnSOD*) is a candidate gene to explain susceptibility at the

IDDM5 locus. Polymorphisms affecting the function of MnSOD could render ß-cells more susceptible to free oxygen radicals damage.

IDDM6

Linkage with the 18q12-q21 region, and in particular with the Kidd Blood group locus (JK), was suggested almost 20 years ago (37). More recently, linkage to the JK-D18S64 markers on chromosome 18q12-q21 was confirmed by the first genome-wide scan based on the utilization of microsatellites (24). Further studies using the Transmission Disequilibrium Test (TDT) provided evidence for increased transmission of allele 4 of marker D18S487 to affected children. Increased transmission was observed using 1,067 families from four different countries, although the TDT also provided evidence for genetic heterogeneity, which may be a confounding factor when mapping susceptibility genes in complex diseases (38). Additional evidence for the existence of the *IDDM6* susceptibility locus in the D18S487 region was recently provided by another large study of 1,708 families from seven different countries (39). A candidate gene was been recently identified in this region, *ZNF236*, a gene encoding a Kruppel-like zinc-finger protein. *ZNF236* is ubiquitously expressed in all human tissues tested. Expression levels appear highest in skeletal muscle and brain, intermediate in heart, pancreas, and placenta, and lowest in kidney, liver, and lung. Two alternative spliced forms of the *ZNF236* transcript were found to be up-regulated in human mesangial cells in response to elevated levels of glucose (40). The glucose-regulated expression in mesangial cells suggests that *ZNF236* may be a candidate gene for diabetic nephropathy.

IDDM7

Linkage on chromosome 2q near the marker D2S326 was initially reported in U.K. families (24). Linkage in this region was later observed with the D2S152 marker (2q31-q33) in 348 affected sibling pairs and 107 simplex families from three different populations (41). Further analysis and expansion of the above data sets have failed to reproduce convincing evidence for a susceptibility gene in this region (42), and another study of families from the U.S.A. and China did not find significant linkage (23,43). Linkage has been more recently replicated in 241 Danish families (44). The available evidence places *IDDM7* within two centiMorgans of D2S152. This chromosomal region of chromosome 2q is syntenic with the nonobese diabetic (NOD) mouse chromosome 1 region containing the *Idd5* susceptibility gene (27,41). The *HOXD8* gene has been proposed as a possible susceptibility gene in the region (45), and codes for a transcription factor. Another potential candidate gene in this chromosomal region is *NEUROD*, a transcription factor regulating the expression of the insulin gene and playing an important role in the development of pancreatic ß-cells. The *NEUROD* gene has been recently mapped to the long arm of human chromosome 2 (2q32) (46). A polymorphism consisting of a nucleotide G-to-A transition results in the substitution of alanine to threonine at codon 45 (Ala45Thr). Analysis of this polymorphism in 60 Japanese patients and 174 healthy control subjects suggested an association with type 1 but not type 2 diabetes (47). However, a similar case-control study in France did not find a similar association (48). Another candidate gene in this region, *GALNT3*, which encodes a polypeptide N-acetyl-galactosaminyltransferase-T3 (GalNAc-T3) (49), was recently mapped to a region 5-25 cM from D2S152. GalNAc transferases may influence autoimmunity by glycosylating autoantigens. However, both a marker corresponding to *GALNT3* (D2S2363) and a T284A polymorphism in the *GALNT3* 3'UTR were not found to be linked with diabetes in Danish families (44).

IDDM8

A number of studies have provided evidence for the existence of a susceptibility gene on chromosome 6q25-q27 linked to markers D6S264, D6S446 (21,24), and D6S281 (23,35,50). There is no known candidate gene in the 6q25-q27 region.

IDDM9

There is only limited evidence for the existence of this locus on chromosome 3q21-q25 linked to the marker D3S1303 (24). Further studies will be necessary to confirm this region as a susceptibility locus. There is no known candidate gene in the 3q21-q25 region. IDDM9 appears to be distinct from a susceptibility locus for Rheumatoid Arthritis reported on chromosome 3q (51).

IDDM10

A region of linkage to type 1 diabetes has also been found on chromosome 10p11-q11 and termed *IDDM10* (24). Further analysis of 1,159 families with at least one affected child from the U.K., the U.S.A., Norway, Sardinia, and Italy provided additional support for linkage at D10S193 using TDT (52). There is no available candidate gene in the 10p11-q11 region.

IDDM11

A susceptibility locus termed *IDDM11* appears to exist on chromosome 14q24.3-q31 and is linked to the microsatellite D14S67. Linkage was obtained using both maximum likelihood methods and affected sib pair methods. It appears that this represents the strongest reported evidence for linkage to any locus outside the HLA region. Similar to *IDDM3*, the subset of families lacking increased HLA sharing among the affected offspring had the strongest linkage with the D14S67 marker. Thus, *IDDM11* may be an important susceptibility locus in families lacking strong HLA region predisposition (53). Two candidate genes have been recently mapped to the suggested 14q24.3-q31 region. The *ENSA* gene encodes alpha-endosulfine, an endogenous regulator of ß-cell K(ATP) channels (54). The recombinant alpha-endosulfine has been shown to inhibit sulfonylurea binding to ß-cell membranes, to reduce cloned K(ATP) channel currents, and to stimulate insulin secretion from ß-cells. The *SEL-1L* gene codes for a negative regulator of the NOTCH, LIN-12, and GLP-1 receptors, which are required for differentiation and maturation of cells as well as cell-cell interactions during development (55). SEL-1 is abundantly expressed only in the pancreas, and appears to be involved in the down-regulation of mammalian Notch signaling, which has recently shown to be critical for the development of the pancreas and ß-cells (56).

IDDM12

Linkage with markers on chromosome 2q33 was initially reported in a group of Italian families (57). This region contains genes for both CTLA-4 (cytotoxic T lymphocyte associated-4) and CD28, two molecules intimately involved in the regulation of T-cell activation and proliferation. Differential regulation of these molecules could easily affect T-cell function and hence the responsiveness of the immune system. In particular, the *CTLA-4* gene is a strong candidate gene for autoimmune diseases since it encodes a molecule that functions as a key negative regulator of T-cell activation. The linked markers encompass a region containing an (AT)n microsatellite located in the 3' UTR of the *CTLA-4* gene. Moreover, the analysis of an A-G transition in the first exon of the *CTLA-4* gene, coding for a Thr/Ala substitution in the leader peptide, also showed preferential transmission to affected siblings (57). Although linkage was not observed in families from Sardinia, U.K., and U.S.A., preferential transmission was observed considering all of the above families together (n= 818). Further confirmation of linkage with the *IDDM12-CTLA-4* locus came through linkage disequilibrium (association) analysis using a multi-ethnic collection of families with one or more affected children, which included families from Spain, France, China, Korea, and Mexican-Americans. In this study, TDT revealed a highly significant deviation for transmission of alleles at the (AT)n microsatellite marker in the 3' untranslated region as well as the A/G polymorphism in the first exon of the *CTLA-4* gene. The overall evidence for transmission deviation of the *CTLA-4* A/G alleles remained highly significant even combining data sets (669 multiplex and 357 simplex families) from this study and the above families from Italy, U.K., U.S.A., Spain and Sardinia. However, significant heterogeneity was observed. U.K., Sardinian, and Chinese families did not show any deviation for the A/G polymorphism, while the U.S.A. families showed weak transmission deviation. In contrast, strong deviation for transmission was seen in the three Mediterranean-European populations (Italian, Spanish and French), in Mexican-Americans, and in Koreans (58). Linkage has also been reported in Japanese patients with IDDM and patients with autoimmune thyroid disease (59,60), although not in all studies of Japanese patients (61). Further evidence for linkage in the CTLA-4/CD28 region was recently obtained in a large study of 960 families from Italy, Sardinia, U.K., and U.S.A. (42). No evidence for linkage was found in the Danish population (62). The CTLA4 predisposing variant increased diabetes risk in synergy with HLA-DR3 but not with HLA-DR4 in a German population (63).

IDDM13

IDDM13 has been mapped to distal chromosome 2q34 (D2S164) in Caucasian family data sets from Australia and the U.K. (BDA Repository) (64). Similarly to *IDDM3* and *IDDM11*, *IDDM13* may be of particular interest since it was detected in non-HLA identical siblings, suggesting it may be an important susceptibility factor in subjects lacking the typical HLA predisposition. Moreover, *IDDM13* may be active early during the evolution of diabetes since linkage was found also in prediabetic subjects. Another study in Japanese families has confirmed linkage to the D2S137 microsatellite in siblings lacking HLA predisposition (65). In contrast, a recent study found no or little evidence for *IDDM13* in a data set including 352 U.K. families and 94 U.S.A. families (42). Some evidence for linkage and association of the *IDDM13*/D2S137-D2S1471 region (approximately 3.5 cM) was found in Danish families (62). It is of interest that *IDDM13*, *IDDM7*, and *IDDM12*, are all located on chromosome 2q31-35. This region may correspond to the syntenic mouse region on chromosome 1 containing *Idd5*, possibly a multigenic susceptibility locus in the NOD mouse. The *IDDM13* locus may correspond to the insulin growth factor-2 and –5 binding proteins (*IGFBP2, IGFBP5*), that are expressed at decreased levels in patients with type 1 diabetes (66). However, a number of polymorphisms of *IGFBP2*, *IGFBP5* and other genes in the region (including *NEUROD*, *HOXD8*, and *CTLA4*) were not associated with diabetes in a case-control study (67).

IDDM15

Linkage with the microsatellite D6S283 (6q21) has been shown in families from France, Denmark, and the U.S.A.. This locus is linked to HLA in males but not in females (50). *IDDM15* is the third locus localized on 6q together with *IDDM5* and *IDDM8*. There is no evidence that these loci may interact with or be linked to *IDDM1* on chromosome 6p. Multilocus analysis shows that linkage (measured by Lod scores) decreases with increasing distance from *IDDM1* (Lod Score *IDDM15*>*IDDM5*>*IDDM8*) (50). As discussed later in this chapter, parental effects may influence susceptibility at the *IDDM15* locus, and it has been suggested that the susceptibility gene at this locus may correspond to an imprinted gene associated with transient neonatal diabetes mellitus (50,68,69).

IDDM17

Evidence for this locus has been found studying a large Bedouin Arab family (19 affected relatives) (70). All affected relatives in this family carry one or two high-risk HLA-DR3 haplotypes that are rarely found in other family members. *IDDM17* maps to the long arm of chromosome 10 (10q25). Remarkably, one chromosome 10 haplotype, the B haplotype, was transmitted from a heterozygous parent to 13 of 13 affected offspring compared to 10 of 23 unaffected siblings. Recombination events occurring on this haplotype place *IDDM17* within an 8-cM interval between markers D10S1750 and D10S1773. Two other markers, D10S592 and D10S554, showed evidence of linkage disequilibrium with the disease locus. A 273-bp allele at D10S592 was transmitted to 8 of 10 affected offspring compared to 3 of 14 unaffected siblings, and a 151-bp allele at D10S554 was transmitted to 15 of 15 affected offspring compared with 10 of 24 unaffected siblings. It is important to notice that the study of this family suggests the alternative hypothesis that type 1 diabetes may be an oligogenic disease rather than a polygenic one, and that perhaps just two or three genes may suffice to explain all of the inherited susceptibility in a given family.

Other Susceptibility Loci

Linkage has been reported with the glucokinase gene (*GCK*) on chromosome 7 in 339 affected sib-pair families, but this finding has never been reproduced in other studies (71). Linkage was recently reported for the D1S1617 marker on chromosome 1q (D1S1617) (72). Another locus may lie on chromosome X linked to markers DX6678 and DXS1068. This locus may influence the male-female bias in HLA-DR3-positive patients (73). Note that the *IDDM14* and *IDDM16* denominations have not been officially assigned to any locus.

PARENTAL EFFECTS ON INHERITED GENES EXPRESSION

There is evidence that the effects of inherited genes are modulated by parental effects acting on their transmission and expression. Several studies have shown that diabetes risk differs in the offspring of diabetic mothers and fathers, although the results of different studies have been discrepant (74-76). It is also controversial whether parent of origin effects influence the transmission of *IDDM1* alleles to diabetic offspring (77-79). Recent evidence also suggests that parental influences may be operative at the *IDDM15* locus (50). There is solid evidence, however, that parental effects influence the transmission of the VNTR alleles at the *IDDM2* locus. Studies of Caucasian families from France (11), U.S.A. (14,15,80), and Canada (81) suggested that class III VNTR alleles conferred protection from Type 1 diabetes only when paternally inherited. Parental effects from the opposite germline were instead observed in families from the U.K., Denmark, and Sardinia (15,82). Such parental influences may be explained by genomic imprinting, a regulatory mechanism allowing the phenotypic expression of only one parental copy of a gene, while the other allele is repressed (83). A more complete discussion of imprinting and parental affects at the *IDDM2* locus and its functional effects on *IDDM2*-encoded susceptibility can be found in Chapter 4. Overall, parental effects can influence the transmission and expression of susceptibility alleles at certain loci and significantly contribute to the complexity of the genetics of Type 1 diabetes.

ACQUIRED GENES

The modest disease concordance rates observed in monozygotic twins suggest that factors other than inherited genes must play a role in determining progression to overt disease in those individuals carrying predisposing genes. Environmental factors (viruses, diet) are suspected to be such determinants (84). Viruses could trigger specific autoimmune responses through mechanisms of molecular mimicry or by mediating a direct insult to ß-cells. It is also an intriguing and yet unproven possibility that novel genes may be acquired through, or their expression stimulated by, environmental factors (viruses or diet) after birth. Unlike more common viruses, retroviruses can integrate into the human genome. Retroviral genes can be either inherited or acquired after birth, and common viral infections and/or sex hormone changes associated with puberty may activate quiescent retroviruses. Such acquired expression may trigger the development of diabetes in genetically predisposed individuals either via cross-reactivity or immunity against novel viral antigens previously unknown to the immune system. This could drive immunity against the tissue that is expressing the novel gene, or to any tissue expressing molecules with significant cross-reactivity. Thus, environmental factors may provide or activate genes that could act as "disease genes". This hypothesis was recently supported by the finding that a human endogenous retrovirus, termed $IDDMK_{1,2}22$, is apparently expressed in and released from leukocytes in patients with Type 1 diabetes but not in controls (85). It is unclear whether this or similar retroviruses could be expressed in the endocrine pancreas, but it was suggested that $IDDMK_{1,2}22$ could drive the same T-cell receptor restriction observed in T-lymphocytes infiltrating the endocrine pancreas of two children who died at the onset of diabetes (86). However, the role of $IDDMK_{1,2}22$ has been seriously questioned by later studies. In fact, $IDDMK_{1,2}22$ was found to be expressed at similar frequencies in patients and controls in several studies, and no evidence for auto-reactivity against this virus has been reported (87-95).

CONCLUSION

A large body of evidence indicates that genetic factors influence both susceptibility to and resistance from type 1 diabetes. Several chromosomal regions have been linked with the disease, suggesting that this is a polygenic disorder, and there is evidence that certain alleles provide genetic protection from diabetes, as clearly shown for the *IDDM1* (HLA-DQB1*0602) and *IDDM2* (*INS*-VNTR class III) loci. A protective allele may also exist at the *IDDM4* locus. Nine of the susceptibility loci reported lie in just three chromosomes (6, 2, and 11). Chromosome 6 contains *IDDM1* on 6p21.3, *IDDM5* on 6q25, *IDDM8* on 6q25-27, and *IDDM15* on 6q21. Chromosome 2 contains *IDDM7* on 2q31-q33, *IDDM12* on 2q33, and *IDDM13* on 2q34. Chromosome 11 contains *IDDM2* on 11p15.5 and *IDDM4* on 11q13.3. Moreover, susceptibility loci on chromosomes 2 and 6 seem to cluster within fairly small regions. This may facilitate co-inheritance of susceptibility and epistatic interactions. Most of the loci identified through linkage analysis, however, provide only modest contribution to the familial clustering of diabetes, and no other major susceptibility loci have been reported besides *IDDM1*. However, significant genetic heterogeneity has been consistently reported among and within different data sets, and this could decrease the probability that other major susceptibility genes, if heterogeneous and occurring in a minority of families, could be identified with the current analytical power and study design. The identification of *IDDM17* in a large pedigree may reflect this phenomenon, and also suggests the alternative hypothesis that type 1 diabetes may be oligogenic rather than polygenic. Most of the susceptibility genes lying in the chromosomal regions linked to diabetes remain unknown. A few candidate genes are available at some loci, but it is expected that significant progress will be made soon with the availability of sequence data from the Human Genome Project. Some progress is also being made in dissecting the molecular mechanisms controlling diabetes susceptibility. It is a fair speculation that *IDDM1* may be involved in antigen presentation and control immune responsiveness to one or more islet cell antigens, either in the thymus or in the periphery, or both. With respect to *IDDM2*, VNTR alleles appear to influence *INS* expression in the thymus, and thus may affect the development of tolerance to insulin. Thus, *IDDM1* and *IDDM2* may influence basic immunological functions such as antigen presentation and thymic selection, and appear to control the specificity of the immune response rather than mediate a generic predisposition to autoimmunity. It is important to note that the susceptibility alleles identified at the best characterized loci (*IDDM1*, *IDDM2, and IDDM12*) are commonly observed in the population and all appear to have normal sequence. This suggests that susceptibility may simply derive from polymorphisms affecting the function and expression of certain proteins. It is plausible that a number of loci may map to regulatory sequences (such as

VNTRs) and act as quantitative traits. Complex parental effects reportedly modifying the transmission and expression of inherited genes further complicate the genetics of diabetes. Parental effects may significantly influence susceptibility, for instance inhibiting the expression and function of certain genes. It is also an intriguing possibility that additional genetic factors or their expression may be acquired after birth, perhaps through environmental exposures. Such factors may play a key role in triggering the process leading to ß-cell destruction. Future studies are expected to lead to the full identification and characterization of susceptibility and, perhaps, disease genes. This will improve the ability to predict disease risk by genetic testing and enhance understanding of the key mechanisms leading to Type 1 diabetes.

REFERENCES

1. Schranz, D.B. and A. Lernmark. 1998. Immunology in diabetes: An update. *Diabetes-Metabolism Rev* 14:3-29.
2. Hearne, C.M. and J.A. Todd. 1992. Microsatellites for linkage analysis of genetic traits. *Trends Genet* 8:288-294.
3. Johnson, A.H., C.K. Hurley, R.J. Hartzman, C.A. Alper, and E.J. Yunis. 1991. HLA: The major histocompatibility complex of man. In 18th edition Clinical Diagnosis & Management by Laboratory Methods. J.B. Henry, editor. WB Saunders, Philadelphia. 761-794.
4. Thomson, G., W.P. Robinson, M.K. Kuhner, S. Joe, M.J. MacDonald, J.L. Gottschall, J. Barbosa, S.S. Rich , J. Bertrams, M.P. Baur, J. Partanen, B.D. Tait, E. Schober, W.R. Mayr, J. Ludvigsson, B. Linblom, N.R. Farid, C. Thompson, and I. Deschamps. 1988. Genetic heterogeneity, modes of inheritance, and risk estimates; a joint study of caucasians with insulin-dependent diabetes mellitus. *Am.J.Hum.Genet.* 43:799-816.
5. Todd, J.A., J.I. Bell, and H.O. McDevitt. 1987. HLA-DQ beta gene contribution to susceptibility and resistance to insulin dependent diabetes mellitus. *Nature* 329:599-604.
6. Horn, G.T., T.L. Bugawan, C.M. Long, and H.A. Erlich. 1988. Allelic sequence variation of the HLA-DQ loci: Relationship to serology and to insulin-dependent diabetes mellitus susceptibility. *Proc Natl Acad Sci USA* 85:6012-6016.
7. Baisch, J.M., T. Week, R. Giles, M. Hoover, P. Stastny, and D. Capra. 1990. Analysis of HLA-DQ genotypes and susceptibility in insulin-dependent diabetes mellitus. *N Eng J Med* 322:1836-1841.
8. Pugliese, A., R. Gianani, R. Moromisato, Z.L. Awdeh, C.A. Alper, H.A. Erlich, R.A. Jackson, and G.S. Eisenbarth. 1995. HLA-DQB1*0602 is associated with dominant protection from diabetes even among islet cell antibody-positive first-degree relatives of patients with IDDM. *Diabetes* 44:608-613.
9. Pugliese, A., E. Kawasaki, M. Zeller, L. Yu, S. Babu, M. Solimena, C.T. Moraes, M. Pietropaolo, R.P. Friday, M. Trucco, C. Ricordi, M. Allen, J.A. Noble, H.A. Erlich, and G.S. Eisenbarth. 1999. Sequence analysis of the diabetes-protective human leukocyte antigen- DQB1*0602 allele in unaffected, islet cell antibody-positive first degree relatives and in rare patients with type 1 diabetes. *J.Clin.Endocrinol.Metab.* 84:1722-1728.
10. Bell, G.I., S. Horita, and J.H. Karam. 1984. A polymorphic locus near the human insulin gene is associated with insulin dependent diabetes mellitus. *Diabetes* 33:176-183.
11. Julier, C., R.N. Hyer, J. Davies, F. Merlin, P. Soularue, L. Briant, G. Cathelineau, I. Deschamps, J.I. Rotter, P. Froguel, C. Boitard, J.I. Bell, and G.M. Lathrop. 1991. Insulin-

IGF2 region encodes a gene implicated in HLA-DR4-dependent diabetes susceptibility. *Nature* 354:155-159.

12. Lucassen, A., C. Julier, J.-P. Beressi, C. Boitard, P. Froguel, M. Lathrop, and J.I. Bell. 1993. Susceptibility to insulin dependent diabetes mellitus maps to a 4.1 kb segment of DNA spanning the insulin gene and associated VNTR. *Nat Genetics* 4:305-310.
13. Owerbach, D. and K.H. Gabbay. 1993. Localization of a Type I diabetes susceptibility locus to the variable tandem repeat region flanking the insulin gene. *Diabetes* 42:1708-1714.
14. Pugliese, A., Z.L. Awdeh, C.A. Alper, R.A. Jackson, and G.S. Eisenbarth. 1994. The paternally inherited insulin gene B allele (1,428 FokI site) confers protection from insulin-dependent diabetes in families. *Journal of Autoimmunity* 7:687-694.
15. Bennett, S.T., A.M. Lucassen, S.C.L. Gough, E.E. Powell, D.E. Undlien, L.E. Pritchard, M.E. Merriman, Y. Kawaguchi, M.J. Dronsfield, F. Pociot, J. Nerup, N. Bouzekri, A. Cambot-Thomsen, K.S. Ronningen, A.H. Barnett, S.C. Bain, and J.A. Todd. 1995. Susceptibility to human type 1 diabetes at IDDM2 is determined by tandem repeat variation at the insulin gene minisatellite locus. *Nature Genetics* 9:284-292.
16. Undlien, D.E., S.T. Bennett, J.A. Todd, H.E. Akselsen, I. Ikaheimo, H. Reijonen, M. Knip, E. Thorsby, and K.S. Ronningen. 1995. Insulin gene region-encoded susceptibility to IDDM maps upstream of the insulin gene. *Diabetes* 44:620-625.
17. Julier, C., A. Lucassen, P. Villedieu, M. Delepine, C. Levy-Marchal, P.M. Danze, F. Bianchi, C. Boitard, P. Froguel, J. Bell, and G.M. Lathrop. 1994. Multiple DNA variant association analysis: application to the insulin gene region in type I diabetes. *Am.J.Hum.Genet.* 55:1247-1254.
18. Pugliese, A., M. Zeller, A.J. Fernandez, L.J. Zalcberg, R.J. Bartlett, C. Ricordi, M. Pietropaolo, G.S. Eisenbarth, S.T. Bennett, and D.D. Patel. 1997. The insulin gene is transcribed in the human thymus and transcription levels correlated with allelic variation at the INS VNTR-IDDM2 susceptibility locus for type 1 diabetes. *Nat.Genet.* 15:293-297.
19. Vafiadis, P., S.T. Bennett, J.A. Todd, J. Nadeau, R. Grabs, C.G. Goodyear, S. Wickramasinghe, E. Colle, and C. Polychronakos. 1997. Insulin expression in the thymus is modulated by *INS* VNTR alleles at the *IDDM2* locus. *Nature Genetics* 15:289-292.
20. Field, L.L., R. Tobias, and T. Magnus. 1994. A locus on chromosome 15q26 (IDDM3) produces susceptibility to insulin- dependent diabetes mellitus [see comments]. *Nat.Genet.* 8:189-194.
21. Luo, D.F., M.M. Bui, A. Muir, N.K. Maclaren, G. Thomson, and J.X. She. 1995. Affected-sib-pair mapping of a novel susceptibility gene to insulin- dependent diabetes mellitus (IDDM8) on chromosome 6q25-q27. *Am.J.Hum.Genet.* 57:911-919.
22. Zamani, M., F. Pociot, P. Raeymaekers, J. Nerup, and J.J. Cassiman. 1996. Linkage of type I diabetes to 15q26 (IDDM3) in the Danish population. *Hum.Genet.* 98:491-496.
23. Luo, D.F., R. Buzzetti, J.I. Rotter, N.K. Maclaren, L.J. Raffel, L. Nistico, C. Giovannini, P. Pozzilli, G. Thomson, and J.X. She. 1996. Confirmation of three susceptibility genes to insulin-dependent diabetes mellitus: IDDM4, IDDM5 and IDDM8. *Hum.Mol.Genet.* 5:693-698.
24. Davies, J.L., Y. Kawaguchi, S.T. Bennett, J.B. Copeman, H.J. Cordell, L.E. Pritchard, P.W. Reed, S.C. Gough , S.C. Jenkins, and S.M. Palmer. 1994. A genome-wide search for human type 1 diabetes susceptibility genes [see comments]. *Nature* 371:130-136.
25. Hashimoto, L., C. Habita, J.P. Beressi, M. Delepine, C. Besse, A. Cambon-Thomsen, I. Deschamps, J.I. Rotter, S. Djoulah, M.R. James, P. Froguel, J. Weissenbach, G.M. Lathrop, and C. Julier. 1994. Genetic mapping of a susceptibility locus for insulin-dependent diabetes mellitus on chromosome 11q. *Nature* 371:161-164.
26. Cordell, H.J., J.A. Todd, S.T. Bennett, Y. Kawaguchi, and M. Farrall. 1995. Two-locus maximum lod score analysis of a multifactorial trait: joint consideration of IDDM2 and IDDM4 with IDDM1 in type 1 diabetes. *Am.J.Hum.Genet.* 57:920-934.

27. Buhler, J., D. Owerbach, A.A. Schaffer, M. Kimmel, and K.H. Gabbay. 1997. Linkage analyses in type I diabetes mellitus using CASPAR, a software and statistical program for conditional analysis of polygenic diseases. *Hum.Hered.* 47:211-222.
28. Pritchard, L.E., Y. Kawaguchi, P.W. Reed, J.B. Copeman, J.L. Davies, A.H. Barnett, S.C. Bain, and J.A. Todd. 1995. Analysis of the CD3 gene region and type 1 diabetes: application of fluorescence-based technology to linkage disequilibrium mapping. *Hum.Mol.Genet.* 4:197-202.
29. Wong, S., S. Moore, S. Orisio, A. Millward, and A.G. Demaine. 1991. Susceptibility to type I diabetes in women is associated with the CD3 epsilon locus on chromosome 11. *Clin.exp.Immunol.* 83:69-73.
30. Hey, P.J., R.C. Twells, M.S. Phillips, N. Yusuke, S.D. Brown, Y. Kawaguchi, R. Cox, X. Guochun, V. Dugan, H. Hammond, M.L. Metzker, J.A. Todd, and J.F. Hess. 1998. Cloning of a novel member of the low-density lipoprotein receptor family. *Gene* 216:103-111.
31. Kim, P.K., A.S. Dutra, S.C. Chandrasekharappa, and J.M. Puck. 1996. Genomic structure and mapping of human FADD, an intracellular mediator of lymphocyte apoptosis. *J.Immunol.* 157:5461-5466.
32. Chervonsky, A.V., Y. Wang, F.S. Wong, I. Visintin, R.A. Flavell, C.A.J. Janeway, and L.A. Matis. 1997. The role of Fas in autoimmune diabetes. *Cell* 89:17-24.
33. Stassi, G., R.D. Maria, G. Trucco, W. Rudert, R. Testi, A. Galluzzo, C. Giordano, and M. Trucco. 1997. Nitric oxide primes pancreatic beta cells for Fas-mediated destruction in insulin-dependent diabetes mellitus. *J.Exp.Med.* 186:1193-1200.
34. Nakagawa, Y., Y. Kawaguchi, R.C. Twells, C. Muxworthy, K.M. Hunter, A. Wilson, M.E. Merriman, R.D. Cox, T. Merriman, F. Cucca, P.A. McKinney, J.P. Shield, J. Tuomilehto, E. Tuomilehto-Wolf, C. Ionesco-Tirgoviste, Nistic, R. Buzzetti, P. Pozzilli, F. San-Raffaele, G. Joner, E. Thorsby, D.E. Undlien, F. Pociot, J. Nerup, K.S. nningen, F.S.G. Bart's-Oxford, S.C. Bain, J.A. Todd, and IDDM4 . 1998. Fine mapping of the diabetes-susceptibility locus, IDDM4, on chromosome 11q13. *Am.J.Hum.Genet.* 63:547-556.
35. Davies, J.L., F. Cucca, J.V. Goy, Z.A. Atta, M.E. Merriman, A. Wilson, A.H. Barnett, S.C. Bain, and J.A. Todd. 1996. Saturation multipoint linkage mapping of chromosome 6q in type 1 diabetes. *Hum.Mol.Genet.* 5:1071-1074.
36. Delepine, M., F. Pociot, C. Habita, L. Hashimoto, P. Froguel, J. Rotter, A. Cambon-Thomsen, I. Deschamps, S. Djoulah, J. Weissenbach, J. Nerup, M. Lathrop, and C. Julier. 1997. Evidence of a non-MHC susceptibility locus in type I diabetes linked to HLA on chromosome 6. *Am.J.Hum.Genet.* 60:174-187.
37. Hodge, S.E., C.E. Anderson, K. Neiswanger, L.L. Field, M.A. Spence, R.S. Sparkes, M. Christ, P.I. Terasaki, D.L. Rimoin, and J.I. Rotter. 1982. Close genetic linkage between diabetes mellitus and Kidd Blood group. *Lancet* ii:893
38. Merriman, T., R. Twells, M. Merriman, I. Eaves, R. Cox, F. Cucca, P. McKinney, J. Shield, D. Baum, E. Bosi, P. Pozzilli, L. Nistico, R. Buzzetti, G. Joner, K. Ronningen, E. Thorsby, D. Undlien, F. Pociot, J. Nerup, S. Bain, A. Barnett, and J. Todd. 1997. Evidence by allelic association-dependent methods for a type 1 diabetes polygene (IDDM6) on chromosome 18q21. *Hum.Mol.Genet.* 6:1003-1010.
39. Merriman, T.R., I.A. Eaves, R.C. Twells, M.E. Merriman, P.A. Danoy, C.E. Muxworthy, K.M. Hunter, R.D. Cox, F. Cucca, P.A. McKinney, J.P. Shield, J.D. Baum, J. Tuomilehto, E. Tuomilehto-Wolf, C. Ionesco-Tirgoviste, G. Joner, E. Thorsby, D.E. Undlien, F. Pociot, J. Nerup, K.S. Ronningen, S.C. Bain, and J.A. Todd. 1998. Transmission of haplotypes of microsatellite markers rather than single marker alleles in the mapping of a putative type 1 diabetes susceptibility gene (IDDM6). *Hum.Mol.Genet.* 7:517-524.
40. Holmes, D.I., N.A. Wahab, and R.M. Mason. 1999. Cloning and characterization of ZNF236, a glucose-regulated Kruppel-like zinc-finger gene mapping to human chromosome 18q22-q23. *Genomics* 60:105-109.

41. Copeman, J.B., F. Cucca, C.M. Hearne, R.J. Cornall, P.W. Reed, K.S. Ronningen , D.E. Undlien, L. Nistico, R. Buzzetti, and R. Tosi. 1995. Linkage disequilibrium mapping of a type 1 diabetes susceptibility gene (IDDM7) to chromosome 2q31-q33. *Nat.Genet.* 9:80-85.
42. Esposito, L., N.J. Hill, L.E. Pritchard, F. Cucca, C. Muxworthy, M.E. Merriman, A. Wilson, C. Julier, M. Delepine, J. Tuomilehto, E. Tuomilehto-Wolf, C. Ionesco-Tirgoviste, L. Nistico', R. Buzzetti, P. Pozzilli, M. Ferrari, E. Bosi, F. Pociot, J. Nerup, S.C. Bain, and J.A. Todd. 1998. Genetic analysis of chromosome 2 in type 1 diabetes: analysis of putative loci IDDM7, IDDM12, and IDDM13 and candidate genes NRAMP1 and IA-2 and the interleukin-1 gene cluster. IMDIAB Group [In Process Citation]. *Diabetes* 47:1797-1799.
43. Luo, D.F., N.K. Maclaren, H.S. Huang, A. Muir , and J.X. She. 1995. Intrafamilial and case-control association analysis of D2S152 in insulin-dependent diabetes. *Autoimmunity.* 21:143-147.
44. Kristiansen, O.P., F. Pociot, E.P. Bennett, H. Clausen, J. Johannesen, J. Nerup, and T. Mandrup-Poulsen. IDDM7 links to insulin-dependent diabetes mellitus in Danish multiplex families but linkage is not explained by novel polymorphisms in the candidate gene GALNT3. The Danish Study Group of Diabetes in Childhood and The Danish IDDM Epidemiology and Genetics Group. *Hum.Mutat.(Online.) 2000.Mar.;15.(3.):295.-6.* 15:295-296.
45. Owerbach, D. and Gabbay, K. H. 1995. The HOXD8 locus (2q31) is linked to type I diabetes. Interaction with chromosome 6 and 11 disease susceptibility genes. *Diabetes* 44, 132-136.
46. Tamimi, R., E. Steingrimsson, N.G. Copeland, K. Dyer-Montgomery, J.E. Lee, R. Hernandez, N.A. Jenkins, and S.J. Tapscott. 1996. The NEUROD gene maps to human chromosome 2q32 and mouse chromosome 2. *Genomics* 34:418-421.
47. Iwata, I., S. Nagafuchi, H. Nakashima, S. Kondo, T. Koga, Y. Yokogawa, T. Akashi, T. Shibuya, Y. Umeno, T. Okeda, S. Shibata, S. Kono, M. Yasunami , H. Ohkubo, and Y. Niho. 1999. Association of polymorphism in the NeuroD/BETA2 gene with type 1 diabetes in the Japanese. *Diabetes* 48:416-419.
48. Dupont, S., C. Dina, E.H. Hani, and P. Froguel. 1999. Absence of replication in the French population of the association between beta 2/NEUROD-A45T polymorphism and type 1 diabetes. *Diabetes Metab.* 25:516-517.
49. Bennett, E.P., H. Hassan, U. Mandel, M.A. Hollingsworth, N. Akisawa, Y. Ikematsu, G. Merkx, A.G. van Kessel , S. Olofsson, and H. Clausen. 1999. Cloning and characterization of a close homologue of human UDP-N-acetyl-alpha-D-galactosamine:Polypeptide N-acetylgalactosaminyltransferase-T3, designated GalNAc-T6. Evidence for genetic but not functional redundancy. *J.Biol.Chem.* 274:25362-25370.
50. Delepine, M., F. Pociot, C. Habita, L. Hashimoto, P. Froguel, J. Rotter, A. Cambon-Thomsen, I. Deschamps, S. Djoulah, J. Weissenbach, J. Nerup, M. Lathrop, and C. Julier. 1997. Evidence for a non-MHC susceptibility locus in type I diabetes linked to HLA on chromosome 6. *Am.J.Hum.Genet.* 60:174-187.
51. Paterson, A.D., P. Rahman, and A. Petronis. 1999. IDDM9 and a locus for rheumatoid arthritis on chromosome 3q appear to be distinct. *Hum.Immunol.* 60:883-885.
52. Reed, P., F. Cucca, S. Jenkins, M. Merriman, A. Wilson, P. McKinney, E. Bosi, G. Joner, K. Ronningen, E. Thorsby, D. Undlien, T. Merriman, A. Barnett, S. Bain, and J. Todd. 1997. Evidence for a type 1 diabetes susceptibility locus (IDDM10) on human chromosome 10p11-q11. *Hum.Mol.Genet.* 6:1011-1016.
53. Field, L.L., R. Tobias, G. Thomson, and S. Plon. 1996. Susceptibility to insulin-dependent diabetes mellitus maps to a locus (IDDM11) on human chromosome 14q24.3-q31. *Genomics* 33:1-8.
54. Heron, L., A. Virsolvy, F. Apiou, A. Le Cam, and D. Bataille. 1999. Isolation, characterization, and chromosomal localization of the human ENSA gene that encodes alpha-endosulfine, a regulator of beta-cell K(ATP) channels. *Diabetes* 48:1873-1876.

55. Harada, Y., K. Ozaki, M. Suzuki, T. Fujiwara, E. Takahashi, Y. Nakamura , and A. Tanigami. 1999. Complete cDNA sequence and genomic organization of a human pancreas-specific gene homologous to Caenorhabditis elegans sel-1. *J.Hum.Genet.* 44:330-336.
56. Apelqvist, A., H. Li, L. Sommer, P. Beatus, D.J. Anderson, T. Honjo, d.A. Hrabe, U. Lendahl, and H. Edlund. 1999. Notch signalling controls pancreatic cell differentiation. *Nature* 400:877-881.
57. Nistico, L., R. Buzzetti, L.E. Pritchard, B. Van der Auwera, C. Giovannini, E. Bosi, M.T. Larrad, M.S. Rios, C.C. Chow, C.S. Cockram, K. Jacobs, C. Mijovic, S.C. Bain, A.H. Barnett, C.L. Vandewalle, F. Schuit, F.K. Gorus, R. Tosi, P. Pozzilli, and J.A. Todd. 1996. The CTLA-4 gene region of chromosome 2q33 is linked to, and associated with, type 1 diabetes. Belgian Diabetes Registry. *Hum.Mol.Genet.* 5:1075-1080.
58. Marron, M.P., L.J. Raffel, H.J. Garchon, C.O. Jacob, M. Serrano-Rios, L.M. Martinez, W.P. Teng, Y. Park, Z.X. Zhang, D.R. Goldstein, Y.W. Tao, G. Beaurain, J.F. Bach, H.S. Huang, D.F. Luo, A. Zeidler, J.I. Rotter, M.C. Yang, T. Modilevsky, N.K. Maclaren, and J.X. She. 1997. Insulin-dependent diabetes mellitus (IDDM) is associated with CTLA4 polymorphisms in multiple ethnic groups. *Hum.Mol.Genet.* 6:1275-1282.
59. Awata, T., S. Kurihara, M. Iitaka, S. Takei, I. Inoue, C. Ishii, K. Negishi, T. Izumida, Y. Yoshida, R. Hagura, N. Kuzuya, Y. Kanazawa, and S. Katayama. 1998. Association of CTLA-4 gene A-G polymorphism (IDDM12 locus) with acute- onset and insulin-depleted IDDM as well as autoimmune thyroid disease (Graves' disease and Hashimoto's thyroiditis) in the Japanese population. *Diabetes* 47:128-129.
60. Hayashi, H., I. Kusaka, S. Nagasaka, A. Kawakami, K. Rokkaku, T. Nakamura, T. Saito, M. Higashiyama, K. Honda, and S.E. Ishikawa. 1999. Association of CTLA-4 polymorphism with positive anti-GAD antibody in Japanese subjects with type 1 diabetes mellitus. *Clin.Endocrinol.(Oxf.)* 51:793-799.
61. Yanagawa, T., T. Maruyama, K. Gomi, M. Taniyama, A. Kasuga, Y. Ozawa, M. Terauchi, H. Hirose, H. Maruyama, and T. Saruta. 1999. Lack of association between CTLA-4 gene polymorphism and IDDM in Japanese subjects. *Autoimmunity.* 29:53-56.
62. Larsen, Z.M., O.P. Kristiansen, E. Mato, J. Johannesen, M. Puig-Domingo, A. de Leiva, J. Nerup, and F. Pociot. 1999. IDDM12 (CTLA4) on 2q33 and IDDM13 on 2q34 in genetic susceptibility to type 1 diabetes (insulin-dependent). *Autoimmunity.* 31:35-42.
63. Badenhoop, K., H. Donner, M. Pani, H. Rau, T. Siegmund, and J. Braun. 1999. Genetic susceptibility to type 1 diabetes: clinical and molecular heterogeneity of IDDM1 and IDDM12 in a german population. *Exp.Clin.Endocrinol.Diabetes* 107 Suppl 3:S89-92:S89-S92
64. Morahan, G., D. Huang, B.D. Tait, P.G. Colman, and L.C. Harrison. 1996. Markers on distal chromosome 2q linked to insulin-dependent diabetes mellitus. *Science* 272:1811-1813.
65. Fu, J., H. Ikegami, Y. Kawaguchi, T. Fujisawa , Y. Kawabata, Y. Hamada, H. Ueda, M. Shintani, K. Nojima, N. Babaya, Q.J. Shen, Y. Uchigata, T. Urakami, Y. Omori, K. Shima, and T. Ogihara. 1998. Association of distal chromosome 2q with IDDM in Japanese subjects. *Diabetologia* 41:228-232.
66. Giannini, S., S. Mohan, J. Kasuya, G. Galli, C.M. Rotella, T.R. LeBon, and Y. Fujita-Yamaguichi. 1994. Characterization of insulin-like growth factor-binding proteins produced by cultured fibroblasts from patients with noninsulin-dependent diabetes mellitus, insulin-dependent diabetes mellitus, or obesity. *J.Clin.Endocrinol.Metab.* 79:1824-1830.
67. Owerbach, D., F.J. Naya, M.J. Tsai, S.V. Allander, D.R. Powell, and K.H. Gabbay. 1997. Analysis of candidate genes for susceptibility to type I diabetes: a case-control and family-association study of genes on chromosome 2q31-35. *Diabetes* 46:1069-1074.
68. Temple, I.K., R.S. James, J.A. Crolla, F.L. Sitch, P.A. Jacobs, W.M. Howell, P. Betts, J.D. Baum, and J.P.H. Shield. 1995. An imprinted gene(s) for diabetes? *Nat Genet* 9:110-112.

69. Haig, D. 1995. Is human insulin imprinted? *Nat Genet* 7:10
70. Verge, C.F., P. Vardi, S. Babu, F. Bao, H.A. Erlich, T. Bugawan, D. Tiosano, L. Yu, G.S. Eisenbarth, and P.R. Fain. 1998. Evidence for oligogenic inheritance of type 1 diabetes in a large Bedouin Arab family. *J.Clin.Invest.* 102:1569-1575.
71. Rowe, R.E., B. Wapelhorst, G.I. Bell, N. Risch, R.S. Spielman, and P. Concannon. 1995. Linkage and association between insulin-dependent diabetes mellitus (IDDM) susceptibility and markers near the glucokinase gene on chromosome 7. *Nat.Genet.* 10:240-242.
72. Concannon, P., K.J. Gogolin-Ewens, D.A. Hinds, B. Wapelhorst, V.A. Morrison, B. Stirling, M. Mitra, J. Farmer , S.R. Williams, N.J. Cox, G.I. Bell, N. Risch, and R.S. Spielman. 1998. A second-generation screen of the human genome for susceptibility to insulin-dependent diabetes mellitus [see comments]. *Nat.Genet.* 19:292-296.
73. Cucca, F., J.V. Goy, Y. Kawaguchi, L. Esposito, M.E. Merriman, A.J. Wilson, H.J. ordell, S.C. in, and J.A. odd. 1998. A male-female bias in type 1 diabetes and linkage to chromosome Xp in MHC HLA-DR3-positive patients. *Nat Genet* 19:301-302.
74. Warram, J.H., A.S. Krolewski, M.S. Gottlieb, and C.R. Kahn. 1984. Differences in risk of insulin-dependent diabetes in offspring of diabetic mothers and diabetic fathers. *New England Journal of Medicine* 311, No.3:149-152.
75. Warram, J.H., C.M. Blaise, and A.S. Krolewski. 1991. Risk of IDDM in children of diabetic mothers decreases with increasing maternal age at pregnancy. *Diabetes* 40:1679-1684.
76. Bleich, D., M. Polak, G.S. Eisenbarth, and R.A. Jackson. 1993. Decreased risk of type I diabetes in offspring of mothers who acquire diabetes during adrenarchy. *Diabetes* 42:1433-1439.
77. Vadheim, C.M., J.I. Rotter, N.K. Maclaren, W.J. Riley, and C.E. Anderson. 1986. Preferential transmission of diabetic alleles within the HLA gene complex. *New England Journal of Medicine* 315:1314-1318.
78. Deschamps, I., J. Hors, F. Clerget-Darpoux, E. Gardais, J.J. Robert, A. Marcelli-Berge, H. Lestradet, and J. Dausset. 1990. Excess of maternal HLA-DR3 antigens in HLA DR3,4 positive type 1 (insulin-dependent) diabetic patients. *Diabetologia* 33:425-439.
79. Bain, S.C., B.R. Rowe, and A.H.T.J.A. Barnett. 1994. Parental origin of diabetes-associated HLA types in sibling pairs with type I diabetes. *Diabetes* 43:1462-1468.
80. Bui, M.M., D.-F. Luo, J.Y. She, N.K. Maclaren, A. Muir, G. Thomson, and J.-X. She. 1996. Paternally transmitted IDDM2 influences diabetes susceptibility despite biallelic expression of the insulin gene in human pancreas. *Journal of Autoimmunity* 9:97-103.
81. Polychronakos, C., A. Kukuvitis, N. Giannoukakis, and E. Colle. 1995. Parental Imprinting effect at the INS-IGF2 diabetes susceptibility locus. *Diabetologia* 38:715-719.
82. Bennett, S.T., A.J. Wilson, F. Cucca, J. Nerup, F. Pociot, P.A. McKinney, A.H. Barnett, S.C. Bain, and J.A. Todd. 1996. *IDDM2*-VNTR-encoded susceptibility to type 1 diabetes: dominant protection and parental transmission of alleles of the insulin gene-linked minisatellite locus. *Journal of Autoimmunity* 9:415-421.
83. Hoffman, A.R. and T.H. Vu. 1996. Genomic Imprinting. *Scientific American* 1:52-61.
84. Akerblom, H.K. and M. Knip. 1998. Putative environmental factors in Type 1 Diabetes. *Diabetes-Metabolism Reviews* 14:31-67.
85. Conrad, B., R.N. Weissmahr, J. Boni, R. Arcari, J. Schupbach, and B. Mach . 1997. A human endogenous retroviral superantigen as candidate autoimmune gene in type I diabetes. *Cell* 90:303-313.
86. Conrad, B., E. Weldmann, G. Trucco, W.A. Rudert, R. Behboo, C. Ricordi, H. Rodriquez-Rilo, D. Finegold, and M. Trucco. 1994. Evidence for superantigen involvement in insulin-dependent diabetes mellitus aetiology. *Nature* 371:351-355.
87. Knerr, I., R. Repp, J. Dotsch, N. Gratzki, J. Hanze, T. Kapellen, and W. Rascher. 1999. Quantitation of gene expression by real-time PCR disproves a "retroviral hypothesis" for childhood-onset diabetes mellitus. *Pediatr.Res.* 46:57-60.

88. Kim, A., H.S. Jun, L. Wong, D. Stephure, D. Pacaud, R.A. Trussell, and J.W. Yoon. 1999. Human endogenous retrovirus with a high genomic sequence homology with IDDMK(1,2)22 is not specific for Type I (insulin-dependent) diabetic patients but ubiquitous. *Diabetologia* 42:413-418.
89. Jaeckel, E., S. Heringlake, D. Berger, G. Brabant, G. Hunsmann, and M.P. Manns. 1999. No evidence for association between IDDMK(1,2)22, a novel isolated retrovirus, and IDDM. *Diabetes* 48:209-214.
90. Murphy, V.J., L.C. Harrison, W.A. Rudert, P. Luppi, M. Trucco, A. Fierabracci , P.A. Biro, and G.F. Bottazzo. 1998. Retroviral superantigens and type 1 diabetes mellitus. *Cell* 95:9-11.
91. Kim, A., H.S. Jun, L. Wong, D. Stephure, D. Pacaud, R.A. Trussell, and J.W. Yoon. 1999. Human endogenous retrovirus with a high genomic sequence homology with IDDMK(1,2)22 is not specific for Type I (insulin-dependent) diabetic patients but ubiquitous. *Diabetologia* 42:413-418.
92. Muir, A., Q.G. Ruan, M.P. Marron, and J.X. She. 1999. The IDDMK(1,2)22 retrovirus is not detectable in either mRNA or genomic DNA from patients with type 1 diabetes. *Diabetes* 48:219-222.
93. Badenhoop, K., H. Donner, J. Neumann, J. Herwig, R. Kurth, K.H. Usadel, and R.R. Tonjes. 1999. IDDM patients neither show humoral reactivities against endogenous retroviral envelope protein nor do they differ in retroviral mRNA expression from healthy relatives or normal individuals. *Diabetes* 48:215-218.
94. Lan, M.S., A. Mason, R. Coutant, Q.Y. Chen , A. Vargas, J. Rao, R. Gomez, S. Chalew, R. Garry, and N.K. Maclaren. 1998. HERV-K10s and immune-mediated (type 1) diabetes. *Cell* 95:14-16.
95. Lower, R., R.R. Tonjes, K. Boller, J. Denner, B. Kaiser, R.C. Phelps, J. Lower, R. Kurth, K. Badenhoop, H. Donner, K.H. Usadel, T. Miethke, M. Lapatschek, and H. Wagner. 1998. Development of insulin-dependent diabetes mellitus does not depend on specific expression of the human endogenous retrovirus HERV-K. *Cell* 95:11-14.

3
TYPE 1 DIABETES, AUTOIMMUNITY, AND THE MHC

Pamela R. Fain, Ph.D. and George S. Eisenbarth, M.D., Ph.D.
Barbara Davis Center for Childhood Diabetes, Denver, CO 80262 USA

INTRODUCTION

Diabetes mellitus is a phenotypically and genetically heterogeneous group of disorders that share chronic hyperglycemia as the predominant feature. Once considered a geneticist's nightmare (1), diabetes mellitus has recently emerged as a prototype for genetic studies of complex diseases. The ultimate goal of genetic studies is to define etiological subtypes by resolving genetic heterogeneity. The transition of diabetes from a geneticist's nightmare to a prototype for study is a sign of significant progress in resolving genetic heterogeneity. The first step was to use family studies to explore the relationship between phenotypic heterogeneity and genetic heterogeneity. The existence of two clinically distinct forms of diabetes has been known for centuries, with one form characterized by abrupt onset of severe hyperglycemia in a child (juvenile diabetes) or lean adult, and the other form characterized by a more gradual onset of mild to severe hyperglycemia, typically in an obese adult (maturity onset diabetes). The vast majority (>90%) of patients with juvenile diabetes are dependent on exogenous insulin for survival (insulin-dependent diabetes, IDDM); while the vast majority (>80%) of patients with maturity onset diabetes are treated initially by diet or oral agents (non-insulin-dependent diabetes, NIDDM). Studies demonstrating familial clustering for age of onset, clinical presentation, and type of treatment provided critical evidence for the etiological distinction between juvenile diabetes and maturity onset diabetes (2,3).

IDDM accounts for the majority of children who develop diabetes. However, the disease can occur at any age, and, in fact, over half of affected cases develop the disease after the age of 15 years (4-6). About 1/200 children and 1/20 adults develop diabetes. Although only a small (10-20%) fraction of adult patients with diabetes present with the classical symptoms of IDDM, patients who develop symptoms after age 15 actually outnumber patients who develop symptoms before age 15. Recognizing the importance of distinguishing etiological subtypes of diabetes for future genetic, clinical, and epidemiological research, the National Diabetes Data Group (NDDG) in the US (7), and later the World Health Organization (WHO) (8), developed a formal framework for categorizing etiological subtypes of diabetes mellitus in which age of onset of symptoms was considered an inappropriate tool for diagnosis and classification. As further justification for an etiological distinction between IDDM and NIDDM, the NDDG and WHO recommendations, made public in 1979 and 1980, respectively, commented briefly on the increased or decreased frequency of certain genetic variants of human leukocyte antigens (HLA-B8 and -B15) and the frequent presence of islet cell antibodies (ICA) at diagnosis in patients with IDDM, but not in patients with NIDDM.

Subsequent research has strengthened the hypothesis that the majority of patients who present with classical symptoms of IDDM have an immune-mediated form of diabetes characterized by specific clinical, immunological, and immunogenetic features that can be used to predict current and future insulin dependency. Over 80% of children who develop hyperglycemia, and over 90% of children who present with classical symptoms of IDDM have one or more, and often two or more, of four immunological markers (ICA, insulin autoantibodies (IAA), antibodies to glutamic acid decarboxylase (GAD65 Ab), and/or antibodies to the tyrosine phosphatase protein, IA-2Ab) of immune-mediated diabetes. A similarly high fraction of patients with juvenile onset IDDM carry one or both of two high risk HLA alleles (HLA-DR3 and/or -DR4). Studies of IDDM in adolescents or adults have been less conclusive, due in part to difficulties in distinguishing true insulin-dependency from insulin-treated NIDDM, the latter of which is very common at older ages. In recognition of the inadequacies of a classification system based on method of treatment, an Expert Committee of the American Diabetes Association recently recommended eliminating the terms IDDM and NIDDM in favor of the terms type 1 and type 2 diabetes, respectively (9). According to the current classification system, the main distinction between type 1 and type 2 diabetes is that patients with type 1 diabetes have an absolute deficiency of insulin secretion, while patients with type 2 diabetes, have insulin resistance with relative, as opposed to absolute, insulin deficiency. Type 1 diabetes is further subdivided into two subtypes designated type 1a, or immune-mediated diabetes, and type 1b, or idiopathic IDDM.

Type 1 diabetes probably accounts for over 95% of patients with IDDM. The remaining cases are due to clearly-defined causes (many representing poorly defined syndromes), most of which are very rare. These include two uncommon immune-mediated forms of diabetes that are also characterized by the presence of GAD antibodies. One of these is the stiff-man syndrome, a rare autoimmune disorder of the central nervous system (10). The other is autoimmune polyendocrinopathy-candidiasis-ectodermal dystrophy (APECED; also known as APS-I or autoimmune polyendocrine syndrome type I), a rare autosomal recessive disease caused by mutations in the autoimmune regulator gene (AIRE) on chromosome 21 (11,12). Over 70 other, mostly rare genetic syndromes are associated with an increased risk for glucose intolerance and diabetes mellitus (13). Most, but not all of these syndromes can be distinguished from type 1 diabetes on the basis of other clinical manifestations. Important exceptions are maturity onset diabetes of the young (MODY), an autosomal dominant disorder that may be caused by a mutation in any one of five different genes (see Chapter 5) (14); and maternally inherited diabetes and deafness (MIDD) (see Chapter 6), which is caused by a mutation in mitochondrial DNA (15). Recent studies suggest that MODY or MIDD mutations may account for a small, but significant fraction of patients initially classified as idiopathic (type 1b) IDDM, a category reserved for patients who present with insulin deficiency in the absence of evidence for β-cell autoimmunity (16-18).

GENETIC STUDIES OF TYPE 1 DIABETES

Type 1 diabetes is a multifactorial disease caused by a combination of genetic and environmental factors. The contribution of genetic factors to the risk for a multifactorial disease is often measured by λ, which is simply the frequency of the disease among relatives of patients divided by the frequency of the disease in the population. The frequency of juvenile onset IDDM among siblings (including dizygous twins) of patients is ~6%, compared to a frequency in the population of ~0.4%, corresponding to a λ of ~15 (19). The frequency of IDDM among offspring of patients is lower than the frequency of IDDM among siblings of patients, and several studies have confirmed higher risks for offspring of affected fathers compared to offspring of affected mothers (20-23). About 1/3 of monozygous twins are concordant for IDDM or become concordant for IDDM within a few years after initial ascertainment (24). However, about 2/3 of long-term disease discordant twin pairs are concordant for the immunological markers of autoimmune diabetes (25). Several studies have shown that the lifetime risk for IDDM among relatives of patients may be at least 2-fold higher than the risk for juvenile onset IDDM (26,27). However, accurate estimates of the lifetime risk for IDDM in the population are currently unavailable for comparison. There are also indications for familial aggregation for the age of diagnosis of type 1 diabetes (28,29).

At least part of the increased risk for diabetes among siblings of patients can be attributed to HLA haplotype sharing. Basic Mendelian principles predict that 50% of siblings will inherit the same haplotype from one of their two parents (1 haplotype shared), 25% of siblings will inherit the same haplotypes from both parents (2 haplotypes shared), and only 25% of siblings inherit different haplotypes from both parents (0 haplotypes shared). The increased risk to siblings attributable to HLA-linked susceptibility loci can be measured by comparing the observed percentage of affected siblings who inherit a different HLA haplotype from both parents with the theoretical expectation of 25% (19). Based on empirical data from multiple studies, about 7% of affected siblings inherited a different HLA haplotype from both parents (30,31). Therefore, the increased risk to siblings due to HLA haplotype sharing is about 3.6 (0.25/0.07), well below the 15-fold overall increased risk to siblings. These results indicate that HLA haplotype sharing accounts for some, but not all of the increased risk for diabetes in siblings of patients, and that other non-HLA familial risk factors are important. Interestingly, it has been reported that the frequencies of the highest risk alleles DR3 and DR4 are higher than expected among many affected sib pairs who do not share HLA haplotypes from their parents (31). These data suggest that the familial aggregation attributable to HLA allele sharing may understate the role of HLA in diabetes susceptibility.

Recurrence risks for different siblings vary from a low of 1% for siblings who share 0 HLA haplotypes with a diabetic sibling to over 20% for siblings who share both of the two highest risk haplotypes (DR3-DQ2 and DR4-DQ8) with a diabetic sibling (13). In the absence of other information, three very different, but equally plausible, genetic hypotheses could account for the observed family data: (1) a simple 2-locus model, in which the interaction(s) between a single non-HLA-linked susceptibility locus (or tightly linked loci) and one or more HLA-linked susceptibility loci determines genetic susceptibility to autoimmune diabetes in the majority patients; (2) a genetic heterogeneity model, which is the same as the 2-locus model, except that the specific loci and interactions that determine genetic susceptibility differ in different patients; or (3) a polygenic model, in which the major effect of HLA-linked genetic susceptibility is modified by many different non-HLA-linked susceptibility loci, with each modifier gene having a relatively small effect. The results of three large studies argue against a simple 2-locus model for genetic susceptibility in consistently demonstrating that no single region of the human genome can account for the increased risk to relatives that remains unexplained (32-34). The distinction between the genetic heterogeneity model and the polygenic model is more difficult, and neither model can be excluded by the empirical data.

TYPE 1 DIABETES AND AUTOIMMUNITY

Autoimmune destruction of the insulin-secreting β-cells of the islets of Langerhans is the major cause of insulin deficiency, accounting for over

95% of patients with type 1 diabetes. One of the first indications that type 1 diabetes is an autoimmune disease came from histopathological studies demonstrating highly selective and nearly complete elimination of insulin-secreting β-cells in pancreatic tissue from patients with long-standing IDDM (35). Varying degrees of β-cell loss are seen in pancreatic tissue from patients with recent-onset IDDM, and many of the residual β-cells are affected by a chronic inflammatory cell infiltrate (insulitis) (36-38). The metabolic consequences of the reduction in β-cell mass are increased insulin sensitivity, reduced insulin secretion, and insulin deficiency, as indicated by an intravenous glucose tolerance test (IVGTT), first-phase insulin response to IVGTT (FPIR), and C-peptide levels.

Patients with type 1 diabetes are at increased risk for other autoimmune endocrine deficiency disorders, notably autoimmune thyroid disease (AITD), Addison's disease, and celiac disease. Conversely, patients with other autoimmune endocrine deficiency disorders are at increased risk for type 1 diabetes. ICA were initially discovered in diabetic patients with multiple autoimmune endocrinopathies (39), but it is now clear that ICA are a relatively specific marker for the current or future development of insulin-dependency. ICA are a heterogeneous family of antibodies (40,41), comprised primarily of antibodies to two major autoantigens, glutamic acid decarboxylase (GAD65) and a tyrosine phosphatase protein (ICA512/IA-2) (42,43). Other studies have shown that antibodies to insulin (IAA), the only β-cell-specific autoantigen, are also present in about 50% of IDDM patients prior to the initiation of insulin treatment (44). ICA, IAA, and/or antibodies to GAD65 or ICA512/IA-2 are present in the vast majority of children who present with classical symptoms of type 1 diabetes (Table 1). Most of these children present with no evidence for other autoimmune endocrine deficiencies, confirming that the combination of immunological markers is relatively specific for autoimmune diabetes.

Table 1. Prevalence of antibodies to major autoantigens in newly diagnosed children with type 1 diabetes (45-49).

ICA	IAA	GAD65	IA-2	>= 1 antibody	>= 2 antibodies
82%	55%	75%	76%	95%	87%

Parallel efforts have led to the discovery of thyroid peroxidase (TPO) as the major autoantigen in AITD (50,51), 21-hydroxylase (21OH) as the major autoantigen in autoimmune adrenal insufficiency (Addison's disease) (52-54), and transglutaminase (Tg) as the major autoantigen in gastric autoimmunity (celiac disease) (55). The development of convenient radioimmunoassays for detecting antibodies to specific autoantigens has made it possible to perform large-scale studies of the prevalence of other organ-specific autoimmunity in patients with diabetes (Table 2). The results of these studies emphasize the importance of antibody screening in patient populations to identify individuals at highest risk for developing multiple autoimmune diseases.

Table 2. Prevalence of other autoimmune disease and antibodies to disease-specific autoantigens in children with type 1 diabetes (56-64).

Addison's disease	21OH antibodies	Celiac disease	Tg antibodies	AITD	TPO antibodies
0.5%	1.5%	5%	12%	15%	25%

AUTOIMMUNITY AND THE MHC

The human major histocompatibility complex (MHC) occupies a 3.6 megabase (Mb) region on the short arm of chromosome 6 (6p21.31), the entire sequence of which is now known (Figure 1) (65). Over 200 known or predicted transcripts are contained in this region, with nearly half of these transcripts corresponding to known genes. The products of an estimated 40% of genes within the MHC have an immune-related function, and many of these genes are involved in the processing and presentation of foreign antigens, and presumably autoantigens.

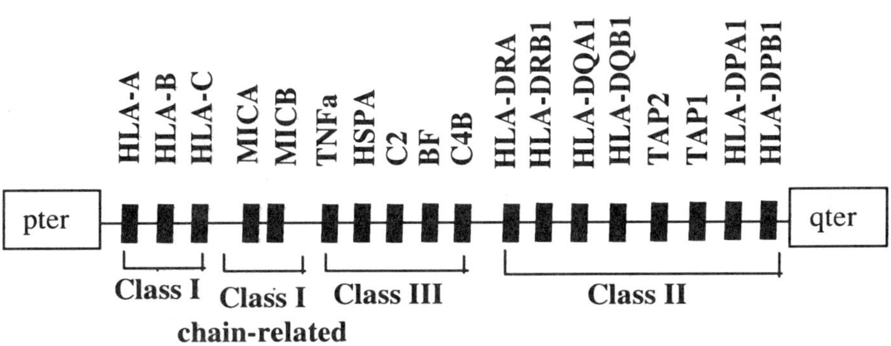

Figure 1. The human major histocompatibility complex (MHC) on chromosome 6.

The MHC is divided into 3 regions designated class I, class II, and class III. The telomeric class I region contains the genes encoding the classical transplantation antigens HLA-A, HLA-B, and HLA-C. The centromeric class II region contains the classical immune-response genes, collectively known as HLA-D, and eventually distinguished as HLA-DR, -

DQ, and -DP. The class III region contains the genes encoding components of the complement system (C4, C2, Bf), the tumor necrosis factor (TNF) cytokines, and other molecules with a variety of immune-related functions. A new family of class I-related sequences, including the MICA and MICB genes, has been localized to the telomeric end of the class III region (66). Most of the well-characterized class I and class II MHC molecules are members of the immunoglobulin superfamily. The primary function of both class I and class II molecules is to present peptide antigens to T-cell receptors. The class I and class II regions are also structurally similar, and differ from the class III regions in showing evidence of frequent duplication with a strong clustering of genes of related function in addition to many pseudogenes (65).

Despite the similarities of class I and class II molecules, there are fundamental structural and functional differences. Class I molecules are expressed on the majority of nucleated cells, and typically present intracellular antigens to CD8+ cytotoxic T lymphocytes. CD8+ T cells recognize peptides bound to the groove of a class I molecule, and initiate a response that eventually kills the offending cell. The expression of class II molecules is somewhat restricted to highly specialized antigen presenting cells such as macrophages and dendritic cells, although class II expression can be induced in many cells with cytokine stimulation. Class II molecules typically present extracellular antigens to CD4+ helper T cells. After engaging the T cell receptor, a second signal provided by other molecules interacting with the class II molecule and T lymphocyte complex leads to activation, proliferation, and cytokine production by the T lymphocyte. CD4+ T cells in turn activate B lymphocytes and CD8+ T lymphocytes (hence the term "helper T cell"). Cytokines produced by T cells can function either as regulators or effectors of delayed type hypersensitivity. CD4+ T lymphocytes are termed Th1 if they produce primarily inflammatory cytokines (e.g. interferon-gamma, IL-2), or Th2 if they produce primary IL-4 and IL-10. Given this central role in immune regulation, it is clear that HLA molecules could have a direct influence on the development of autoimmunity.

HLA class I and class II molecules represent the extremes of inherited variation (in contrast to T cell receptors and immunoglobulin genes, which often vary due to random somatic rearrangements of segments of genes). The main functional genes, HLA-A, HLA-B, and HLA-C, each encode an α-chain of a class I molecule. β-2 microglobulin, which is encoded by a monomorphic non-MHC gene on chromosome 15, is the second of the two polypeptide chains that comprise the class I molecule. The main class II molecules, HLA-DP, -DQ, and –DR, each consist of an α-chain and β-chain. All of the six genes encoding the α- and β-chains of the three main class II molecules are contained within the MHC, and are designated HLA-DPA1, -DPB1, -DQA1, -DQB1, -DRB1, and -DRA1. Four of these six genes are highly polymorphic, the exceptions being DRA1 and DPA1, for which only a few sequence variants have been found.

Historically, allelic variants for HLA molecules were detected serologically, primarily using microcytoxicity and mixed lymphocyte reaction assays. Subsequent studies using molecular genetic techniques have shown that serologic methods were able to detect a relatively small subset of the total number of HLA alleles. For example, over 165 DNA sequence variants have now been reported for DRB1, about 3/4 of which encode unique amino acid sequences. However, only 10-15% of the unique amino acid sequences can be detected using serologic reagents (67). The resolution of serologic typing methods varies for different HLA alleles. For example, the serologically defined DR4 allele includes over twenty unique amino acid sequences that can be distinguished at the DNA level. On the other hand, the DR3 serologic specificity includes only a few different DNA variants.

The alleles at different HLA loci that are present on the same chromosome are called the extended HLA haplotype. Given the large number of allelic variants at each of the seven highly polymorphic HLA loci (HLA-A, -B, -C, -DPB1, DQB1, DQA1, and DRB1), there are hundreds of billions of possible extended haplotypes. Considering the extraordinary number of possible allelic combinations, it seems unlikely that any extended haplotype would be represented more than once in a sample of unrelated haplotypes. However, this is rarely the case in practice, due to strong linkage disequilibrium across the MHC. Linkage disequilibrium between loci is apparent as an increased frequency of specific combinations of alleles compared to what would be expected if alleles were combined at random (linkage equilibrium). For example, in one study of 256 haplotypes from unrelated individuals, 28, 7, and 12 allelic variants were found at the DRB1, DQA1, and DQB1 loci, respectively. Based on these data, there are 2,352 possible 3-locus haplotypes. However, only 30 unique 3-locus haplotypes were found, one of which (DRB1*1501-DQA1*0102-DQB1*0602) accounted for 15% of the 256 haplotypes (68).

The pattern of linkage disequilibrium often reflects the population genetics history of a population, but may also be influenced by selective forces that favor certain combinations of alleles over others. In particular, the combination of alleles carried on the extended haplotypes of the original population founders can be conserved for many generations, depending on the frequency of recombination between the loci involved. In the absence of other forces, a regular pattern of linkage disequilibrium is expected, with the strength of linkage disequilibrium between loci decreasing with increasing recombination distance. However, the pattern of linkage disequilibrium across the MHC does not conform to these predictions. For example, there is significant linkage disequilibrium between the HLA-DRB1 and HLA-DP loci, which are separated by a distance of over 500 kb. However, there is little or no disequilibrium between the peptide-transporter loci (TAP1 and TAP2), which lie between HLA-DRB1 and HLA-DP, and are separated by less than 15 kb. These results suggest selective forces operate to maintain the association between alleles at HLA-DRB1 and HLA-DP and/or to disrupt the allelic association between TAP1 and TAP2 (69).

The strong and irregular pattern of linkage disequilibrium across the MHC has made it difficult to pinpoint the precise sequences responsible for diabetes susceptibility and résistance. However, many studies have confirmed that the original associations between diabetes and HLA class I alleles were most likely due to linkage disequilibrium between the HLA class I and class II loci (70-72). The strongest associations between diabetes and HLA class II loci were initially observed for the serologically defined alleles DR3 and DR4, and later for DQ2 and DQ8. Overall, the results reflect the frequent presence of DR3 and DQ2 on haplotypes also carrying B8, and the frequent presence of DR4 and DQ8 on haplotypes also carrying B15. DNA typing has since shown that the B8-DR3-associated DQ2 allele typically corresponds to DQA1*0501-DQB1*0201, while the B15-DR4-associated DQ8 allele typically corresponds to DQA1*0301-DQB1*0302.

DQ2/DQ8 heterozygotes are at highest risk for diabetes in the majority of Caucasian populations studied. For example, DQ2/DQ8 individuals represent about 2.4% of the population of Denver, Colorado, and about 30% of children with type 1 diabetes. Over 90% of children with diabetes have one or both high risk alleles compared to over 30% of the population. While these data clearly demonstrate a strong association between HLA-DQ and susceptibility to diabetes, the highest risk alleles are also very common in the population. As a result, the HLA-DQ association with diabetes susceptibility may be of limited value in predicting those members of the population who will eventually develop the type 1 diabetes.

The high population frequencies of DQ8 and DQ2 and their strong association with type 1 diabetes has a tendency to obscure the effects of other HLA alleles. One method of overcoming this problem is to determine how often a specific allele is transmitted to affected offspring from a heterozygous

Table 3. Transmission frequencies of DQA1 and DQB1 haplotypes to affected and unaffected offspring of heterozygous parents (73).

Haplotype	Affected offspring	Unaffected offspring
DQA1*03-DQB1*0302	0.87	0.43
DQA1*0501-DQB1*02	0.82	0.48
DQA1*0401-DQB1*0402	0.82	0.44
DQA1*0102-DQB1*0502	0.79	0.57
DQA1*0101-DQB1*0501	0.72	0.47
DQA1*0103-DQB1*0603	0.29	0.89
DQA1*0102-DQB1*0602	0.03	0.60

parent. A transmission disequilibrium test (TDT) is used to test if the frequency of transmission is greater than the Mendelian expectation of 50%. A similar test applied to unaffected offspring is used to rule out the possibility of segregation distortion due to factors unrelated to disease. The results of applying the TDT reveal a hierarchy of transmission frequencies, with indications for high risk, moderate risk, and protective HLA alleles (Table 3).

One of the most consistent results from studies of the association between HLA and diabetes is the protective effect of haplotypes carrying DR2, or more specifically the extended haplotype DRB1*1501-DQA1*0102-DQB1*0602 (31,71,74-77). Less than 1% of children with diabetes carry this haplotype compared to about 20% of the population. Individuals carrying this haplotype in addition to one of the high risk haplotypes are also at low risk for developing diabetes, suggesting a dominant mode of inheritance for protection against diabetes. Interestingly, the frequency of the DQA1*0102-DQB1*0602 is not decreased as dramatically in family members who are β-cell antibody positive compared to family members who are antibody-negative (78,79). Thus, the protective effect of the low risk haplotype HLA applies to the progression to diabetes, and may not extend to the development of autoimmunity.

The results of several studies point to DRB1*0301-DQA1*0501-DQB1*0201 as one of the common denominators explaining the increased risk for other organ-specific autoimmunity in patients with autoimmune diabetes (80,81). This haplotype is found in increased frequency in Addison's disease, Graves disease, and celiac disease with or without diabetes. One of the most dramatic findings is the greatly increased prevalence (~1/3) of celiac disease-associated transglutaminase antibodies in DR3-homozygous patients with type 1 diabetes (61). There are also reports of an increased frequency of DR4, and in particular, DRB1*0404-DQA1*0301-DQB1*0302, in patients with Addison's disease (58). However, the association between Addison's disease and DR4 may be specific to Addison's disease patients who are also affected with type 1 diabetes and/or rare cases of familial Addison's disease (82). It has been suggested that DR4 protects against a severe course of Graves disease (80) and that the protective effects of DR2 (DQB1*0602) may apply to Graves disease as well as to type 1 diabetes (81).

Although there is general agreement that the major component of diabetes susceptibility maps to the class II region of the MHC, there are also indications for other susceptibility loci within or near the MHC. One method for assessing the global influence of other MHC loci after correcting for the effect of the class II susceptibility loci is to examine extended haplotype sharing among pairs of affected offspring of parents who are homozygous for the high risk class II alleles. A significant deviation from expected sharing has been found in such studies, indicating that variation at non-class II MHC loci also contributes to individual differences in diabetes susceptibility. In particular, it has been found that HLA class I alleles may influence the progression of autoimmunity, including the rate of β-cell destruction and the age of onset of clinical symptoms (83-85).

One or more genes mapping to the class III region of the MHC may also contribute to diabetes susceptibility independently of class II or class I genes. Two independent studies have implicated one or more susceptibility loci near the microsatellite D6S273, which lies between the genes encoding tumor necrosis factor (TNF) and heat shock protein (HSP70) (86,87). The MHC class I chain-related MICA and MICB genes have also been localized to this region. A short tandem repeat (STR) polymorphism within the MICA gene results in a variable number of alanine residues in a transmembrane region of the protein (66). One of the STR alleles is a frameshift variant that produces a truncated and less hydrophobic transmembrane segment, potentially leading to a soluble MICA molecule and a deficiency of the membrane-bound MICA molecule. Interestingly, this allele, designated A5.1, is strongly associated with HLA-B8, the HLA-B allele often found on DR3 haplotypes. Subsequent studies have reported an increased frequency of the A5.1 allele in patients with Addison's disease (88). However, other studies have reported an association between MICA and type 1 diabetes involving a different MICA allele (A5) (89). Additional studies are needed to confirm these observations and to further characterize MHC-linked diabetes susceptibility genes.

ANIMAL MODELS OF TYPE 1 DIABETES

Given the complex genetics of the non-obese diabetic (NOD) mouse, it is remarkable that this spontaneously diabetic strain arose at all. The NOD mouse was derived from a control strain of a breeding program designed to produce a diabetic mouse (presumably type 2) from a strain that developed cataracts. Genetic studies of the autoimmune diabetes phenotype suggest over fifteen loci contribute to diabetes susceptibility, of which at least three loci reside within the mouse MHC (H-2). Mouse MHC genes encode two class II molecules, known as I-E and I-A, which correspond to the human class II molecules, HLA-DR and HLA-DQ, respectively. The NOD mouse does not produce I-Eα, due to a deletion in the promoter region of the I-Eα gene, an anomaly that is also seen in many normal mouse strains. However, there is significant evidence that expression of I-Eα provides dominant protection from diabetes, and its absence in NOD mice could in part explain their unique susceptibility to autoimmune diabetes. In addition, the I-Aβ chain produced by NOD mice has a relatively unique sequence, and alternative I-Aβ alleles have been shown to prevent diabetes in transgenic mice. There is also evidence for the importance of class I HLA alleles in the development of diabetes in NOD mice (90,91). Although transgenic studies clearly indicate that specific MHC alleles influence diabetes susceptibility in the mouse, the precise mechanisms remain unclear.

The BB rat does not conform to the NOD mouse model of polygenic inheritance of type 1 diabetes (92). Instead, the BB rat model involves a major autosomal recessive locus associated with T cell lymphopenia. NOD mice and BB rats do not differ in terms of the importance of the MHC (RT in rats) on diabetes susceptibility. In particular, it appears that a specific rat MHC haplotype, RT1-U, is necessary, but not sufficient for the development of diabetes (93). A similar, oligogenic model of type 1 diabetes has also been reported for the Long-Evans Tokoshima rat (94).

Despite the dramatic effects of the MHC on the development of type 1 diabetes in humans and other organisms, the mechanisms that determine diabetes susceptibility and resistance are poorly understood. There are, however, three major hypotheses: (1) the structural properties of certain allelic forms of class I and/or class II molecules favor the development of autoimmunity; (2) the unique peptide binding properties of specific HLA molecules alters the T cell repertoire; and (3) the molecules encoded by susceptibility alleles favor the binding and presentation of specific peptides, while the molecules encoded by protective alleles compete for immunodominant autoantigenic peptides (95). The three hypotheses are not mutually exclusive, and different hypotheses may apply to different alleles and different peptides.

The hypothesis that structural abnormalities may determine differences in the effects of HLA class II molecules on diabetes susceptibility and resistance is derived from studies of I-A^{g7} in the NOD mouse, and from comparisons of the high risk DQ8 allele and protective DQ6 allele (DQA1*0102-DQB1*0602) allele in humans (96). I-A^{g7} is reportedly unstable on gel chromatography, and the instability of the molecule may correlate with the absence of negative selection of autoreactive T lymphocytes within the thymus (97-99). Similarly, DQ8 is reportedly less stable than DQ6. However, these global anomalies of HLA molecules are difficult to reconcile with disease-specific allelic associations. For example, DQ6 is associated with dominant protection from type 1 diabetes in humans, but the same allele is associated with an increased risk for multiple sclerosis. In addition, the crystalline structure of I-A^{g7} is inconsistent with its reported molecular instability, but the molecule does have a fairly wide peptide binding groove at pocket P9 (100).

With multiple animal models available for detailed study, knockout and transgenic mice are providing interesting, albeit often conflicting information. NOD mice lacking β-2 microglobulin do not develop diabetes, which points to the importance of class I HLA molecules and CD8+ T lymphocytes. Slattery and coworkers produced mice lacking β-2 microglobulin only within islet β-cells (101). These mice developed type 1 diabetes, indicating that diabetes susceptibility does not depend on direct

CD8-mediated cytotoxicity with T lymphocytes recognizing class I-bound autoantigenic peptides. It is likely that CD8+ T lymphocytes and class I molecules play multiple roles in the initiation of autoimmune islet destruction and that presentation of islet autoantigens by "professional" antigen-presenting cells is sufficient for β-cell destruction. Several NOD CD8+ T cell clones capable of transferring diabetes have recently been characterized, and have been found to be directly cytotoxic to islet β-cells. One of these clones is especially interesting in recognizing the insulin B chain peptide B:15-23, a B chain region which is also a prominent target (B:9-23) of CD4+ T lymphocytes. Using the class I K^d molecule with the B:15-23 peptide, Wong and coworkers produced labeled tetramers to quantitate T lymphocytes reacting with this peptide. This technology, which enables characterization of antigen-specific T lymphocytes, is likely to have a dramatic influence on the understanding of the development of diabetes.

Mice lacking class II molecules also do not develop diabetes (102). Islet β-cells may express class II molecules, a finding that could be important for antigen recognition. However, in general, class II molecules have a restricted pattern of expression, but their expression can be induced. Animal models provide convincing evidence that diabetes does not develop when class II expression is induced and that, in the absence of islet class II molecules, autoreactive T lymphocyte clones readily destroy islet β-cells (103).

A large series of transgenic mouse models have been created to explore whether and how the expression of class II alleles influences the development of diabetes (104,105). Transgenic NOD mice with class II alleles other than I-A^{g7} (e.g., I-A^k) are protected from diabetes, as are mice with mutations in the β-chain of I-A^{g7}(e.g., position 56) (106,107). The protection appears dominant, which is also the case for the DQ6 allele in humans. Santamaria and coworkers showed that transgenic mice which express a T-cell receptor that targets islets develop diabetes but that, with the introduction of multiple class II alleles, the diabetogenic T cell clones are eliminated and the development of diabetes is prevented (104,108,109).

Recent studies indicate that human class II molecules can be successfully introduced into mice (110). The DQ8 molecule by itself does not lead to diabetes when introduced into mice engineered to produce no endogenous murine class II molecules. However, if the mice are engineered to increase their propensity for autoimmunity, for example, by inducing the T cell-activating molecule B7-1 on islet β-cells, then DQ8 mice develop diabetes, while mice carrying protective human DQ alleles do not develop diabetes. Further manipulations, such as introducing a DR4 allele in combination with DQ8, do not enhance the development of diabetes. Despite the tedious complexities of introducing multiple combinations of human MHC alleles into mice, these contemporary mouse models provide an important tool for studying human HLA molecules, and may provide an important resource for developing preventive therapies.

SUMMARY AND CONCLUSIONS

The formal distinction of type 1 and type 2 diabetes has had a major impact on our current understanding of the pathogenesis of chronic hyperglycemia. The preponderance of immune-mediated diabetes among all cases of diabetes in children under 15 years of age, the ease of distinguishing type 1 diabetes from other forms of childhood diabetes on clinical grounds, and the universal use of insulin for treatment of type 1 diabetes in this age group have all contributed to the development of disease registries with complete or nearly complete ascertainment of incident and prevalent cases. Disease registries have made it possible to compare the incidence and prevalence of childhood diabetes in different populations and to validate and quantify previous indications for a strong association with other autoimmune diseases and HLA. Despite this progress, most of what is known about type 1 diabetes is derived from studies of the disease in children. Studies of type 1 diabetes in adolescents and adults is complicated by the increasing prevalence of type 2 diabetes with age, and the decreased sensitivity and specificity of insulin treatment and other clinical variables as markers of type 1 diabetes at older ages. Future progress in unraveling genetic heterogeneity within the two major forms of diabetes is likely to depend on the ability to overcome the barriers of studying type 1 diabetes at any age.

There has also been considerable progress in understanding the nature of the association between specific HLA alleles and type 1 diabetes. It has become clear that the development of diabetes depends on a complex interaction between MHC-linked and non-MHC-linked susceptibility loci. There are also clear indications that environmental factors influence diabetes susceptibility, but there is no consistent evidence for a strong effect of any specific environmental factor. Likewise, the effects of specific HLA molecules is largely speculative. Nevertheless, with an ever-increasing wealth of structural information, basic immunologic studies, and an almost universal influence of class II molecules on diabetes, these molecules provide an important focus for studies aimed at understanding the pathogenesis of type 1 diabetes. Current HLA typing techniques have made it possible to identify individuals in the general population whose risk for diabetes is as high or nearly as high as the risk for diabetes in relatives of patients (111-113). This is especially important since over 85% of patients present with no family history of the disease.

The consistency of the overall effect of the MHC on diabetes susceptibility in genetically diverse populations, including Asians, Africans, and Caucasians suggests the pathways leading to diabetes have a common critical juncture. It is reasonable to hypothesize that this juncture will relate to a critical autoantigen, although many other hypotheses are worthy of exploration. It is now recognized that each T cell receptor reacts with approximately 1 million different peptides, with many of these peptides having no obvious structural relationship. This has led to the production of random peptide libraries of "mimotopes", a term used to describe peptides able to drive T cells, including T cells causing type 1 diabetes. There may be many environmentally-derived (dietary and infectious) mimotopes of important autoantigenic islet peptides, and an encounter with such mimotopes, in an immunogenic setting may initiate the autoimmunity that eventually leads to type 1 diabetes. The mimotopes need not be exogenous agents. Mimotope induction of anti-islet autoimmunity to an important self-antigen such as insulin (114-116) is consistent with a central role of HLA class II molecules in the development of diabetes. As more is learned about the pathogenesis of type 1 diabetes, it should be possible to develop safe and effective strategies for prevention. It is likely that the most efficient and cost-effective form of prevention will utilize forms of "antigen" vaccination (117-119). “Antigen” vaccination can already be accomplished in animal models. However, the development of similarly successful therapies in humans is likely to depend on a more specific understanding of the connection between the MHC and the development of diabetes.

ACKNOWLEDGMENTS

Research was supported by grants from the National Institutes of Health (DK32083, AI39213, DK32493, DK50979, DK55969), the American Diabetes Association (PN907-132), and the Juvenile Diabetes Foundation (198203). Clinical Research Center grants MO1 RR00069 and RR00051 at the Denver Children's Hospital and University Hospital were essential for clinical studies.

REFERENCES

1. Neel, J. 1976. Diabetes mellitus - A geneticist's nightmare. In The Genetics of Diabetes Mellitus. W. Creutzfeldt, J. Kobberling, and J. Neel, eds. Springer-Verlag, New York. 1-11.
2. Pyke, D. 1979. The genetic connections. *Diabetologia.* 17:333-343.
3. Irvine, W., A. Toft, D. Holton, R. Prescott, B. Clarke, and L. Duncan. 1977. Familial studies of type I and type II idiopathic diabetes mellitus. *Lancet.* 2:(8033)325-328.
4. Caillat-Zucman, S., H.-J. Garchon, J. Timsit, R. Assan, C. Boitard, I. Djilali-Saiah, P. Bougnères, and J.F. Bach. 1992. Age-dependent HLA genetic heterogeneity of type 1 insulin- dependent diabetes mellitus. *J. Clin. Invest.* 90:2242-2250.
5. Laakso, M. and K. Pyorala. 1985. Age of onset and type of diabetes. *Diabetes Care.* 8:(2)114-117.

6. Melton, L.3., P. Palumbo, and C. Chu. 1983. Incidence of diabetes mellitus by clinical type. *Diabetes Care.* 6:(1)75-86.
7. National Diabetes Data Group. 1979. Classification and diagnosis of diabtes mellitus and other categories of glucose intolerance. *Diabetes.* 28:1039-1057.
8. World Health Organization. 1980. Second Report on Diabetes Mellitus. Geneva, Switzerland. WHO. Technical Report Series 646.
9. The Expert Committee on the Diagnosis and Classification of Diabetes Mellitus. 1997. Report of the expert committee on the diagnosis and classification of diabetes mellitus. *Diabetes Care.* 20:(7)1183-1197.
10. Ellis, T. and M. Atkinson. 1996. The clinical significance of an autoimmune response against glutamic acid decarboxylase. *Nat. Med.* 2:(2)148-153.
11. Nagamine, K., P. Peterson, H. Scott, J. Kudoh, S. Minoshima, M. Heino, K. Krohn, M. Lalioti, P. Mullis, S. Antonarakis, K. Kawasaki, S. Asakawa, F. Ito, and N. Shimizu. 1997. Positional cloning of the APECED gene. *Nat. Genet.* 17:(4)393-398.
12. Finnish-German APECED Consortium. 1997. An autoimmune disease, APECED, caused by mutations in a novel gene featuring two PHD-type zinc-finger domains. *Nat. Genet.* 17:399-403.
13. Scheuner, M., L. Raffel, and J. Rotter. 1997. Genetics of diabetes. In International Textbook of Diabetes Mellitus. K. Alberti, P. Zimmet, R. DeFronzo, and H.H. Keen, eds. John Wiley & Sons, New York. 37-88.
14. Winter, W., M. Nakamura, and D. House. 1999. Monogenic diabetes mellitus in youth. The MODY syndromes. *Endocrinol. Metab. Clin. North Am.* 28:(4)765-785.
15. Alcolado, J. and A. Thomas. 1995. Maternally inherited diabetes mellitus: the role of mitochondrial DNA defects. *Diabet. Med.* 12:102-108.
16. Boutin, P., L. Gresh, A. Cisse, M. Hara, G. Bell, S. Babu, G. Eisenbarth, and P. Froguel. 1999. Missense mutation Gly574Ser in the transcription factor HNF-1α is a marker of atypical diabetes mellitus in African-American children. *Diabetologia.* 42:(3)380-381.
17. Lehto, M., C. Wipemo, S. Ivarsson, C. Lindgren, M. Lipsanen-Nyman, J. Weng, L. Wibell, E. Widen, T. Tuomi, and L. Groop. 1999. High frequency of mutations in MODY and mitochondrial genes in Scandinavian patients with familial early-onset diabetes. *Diabetologia.* 42:(9)1131-1137.
18. Moller, A., L. Dalgaard, F. Pociot, J. Nerup, T. Hansen, and O. Pedersen. 1998. Mutations in the hepatocyte nuclear factor-1α gene in Caucasian families originally classified as having type I diabetes. *Diabetologia.* 41:(12)1528-1531.
19. Risch, N. 1987. Assessing the role of HLA-linked and unlinked determinants of disease. *Am. J. Hum. Genet.* 40:1-14.
20. Warram, J., A. Krolewski, M. Gottlieb, and C. Kahn. 1984. Differences in risk of insulin-dependent diabetes in offspring of diabetic mothers and diabetic fathers. *N. Engl. J. Med.* 311:(3)149-152.
21. Dahlquist, G., L. Blom, T. Tuvemo, L. Nystrom, A. Sandstrom , and S. Wall. 1989. The Swedish childhood diabetes study - Results from a nine year case register and a one year case-referent study indicating that type 1 (insulin-dependent) diabetes mellitus is associated with type 2 (non-insulin-dependent) diabetes mellitus and autoimmune disorders . *Diabetologia.* 32:(1)2-6.
22. Lorenzen, T., F. Pociot, L. Stilgren, O. Kristiansen, J. Johannesen, P. Olsen, A. Walmar, A. Larsen, N. Albrechtsen, P. Eskildsen, O. Andersen, J. Nerup, and the Danish IDDM Epidemiology and Genetics Group. 1998. Predictors of IDDM recurrence risk in offspring of Danish IDDM patients. *Diabetologia.* 41:(6)666-673.
23. Tuomilehto, J., T. Podar, E. Tuomilehto-Wolf, and E. Virtala. 1995. Evidence for importance of gender and birth cohort for risk of IDDM in offspring of IDDM parents. *Diabetologia.* 38:(8)975-982.
24. Olmos, P., R. A'Hern, D. Heaton, B. Millward, D. Risley, D. Pyke, and R. Leslie. 1988. The significance of the concordance rate for type 1 (insulin-dependent) diabetes in identical twins. *Diabetologia.* 31:(10)747-750.

25. Verge, C., R. Gianani, L. Yu, M. Pietropaolo, T. Smith, R. Jackson, J.S. Soeldner, and G.S. Eisenbarth. 1995. Late progression to diabetes and evidence for chronic β-cell autoimmunity in identical twins of patients with type I diabetes. *Diabetes.* 44:(10)1176-1179.
26. Lorenzen, T., F. Pociot, P. Hougaard, and J. Nerup. 1994. Long-term risk of IDDM in first-degree relatives of patients with IDDM. *Diabetologia.* 37:(3)321-327.
27. Srikanta, S., O.P. Ganda, R.A. Jackson, R.E. Gleason, A. Kaldany, M.R. Garavoy, E.L. Milford, C.B. Carpenter, J.S. Soeldner, and G.S. Eisenbarth. 1983. Type I diabetes mellitus in monozygotic twins: chronic progressive beta cell dysfunction. *Ann. Intern. Med.* 99:320-326.
28. Fava, D., S. Gardner, D. Pyke, and R. Leslie. 1998. Evidence that the age of diagnosis of IDDM is genetically determined. *Diabetes Care.* 21:925-929.
29. Valdes, A., G. Thomson, H. Erlich, and J. Noble. 1999. Association between type 1 diabetes age of onset and HLA among sibling pairs. *Diabetes.* 48:(8)1658-1661.
30. Payami, H., G. Thomson, U. Motro, E. Louis, and E. Hudes. 1985. The affected sib pair method. IV. Sib trios. *Ann. Hum. Genet.* 49:(Pt 4)303-314.
31. Noble, J., A. Valdes, M. Cook, W. Klitz, G. Thomson, and H. Erlich. 1996. The role of HLA class II genes in insulin-dependent diabetes mellitus: Molecular analysis of 180 Caucasian, multiplex families. *Am. J. Hum. Genet.* 59:1134-1148.
32. Field, L., R. Tobias, and T. Magnus. 1994. A locus on chromosome 15q26 (IDDM3) produces susceptibility to insulin-dependent diabetes. *Nat. Genet.* 8:189-194.
33. Davies, J., Y. Kawaguchi, S. Bennett, J. Copeman, H. Cordell , L. Pritchard, P. Reed, S. Gough, S. Jenkins, S. palmer, K. Balfour, B. Rowe, M. Farrall, A. Barnett, S. Bain, and J. Todd. 1994. A genome-wide search for human type 1 diabetes susceptibility genes. *Nature.* 371:130-136.
34. Hashimoto, L., C. Habita, J. Beressi, M. Delepine, C. Besse, A. Cambon-Thomsen, I. Deschamps, J. Rotter, S. Djoulah, M. James, P. Froguel, J. Weissenbach, G. Lathrop, and C. Julier. 1994. Genetic mapping of a susceptibility locus for insulin-dependent diabetes mellitus on chromosome 11q. *Nature.* 371:(6493)161-164.
35. Gepts, W. 1965. Pathologic anatomy of the pancreas in juvenile diabetes mellitus. *Diabetes.* 14:(10)619-633.
36. Bottazzo, G.F., B.M. Dean, J.M. McNally, E.H. Mackay, P.G. Swift, and D.R. Gamble. 1985. In situ characterization of autoimmune phenomena and expression of HLA molecules in the pancreas in diabetic insulitis. *N. Engl. J. Med.* 313:353-360.
37. Foulis, A., C. Liddle, M. Farquharson, J. Richmond, and R. Weir. 1986. The histopathology of the pancreas in type 1 (insulin-dependent) diabetes mellitus: a 25-year review of deaths of patients under 20 years of age in the United Kingdom. *Diabetologia.* 29:(5)267-274.
38. Foulis, A. and J. Stewart. 1984. The pancreas in recent-onset type 1 (insulin-dependent) diabetes mellitus: insulin content of islets, insulitis and associated changes in the exocrine acinar tissue. *Diabetologia.* 26:(6)456-461.
39. Bottazzo, G.F., A. Florin-Christensen, and D. Doniach. 1974. Islet-cell antibodies in diabetes mellitus with autoimmune polyendocrine deficiencies. *Lancet.* 2:1279-1283.
40. Genovese, S., E. Bonifacio, J.M. McNally, B.M. Dean, R. Wagner, E. Bosi, E.A.M. Gale, and G.F. Bottazzo. 1992. Distinct cytoplasmic islet cell antibodies with different risks for type 1 (insulin-dependent) diabetes mellitus. *Diabetologia.* 35:385-388.
41. Gianani, R., A. Pugliese, S. Bonner-Weir, A.J. Shiffrin, J.S. Soeldner, H. Erlich, Z.L. Awdeh, C.A. Alper, R.A. Jackson, and G.S. Eisenbarth . 1992. Prognostically significant heterogeneity of cytoplasmic islet cell antibodies in relatives of patients with type I diabetes. *Diabetes.* 41:347-353.
42. Myers, M., D. Rabin, and M. Rowley. 1995. Pancreatic islet cell cytoplasmic antibody in diabetes is represented by antibodies to islet cell antigen 512 and glutamic acid decarboxylase. *Diabetes.* 44:(11)1290-1295.

43. Lan, M., C. Wasserfall, N. Maclaren, and A. Notkins. 1996. IA-2, a transmembrane protein of the protein tyrosine phosphatase family, is a major autoantigen in insulin-dependent diabetes mellitus. *Proc. Natl. Acad. Sci. USA* 93:(13)6367-6370.
44. Palmer, J., C. Asplin, P. Clemons, K. Lyen, O. Tatpati, P. Raghu, and T. Paguette. 1983. Insulin antibodies in insulin-dependent diabetics before insulin treatment. *Science.* 222:1337-1339.
45. Gorus, F., P. Goubert, C. Semakula, C.L. Vandewalle, J. De Schepper, A. Scheen, M. Christie, D. Pipeleers, and The Belgian Diabetes Registry. 1997. IA-2 autoantibodies complement GAD65-autoantibodies in new-onset IDDM patients and help predict impending diabetes in their siblings. *Diabetologia.* 40:(1)95-99.
46. Bingley, P., E. Bonifacio, A. Williams, S. Genovese, G. Bottazzo, and E. Gale. 1997. Prediction of IDDM in the general population: strategies based on combinations of autoantibody markers. *Diabetes.* 46:(11)1701-1710.
47. Ongagna, J. and C. Levy-Marchal. 1997. Sensitivity at diagnosis of combined beta-cell autoantibodies in insulin-dependent diabetic children. French Registry of IDDM in Children Study Group. *Diabetes Metab.* 23:(2)155-160.
48. Hagopian, W., C. Sanjeevi, I. Kockum, M. Landin-Olsson, A. Karlsen, G. Sundkvist, G. Dahlquist, J. Palmer, and A. Lernmark. 1995. Glutamate decarboxylase-, insulin-, and islet cell-antibodies and HLA typing to detect diabetes in a general population-based study of Swedish children. *J. Clin. Invest.* 95:(4)1505-1511.
49. Sabbah, E., K. Savola, P. Kulmala, R. Veijola, P. Vahasalo , J. Karjalainen, H. Akerblom, and M. Knip. 1999. Diabetes-associated autoantibodies in relation to clinical characteristics and natural course in children with newly diagnosed type 1 diabetes. The Childhood Diabetes In Finland Study Group. *J. Clin. Endocrinol. Metab.* 84:(5)1534-1539.
50. Ruf, J., B. Czarnocka, C. De Micco, C. Dutoit, M. Ferrand, and P. Carayon. 1987. Thyroid peroxidase is the organ-specific 'microsomal' autoantigen involved in thyroid autoimmunity. *Acta Endocrinol. (Copenh).* 281:49-56.
51. Czarnocka, B., J. Ruf, M. Ferrand, P. Carayon, and S. Lissitzky. 1985. Purification of the human thyroid peroxidase and its identification as the microsomal antigen involved in autoimmune thyroid disease. *FEBS Lett.* 190:147-152.
52. Baumann-Antczak, A., N. Wedlock, J. Bednarek, Y. Kiso, H. Krishnan, S. Fowler, B. Smith, and J. Furmaniak. 1992. Autoimmune Addison's disease and 21-hydroxylase. *Lancet.* 340:429-430.
53. Winqvist, O., F. Karlsson, and O. Kampe. 1992. 21-Hydroxylase, a major autoantigen in idiopathic Addison's disease. *Lancet.* 339:1559-1562.
54. Bednarek, J., J. Furmaniak, N. Wedlock, Y. Kiso, A. Baumann-Antczak, S. Fowler, H. Krishnan, J. Craft, and B. Rees Smith. 1992. Steroid 21-hydroxylase is a major autoantigen involved in adult onset autoimmune Addison's disease. *FEBS Lett.* 309:51-55.
55. Dieterich, W., T. Ehnis, M. Bauer, P. Donner, U. Volta, E. Riecken, and D. Schuppan. 1997. Identification of tissue transglutaminase as the autoantigen of coeliac disease . *Nat. Med.* 3:797-801.
56. Peterson, P., H. Salmi, H. Hyoty, A. Miettinen, J. Ilonen, H. Reijonen, M. Knip, H. Akerblom, K. Krohn, and Childhood Diabetes in Finland (DiMe) Study Group. 1997. Steroid 21-hydroxylase autoantibodies in insulin-dependent diabetes mellitus. *Clin. Immunol. Immunopath.* 82:(1)37-42.
57. Brewer, K., V. Parziale, and G. Eisenbarth. 1997. Screening patients with insulin-dependent diabetes mellitus for adrenal insufficiency. *N. Engl. J. Med.* 337:202.
58. Yu, L., K. Brewer, S. Gates, A. Wu, T. Wang, S. Babu, P. Gottlieb, B. Freed, H. Erlich, M. Rewers, and G. Eisenbarth. 1999. DRB1*04 and DQ alleles: expression of 21-hydroxylase autoantibodies and risk of progression to Addison's Disease. *J.Clin..Endocrinol..Metab.* 84:328-335.

59. Seissler, J., M. Schott, S. Boms, U. Wohlrab, B. Ostendorf, N. Morgenthaler, and W. Scherbaum. 1999. Autoantibodies to human tissue transgutaminase identify silent coeliac disease in type I diabetes. *Diabetologia.* 42:(12)1440-1441.
60. Lampasona, V., R. Bonfanti, E. Bazzigaluppi, A. Venerando, G. Chiumello, E. Bosi, and E. Bonifacio. 2000. Antibodies to tissue transglutaminase C in type I diabetes. *Diabetologia.* 42:1195-1198.
61. Bao, F., L. Yu, S. Babu, T. Wang, E. Hoffenberg, M. Rewers, and G. Eisenbarth. 1999. One third of HLA DQ2 homozygous patients with type 1 diabetes express celiac disease-associated transglutaminase autoantibodies. *J. Autoimmun.* 13:(1)143-148.
62. Fernández-Castañer, M., A. Molina, L. López-Jiménez, J.M. Gómez, and J. Soler. 1999. Clinical presentation and early course of type 1 diabetes in patients with and without thyroid autoimmunity. *Diabetes Care.* 22:377-381.
63. Kontiainen, S., A. Schlenzka , S. Koskimies, A. Rilva, and J. Maenpaa. 1990. Autoantibodies and autoimmune diseases in young diabetics. *Diabetes Res.* 13:151-156.
64. Radetti, G., C. Paganini, L. Gentili, S. Bernasconi, C. Beterle, M. Borkenstein, K. Cvijovic, M. Kadrnka-Lovrencic, C. Krzisnic, T. Battelino, and et al. 1995. Frequency of Hashimoto's thyroiditis in children with type 1 diabetes mellitus. *Acta Diabetol.* 32:121-124.
65. The MHC sequencing consortium. 1999. Complete sequence and the gene map of a human major histocompatibility complex. *Nature.* 401:(6756)921-923.
66. Bahram, S., M. Bresnahan, D. Geraghty, and T. Spies. 1994. A second lineage of mammalian major histocompatibility complex class I genes. *Proc. Natl. Acad. Sci. USA* 91:(14)6259-6263.
67. Apple, R. and H. Erlich. 1996. HLA class II genes: structure and diversity. In HLA and MHC: genes, molecules, and function. M. Browning and A. McMichael, eds. BIOS Scientific Publications, Ltd, Oxford. 97-109.
68. Carrington, M., J. Stephens, W. Klitz, A. Begovich, H. Erlich, and D. Mann. 1994. Major histocompatibility complex class II haplotypes and linkage disequilbrium values observed in the CEPH families. *Hum.Immunol.* 41:234-240.
69. Klitz, W., J. Stephens, M. Grote, and M. Carrington. 1995. Discordant patterns of linkage disequilibrium of the peptide-transporter loci within the HLA class II region. *Am. J. Hum. Genet.* 57:(6)1436-1444.
70. Khalil, I., L. d'Auriol, M. Gobet, L. Morin, V. Lepage, I. Deschamps, M. Park, L. Degos, F. Galibert, and J. Hors. 1990. A combination of HLA-DQβ Asp57-negative and HLA DQα Arg52 confers susceptiblity to insulin-dependent diabetes mellitus . *J.Clin.Invest.* 85:(4)1315-1319.
71. Baisch, J., T. Weeks, R. Giles, M. Hoover, P. Stastny, and J. Capra. 1990. Analysis of HLA-DQ genotypes and susceptibility in insulin-dependent diabetes mellitus. *N. Engl. J. Med.* 322:(26)1836-1841.
72. Todd, J.A., J.I. Bell, and H.O. McDevitt. 1987. HLA-DQβ gene contributes to susceptibility and resistence to insulin-dependent diabetes . *Nature.* 329:599-604.
73. Kawasaki, E., J. Noble, H. Erlich, C. Mulgrew, P. Fain, and G. Eisenbarth. 1998. Transmission of DQ haplotypes to patients with type 1 diabetes. *Diabetes.* 47:1971-1973.
74. Kawasaki, E. and S. Nagataki . 1996. Japanese type 1 diabetic syndrome. *Diabetes Metab. Rev.* 12:175-194.
75. Kockum, I., A. Lernmark, G. Dahlquist, A. Falorni, W. Hagopian, M. Landin-Olsson, L. Li, H. Luthman, J. Palmer, C. Sanjeevi, G. Sundkvist, J. Ostman, The Swedish Childhood Diabetes Study group, and The Diabetes Incidence Sweden Study (DISS) Group. 1996. Genetic and immunological findings in patients with newly diagnosed insulin-dependent diabetes mellitus. *Horm. .Metab. Res.* 28:344-347.
76. Buyse, I., L. Sandkuyl, M. Ghabanbasani, X.-X. Gu, R. Bouillon, M. Bex, L. Dooms, M.-P. Emonds, M. Duhamel, P. Marynen, and J.-J. Cassiman. 1994. Association of particular HLA class II alleles, haplotypes and genotypes with susceptibility to IDDM in the Belgium population. *Diabetologia.* 37:(8)808-817.

77. Reijonen, H., J. Ilonen, H. Akerblom, M. Knip, and H. Dosch. 1994. Multi-locus analysis of HLA class II genes in DR2-positive IDDM haplotypes in Finland. The Childhood Diabetes in Finland (DiMe) Study Group. *Tissue Antigens.* 43:(1)1-6.
78. Pugliese, A., R. Gianani, R. Moromisato, Z. Awdeh, C. Alper, H. Erlich, R. Jackson, and G. Eisenbarth. 1995. HLA-DQB1*0602 is associated with dominant protection from diabetes even among islet cell antibody-positive first-degree relatives of patients with IDDM. *Diabetes.* 44:(6)608-613.
79. Grrenbaum, C., D. Schatz, D. Cuthbertson, A. Zeidler, G. Eisenbarth, and J. Krischer. 2000. Islet cell antibody-positive relatives with human leukocyte antigen DQA1*0102, DQB1*0602: Identification by the Diabetes Prevention Trial-type 1. *J. Clin. Endocrinol. Metab.* 85:(3)1255-1260.
80. Bach, J.-F. and S. Caillat-Zucman. 1993. Genetics of autoimmune endocrine diseases. *Springer Semin. Immunopath.* 14:(3)239-252.
81. Badenhoop, K., P. Walfish, H. Rau, S. Fischer, A. Nicolay, U. Bogner, H. Schleusener, and K. Usadel. 1995. Susceptibility and resistance alleles of human leukocyte antigen (HLA) DQA1 and HLA DQB1 are shared in endocrine autoimmune disease. *J. Clin. Endocrinol. Metab.* 80:2112-2117.
82. Huang, W., E. Connor, T. dela Rosa, A. Muir, D. Schatz, J. Silverstein, S. Crockett, J.-X. She, and N.K. Maclaren. 1996. Although DR3-DQB1*0201 may be associated with multiple component diseases of the autoimmune polyglandular syndromes, the human leukocyte antigen DR4-DQB1*0302 haplotype is implicated only in β-cell autoimmunity. *J.Clin. Endocrinol. .Metab.* 81:2559-2560.
83. Demaine, A., M. Hibberd, D. Mangels, and B. Millward. 1995. A new marker in the HLA class I region is associated with the age at onset of IDDM. *Diabetologia.* 38:(5)623-628.
84. Fujisawa, T., H. Ikegami, Y. Kawaguchi, E. Yamato, K. Takekawa, Y. Nakagawa, Y. Hamada, H. Ueda, K. Shima, and T. Ogihara. 1995. Class I HLA is associated with age-at-onset of IDDM, while class II HLA confers susceptibility to IDDM. *Diabetologia.* 38:1493-1495.
85. Tait, B., L. Harrison, B. Drummond, V. Steward, M. Varney, and M. Honeyman. 1995. HLA antigens and age at diagnosis of insulin-dependent diabetes. *Hum.Immunol.* 42:(2)116-122.
86. Lie, B., J. Todd, F. Pociot, J. Nerup, H. Akselsen, G. Joner, K. Dahl-Jorgensen, K. Ronningen, E. Thorsby, and D. Undlien. 1999. The predisposition to type 1 diabetes linked to the human leukocyte antigen complex includes at least one non-class II gene. *Am. J. Hum. Genet.* 64:(3)793-800.
87. Hanifi Moghaddam, P., P. de Knijf, B. Roep, B. Van der Auwera, A. Naipal, F. Gorus, F. Schuit, M. Giphart, and The Belgian Diabetes Registry. 1998. Genetic structure of IDDM1. Two separate regions in the major histocompatibility complex contribute to susceptibility or protection. *Diabetes.* 47:(2)263-269.
88. Gambelunghe, G., A. Falorni, M. Ghaderi, S. Laureti, C. Tortoioli, F. Santeusanio, P. Brunetti, and C. Sanjeevi. 1999. Microsatellite polymorphism of the MHC class I chain-related (MIC-A and MIC-B) genes marks the risk for autoimmune Addison's disease. *J. Clin. Endocrinol. Metab.* 84:(10)3701-3707.
89. Gambelunghe, G., M. Ghaderi, A. Cosentino, A. Falorni, P. Brunetti, A. Falorni, and C. Sanjeevi. 2000. Association of MHC class I chain-related A (*MIC-A)* gene polymorphism with type I diabetes. *Diabetologia.* 43:507-514.
90. Ikegami, H., S. Makino, E. Yamato, Y. Kawaguchi, H. Ueda, T. Sakamoto, K. Takekawa, and T. Ogihara. 1995. Identification of a new susceptibility locus for insulin-dependent diabetes mellitus by ancestral haplotype congenic mapping. *J. Clin. Invest.* 96:1936-1942.
91. Mathews, C.E., R.T. Graser, D.V. Serreze, and E.H. Leiter. 2000. Reevaluation of the major histocompatibility complex genes of the NOD-progenitor CTS/Shi strain. *Diabetes.* 49:131-134.

92. Petterson, A., H. Jacob, and Å. Lernmark. 1996. Lessons from the animal models: the BB rat. In Prediction, prevention, and genetic counseling in IDDM. J.P. Palmer, ed. Wiley, Chichester, England. 181-201.
93. Martin, A.M., M.N. Maxson, J. Leif, J.P. Mordes, D.L. Greiner, and E.P. Blankenhorn. 1999. Diabetes-prone and diabetes-resistant BB rats share a common major diabetes susceptibility locus, iddm4: additional evidence for a "universal autoimmunity locus" on rat chromosome 4. *Diabetes.* 48:2138-2144.
94. Kawano, K., T. Hirashima, S. Moris, Y. Saitoh, M. Kurosumi, and T. Natori. 1991. New inbred strain of Long-Evans Tokushima lean rats with IDDM without lymphopenia. *Diabetes.* 40:1375-1381.
95. Nepom, G.T. and D.M. Robinson. 1992. HLA-DQ and diabetes mellitus: a genetic and structural paradigm for models of disease susceptibility. *Mol. Biol. Autoimmun. Dis.* H 38:251-257.
96. Ettinger, R.A., A.W. Liu, G.T. Nepom, and W.W. Kwok. 1998. Exceptional stability of the HLA-DQA1*0102/DQB1*0602 alpha beta protein dimer, the class II MHC molecule associated with protection from insulin-dependent diabetes mellitus. *J. Immunol.* 161:6439-6445.
97. Carrasco-Marin, E., J. Shimizu, O. Kanagawa, and E.R. Unanue. 1996. The class II MHC I-A^{g7} molecules from non-obese diabetic mice are poor peptide binders. *J. Immunol.* 156:450-458.
98. Carrasco-Marin, E., O. Kanagawa, and E.R. Unanue. 1999. The lack of consensus for I-A(g7)-peptide binding motifs: is there a requirement for anchor amino acid side chains? *Proc. Natl. Acad. Sci. USA.* 96:8621-8626.
99. Ridgway, W.M., M. Fasso, and C.G. Fathman. 1999. A new look at MHC and autoimmune disease. *Science.* 284:749,751.
100. Corper, A.L., T. Stratmann, V. Apostolopoulos, C.A. Scott, K.C. Garcia, A.S. Kang, I.A. Wilson, and L. Teyton. 2000. A structural framework for deciphering the link between I-Ag7 and autoimmune diabetes. *Science.* 288:505-511.
101. Verge, C., D. Stenger, E. Bonifacio, P. Colman, C. Pilcher , P. Bingley, G. Eisenbarth, and participating laboratories. 1998. Combined use of autoantibodies (IA-2 autoantibody, GAD autoantibody, insulin autoantibody, cytoplasmic islet cell antibodies) in type 1 diabetes. Combinatorial Islet Autoantibody Workshop . *Diabetes.* 47:1857-1866.
102. Mora, C., F.S. Wong, C.H. Chang, and R.A. Flavell. 1999. Pancreatic infiltration but not diabetes occurs in the relative absence of MHC class II-restricted CD4 T cells: studies using NOD/CIITA- deficient mice. *J. Immunol.* 162:4576-4588.
103. Crawford, M., D. Daniel, D. Wegmann, H. Yang, and R.G. Gill . 1997. Autoimmune islet damage mediated by insulin-specific T cells. *Transplant. Proc.* 29:758-759.
104. Sarvetnick, N., D. Liggitt, S.L. Pitts, S.E. Hansen, and T.A. Stewart. 1988. Insulin-dependent diabetes mellitus induced in transgenic mice by ectopic expression of class II MHC and interferon-gamma. *Cell.* 52:773-782.
105. Miller, J.F. and A. Basten. 1996. Mechanisms of tolerance to self. *Curr. Opin. Immunol.* 8:815-821.
106. Slattery, R.M., L. Kjer-Nielsen, J. Allison, B. Charlton, T.E. Mandel, and J.F.A.P. Miller. 1990. Prevention of diabetes in non-obese diabetic I-Ak transgenic mice. *Nature.* 345:724-726.
107. Miller, J.F.A.P. 1996. Influence and fate of T lymphocytes in autoimmunity. *J. Autoimmun.* 9:301-304.
108. Verdaguer, J., A. Amrani, B. Anderson, D. Schmidt, and P. Santamaria. 1999. Two mechanisms for the non-MHC-linked resistance to spontaneous autoimmunity. *J. Immunol.* 162:4614-4626.
109. Schmidt, D., J. Verdaguer, N. Averill, and P. Santamaria. 1997. A mechanism for the major histocompatibility complex-linked resistance to autoimmunity. *J. Exp. Med.* 186:1059-1075.

110. Wen, L., F.S. Wong, J. Tang, N.Y. Chen, M. Altieri, C. David, R. Flavell, and R. Sherwin. 2000. In vivo evidence for the contribution of human histocompatibility leukocyte antigen (HLA)-DQ molecules to the development of diabetes. *J. Exp. Med.* 191:97-104.
111. Rewers, M., T.L. Bugawan, J.M. Norris, A. Blair, B. Beaty, M. Hoffman, R.S.Jr. McDuffie, R.F. Hamman, G. Klingensmith, G.S. Eisenbarth, and H.A. Erlich. 1996. Newborn screening for HLA markers associated with IDDM: diabetes autoimmunity study in the young (DAISY). *Diabetologia.* 39:807-812.
112. Schenker, M., M. Hummel, K. Ferber, M. Walter, E. Keller, E.D. Albert, H.U. Janka, C. Kastendiek, M. Sorger, F. Louwen, and A.G. Ziegler. 1999. Early expression and high prevalence of islet autoantibodies for DR3/4 heterozygous and DR4/4 homozygous offspring of parents with Type I diabetes: the German BABYDIAB study. *Diabetologia.* 42:671-677.
113. Naserke, H.E., E. Bonifacio , and A.-G. Ziegler. 1999. Immunoglobulin G insulin autoantibodies in BABYDIAB offspring appear postnatally: sensitive early detection using a protein A/G-based radiobinding assay. *J. Clin. Endocrinol. Metab.* 84:1239-1243.
114. Abiru, N., D. Wegmann, E. Kawasaki, P. Gottlieb, E. Simone , and G.S. Eisenbarth. 2000. Dual overlapping peptides recognized by insulin peptide B:9-23 T cell receptor AV13S3 T cell clones of the NOD mouse. *J. Autoimmun.* 14:231-237.
115. Simone, E., D. Daniel, N. Schloot, P. Gottlieb, S. Babu, E. Kawasaki, D. Wegmann, and G.S. Eisenbarth. 1997. T cell receptor restriction of diabetogenic autoimmune NOD T cells. *Proc. Natl. Acad. Sci. USA* 94:2518-2521.
116. Wegmann, D.R., M. Norbury-Glaser, and D. Daniel. 1994. Insulin-specific T cells are a predominant component of islet infiltrates in pre-diabetic NOD mice. *Eur. J. Immunol.* 24:1853-1857.
117. Simone, E.A., D.R. Wegmann, and G.S. Eisenbarth. 1999. Immunologic "vaccination" for the prevention of autoimmune diabetes (type 1A). *Diabetes Care.* 22:B7-B15
118. Daniel, D. and D.R. Wegmann . 1996. Protection of nonobese diabetic mice from diabetes by intranasal or subcutaneous administration of insulin peptide B-(9-23). *Proc. Natl. Acad. Sci. USA* 93:956-960.
119. Muir, A., R. Luchetta, H.-Y. Song, A. Peck, J. Krischer, and N. Maclaren. 1993. Insulin immunization protects NOD mice from diabetes. *Autoimmunity.* 15:58(Abstr.)

4
THE INSULIN VNTR IN THE GENETICS OF TYPE 1 DIABETES

Constantin Polychronakos M.D.
McGill University, Montréal, Québec, Canada H3H 1P3

Alberto Pugliese, M.D.
University of Miami School of Medicine, Miami, FL 33134 USA

INTRODUCTION

Type 1 diabetes results from the autoimmune destruction of pancreatic insulin-producing ß-cells. Insulin is one of several ß-cell molecules targeted as an autoantigen, but is the only autoantigen for which expression is specifically restricted to ß-cells and the only autoantigen whose gene maps to a locus of genetic predisposition. In this chapter, we will review what is known about this locus and discuss the implications on the role of insulin as an autoantigen in autoimmune diabetes.

Observations of familial clustering and twin studies clearly show that genetic susceptibility to type 1 diabetes is a complex trait, dependent on more than one gene. Specific alleles at the HLA-DQ and -DR loci, which are comprised within the major histocompatibility locus on chromosome 6p21, appear to represent a major susceptibility factor (*IDDM1*) and account for about half of the genetic predisposition to diabetes (see Chapter 3) (1). The remaining half is determined by a still unknown number of loci with smaller individual effects. This makes the determination of the "diabetes genotype(s)" a daunting task, albeit one that is crucial to understanding the pathophysiology of the disease as a basis for the development of effective preventive strategies.

The first step in the identification of loci linked to type 1 diabetes risk involves sib-pair linkage analysis to identify polymorphic markers shared by diabetic siblings significantly more than the expected 50% (2). Using this approach, several chromosomal regions have been linked to disease, each typically consisting of a region of several megabases containing dozens of genes (see Chapter 2). By convention they are named *IDDM* (for insulin-dependent diabetes mellitus), followed by a number (HLA is *IDDM1* and insulin is *IDDM2*). Mapping can be further narrowed down by scanning of these regions for polymorphic markers at which specific alleles are found at higher frequency in diabetic subjects than in healthy controls (3).

The next step, probably the most difficult, is to establish a causal relationship between DNA sequence variant and disease-predisposing functional effect. The spectacular successes of positional cloning over the past two decades have been achieved almost exclusively for Mendelian (monogenic) disorders, where mapping the gene involved to a genomic location is followed by the search for severe, gene-inactivating mutations in a gene encompassed by the region. This paradigm will be of less use in polygenic disorders such as diabetes (3). Here genetic susceptibility is likely determined by commonly occurring DNA sequence variants causing subtle functional alterations rather than inactivation of the gene involved. Identification of these subtle alterations requires detailed functional studies, such as the ones described here for the insulin locus.

THE INSULIN VARIABLE NUMBER OF TANDEM REPEATS

One of the first repeat polymorphisms described in the human genome is located 0.5 kb upstream of the insulin gene (*INS*) and consists of a variable number of tandem repeats (VNTR). The repeats consist of a 14-15 base pair (bp) unit consensus sequence (ACAGGGGTCTGGGG) with slight variations of the unit co-existing on the same chromosome. Any number from 30 to several hundred repeats has been observed, but allele frequencies tend to cluster in the range of 30-60 repeats (class I allele) or 120-170 repeats (class III allele). The intermediate class II allele is rare in Caucasians, and less rare in individuals of African descent (4,5). Shortly after its discovery, the insulin VNTR was found to be associated with type 1 diabetes (6), a finding that has been confirmed in many other studies (7-10). Homozygosity for class I alleles, which is found in ~50-60% of Caucasians, was even more common in patients (~75-85%), indicating that it predisposes to diabetes or, more meaningfully, that the less numerous class III alleles have a dominant protective effect (6-10). The functional determinant of the *IDDM2* locus could be the VNTR itself, or a nearby variant for which the VNTR is merely a marker. Linkage disequilibrium that could account for such marker function extends over 4-5 kb region around *INS* (11), encompassing several single-nucleotide polymorphisms (SNP) in and around the INS gene and the gene encoding insulin-like growth factor II (*IGF2*) (Fig. 1). The contributions of individual polymorphisms was determined by genetic analysis confined to the unusual cases in which the allele at the SNPs was not the one predicted by the *INS* VNTR allele on the basis of the known linkage disequilibrium. In individuals with such "mismatched" haplotypes, it was clearly the VNTR rather than the other polymorphisms that conferred diabetes susceptibility or protection (9,12,13). Thus, it is generally accepted that the VNTR is the mechanistically important DNA variant, although this has not been demonstrated beyond all doubt (14). The relative risk ratio of the I/I genotype

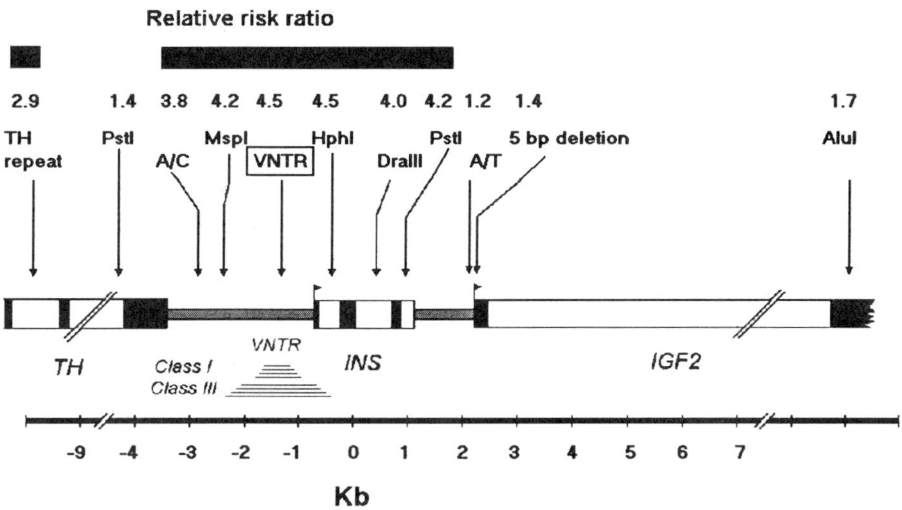

Figure 1. Diabetes-associated haplotype at the *IDDM2* locus. The relative risk ratio associated with each polymorphism is indicated. A bar over the numerical value indicates statistical significance. *TH*: tyrosine hydroxylase; *INS*: insulin; *IGF2*: insulin-like growth factor II. Data adapted from Lucassen *et al.*, 1993, with RR values calculated on the most predisposing allele at each site, so that all values are above 1 for easier comparison.

vs. I/III or III/III has been reported to be in the 3-5 range in various studies, and it accounts for about 10% of the familial clustering of type 1 diabetes (15).

PARENT-OF-ORIGIN EFFECTS AT THE *IDDM2* LOCUS

IDDM2 is situated in one of the few regions in the human genome that is known to be subject to parental imprinting. Parental imprinting refers to the differential behavior of genetic material depending on the sex of the parent from whom it has been inherited (16). Typically, either the maternal or the paternal allele is silenced in somatic cells as a result of some epigenetic modification of the DNA during the passage from the male or the female germline that marks the genetic material as maternal or paternal (parental imprint). *IGF2,* the first human gene found to be imprinted, is expressed exclusively from the paternal chromosome (17), while *H19,* 200 kb downstream, is expressed only from the maternal (18). Several other genes in the region are expressed from the paternal or maternal chromosomes only, at least in some tissues or developmental stages (18). *INS* is expressed from both copies in the pancreas of mice (19), human fetuses of 7-20 weeks gestation (20) and adult humans (10,12), but only from the paternal chromosome in the mouse yolk sack. Thus, imprinted expression can depend on tissue and possibly developmental stage (21), making it possible that human *INS* is also imprinted in an extra-pancreatic site or at some developmental stage not yet examined. Here we shall review preliminary findings from our laboratories consistent with this possibility.

If the gene(s) responsible for the *IDDM2* effect is imprinted, one would expect this to cause a parent-of-origin distortion in the genetic effect. Indeed, the first report of linkage at *IDDM2* found evidence, in a small subset of families that were informative for parental origin, that the excess allele sharing was exclusively paternal (7). Furthermore, studies of intrafamilial association (comparing allele frequency in diabetic children to a control frequency determined by counting the alleles *not transmitted* to the child from his/her non-diabetic parents) at *IDDM2* by us (22,23) and others (24) found it to be statistically significant only for paternally transmitted alleles. Other studies failed to find this effect (8). The presence of genetic differences among the populations studied is one explanation for this discrepancy. It implies that the imprinting that determines this effect may be possible only in the presence of a specific genetic background.

Interestingly, when transmission distortion of individual alleles within class I was examined in a large study of more than 1,300 triads (diabetic child and two parents), an intriguing phenomenon was observed. The most common class I allele among Caucasians, termed I_{814} (in arbitrary electrophoretic mobility units) was transmitted at a frequency higher than the expected 50% from heterozygous I_{814}/III mothers, consistent with the known behavior of class I alleles as a whole (25). Heterozygous I_{814}/III fathers, however, transmitted each allele with equal frequency, suggesting that paternally derived I_{814} may be as diabetes-protective as class III alleles. This would predict that I_{814} is under-transmitted from fathers who were heterozygous for I_{814}/I_{other}, where I_{other} is a class I allele other than I_{814}. This did not turn out to be the case: I_{814}/I_{other} fathers transmitted both alleles equally to their diabetic child (25). Because of the large numbers involved, these results were highly significant statistically, making a strong case for differential function of paternal I_{814} in the offspring, depending on the father's *untransmitted* allele. This unconventional genetic behavior, for which there is a precedent in the phenomenon of paramutation in plants (26), would require some kind of physical interaction of the two copies of the VNTR in the pre-meiotic nucleus of the male germline. Morphological evidence for a similar interaction has been presented for another imprinted locus (the Prader-Willi/Angelman syndrome locus on chromosome 15) in somatic cells (27). This hypothesis finds additional support in the recent finding that both *cis*- and *trans*-allelic interactions influence imprinting at the *Ins2* locus in the mouse (28). Further studies on large, independent DNA data sets and/or transgenic models are required to confirm and further study this intriguing departure from Mendelian genetics.

THE SEARCH FOR A BIOLOGICAL MECHANISM FOR *IDDM2*

What could be the mechanistic basis for the genetic effect at *IDDM2*? The *INS* VNTR (or, for that matter, any of the associated polymorphisms) does not alter the coding sequences in either *INS* or *IGF2*. Therefore, the biological effect must be mediated through effects on transcription control, and such effects could influence the expression of insulin and/or *IGF2*. Because insulin secretion and blood glucose are normal prior to the development of diabetes and both insulin and glucose levels are regulated by metabolic feedback, insulin expression is unlikely to vary significantly in individuals with different VNTR genotypes. Indeed, a recent study found only subtle differences in pancreatic insulin secretion between normal individuals with different *INS* VNTR genotypes (29). Although it has been suggested that differences in the expression of pancreatic insulin, an important autoantigen, might alter the course of autoimmunity to insulin, there is no experimental evidence in support of this hypothesis. On the other hand, IGF-II, the protein product of *IGF2*, is a growth factor with ubiquitous expression that has been implicated in functions that could be relevant to type 1 diabetes. These include inhibition of apoptosis (30) and the stimulation of ß-cell proliferation (31), functions that are of potential importance in resistance to immune injury and regeneration, respectively. Moreover, IGF-II is produced by and acts upon T-lymphocytes (32) in an activation-induced autocrine loop that would amplify clonal expansion of the type of immune cell responsible for ß-cell destruction. Finally, the four promoters of *IGF2*, which encodes a peptide of the insulin family, are situated only 5-20 kb downstream of the *INS* VNTR, a distance consistent with enhancer effects (Fig. 1). Thus, based on theoretical considerations, *IGF2* appears as a better candidate than insulin to explain the biological mechanism mediating *IDDM2*-encoded susceptibility.

FUNCTIONAL EXPLORATION OF THE *IDDM2* EFFECT

In order to dissect the mechanism underlying *IDDM2* susceptibility, we and others evaluated the effect of VNTR alleles on IGF2 and *INS* expression, both *in vitro* and *in vivo*. The possible effects of VNTR alleles were studied on *IGF2* expression in tissues that could affect the development of type 1 diabetes, such as pancreas, thymus, blood leukocytes and activated lymphocytes. *IGF2* is one of the few known genes subject to parental imprinting: only the paternal copy is expressed in most tissues, including thymus and pancreas (38). We, therefore, compared *IGF2* mRNA levels in human pancreas and thymus from fetuses with a paternally derived class I, to those with a paternally derived class III. The results were virtually identical, indicating no significant effect of the *INS* VNTR on *IGF2* transcription in these tissues (39). In leukocytes and activated lymphocytes the results were more complex but still did not support an *IGF2* transcriptional effect. We and others found that in these cells the normally silent maternal copy is reactivated to an extent that is variable among individuals (20,40). VNTR-dependence of this trait would have been a very attractive explanation for the *IDDM2* effect but, again, the data did not support this hypothesis. The paternal/maternal ratio of *IGF2* mRNA levels was variable, but neither the mean value nor its distribution was different between two groups of *INS* VNTR-heterozygous subjects who had paternal I/maternal III vs. those who had the reverse (41). Furthermore, a non-coding single nucleotide polymorphism that was found to be associated with *IGF2* mRNA levels in leukocytes was not associated with type 1 diabetes in large sets of families studied by us and others (11-13,41). The only tissue in which the *INS* VNTR appeared to have a marginal transcriptional effect (class I>III by about 50%) was placenta (35), an organ not known to participate in any obvious way in the pathogenic process of type 1 diabetes. The significance of this finding remains to be understood.

Table 1. Summary of in vitro expression data in b-cell lines of reporter constructs driven by the insulin promoter in conjunction with class I vs. class III INS VNTR alleles.

Report	Relative Expression	Fold Increase	Construct
Kennedy *et al.*, Ref. 34	III > I	~3	CAT and luciferase
Lucassen *et al.*, Ref. 33	I > III	1.5 – 3.5	Native *INS*, whole haplotype
Owerbach and Gabbay, Ref. 61	I > III	2.9 ± 0.4	luciferase
Ounissi *et al.*, unpublished	I ≈ III	0.8 – 1.5	CAT, three class III alleles against I_{814}

The alleles used to represent each class are not necessarily the same between studies

Several studies have evaluated VNTR effects on *INS* transcription. Transfection of rodent ß-cell lines with reporter constructs representing the *INS* promoter flanked by class I vs. class III alleles resulted in three-fold differences going in opposite directions in reports from different laboratories (Ref. 33, 34 and Table 1). In our hands, transfection of cells of the HIT hamster insulinoma line with such constructs did not show a substantial difference between class I and a class III alleles in activating the CAT reporter (Ounissi *et al.*, in preparation).

These discrepant results may be due to species-specificity, differences among specific alleles within each class, or the absence of the genomic context necessary for the VNTR to have its effect (our preferred explanation). We also found a small (~50%) increase in transcriptional activity of constructs of *IGF2* promoters flanked by class I compared to III VNTR in HepG2 cells (35) but, for the same reason, it is difficult to know the significance of these results in the normal context.

More meaningful results were obtained by studies of the transcriptional effect of the *INS* VNTR *in vivo*. This was achieved by comparing steady-state *INS* mRNA levels from each allele in normal fetal and post-natal tissue samples from heterozygous individuals (36). To distinguish mRNA derived from each of the chromosomes, we digested the product of RT-PCR amplification with *Pst*I, an endonuclease recognizing a polymorphic site in the 3' untranslated region of *INS*. Because of tight linkage disequilibrium, this site is virtually always present on the class III chromosome and is absent on the class I chromosome in double heterozygotes. The intensity ratio of the digested over the non-digested bands in genomic DNA was taken as the control representing 1:1 stoichiometry. Comparing this to fetal pancreas RNA, the *INS* transcript in *cis* with the class III VNTR was expressed at lower levels (15-20%) than the class I transcript, a small but statistically significant difference (20). Bennett *et al.* found a somewhat larger difference in adult pancreas (10). Yet, this marginal loss of function is an unsatisfactory explanation for the protective effect of the class III allele, whose dominant nature suggests gain of function.

Thus, the studies described above did not provide data to associate the VNTR effect on diabetes susceptibility with a particular biological mechanism. Yet, such studies were very useful to exclude the mechanisms discussed above. Exploration of all alternative possibilities is a particularly important aspect of the functional dissection of polygenic traits.

THE *INS* VNTR AND EXPRESSION OF INSULIN IN THE THYMUS

The most plausible hypothesis for the mechanism linking DNA sequence variants to the mechanism of diabetes susceptibility at the *IDDM2* locus was formulated following the discovery that *INS* is also transcribed in thymus, in mice (42), rats (43), and humans (36,37). The human thymus expresses low levels of *INS* mRNA throughout fetal development and childhood, but also during adulthood (Pugliese A, personal observation). Messenger RNA for other ß-cell autoantigens, such as glutamic acid decarboxylase (GAD) and the tyrosine-phosphatase-like-protein IA-2, have also been detected (37). *INS* transcription in human thymus also has been reported by others (44) and similarly glucagon, somatostatin, and GAD transcripts have been detected in the mouse thymus (42). Overall, genes encoding several self-molecules have been found to be expressed in the thymus, including pancreatic and thyroid hormones, neuroendocrine molecules, and other peripheral proteins (44-46). Increasing evidence suggests that thymic expression of self-antigens may be crucial for the development of self-tolerance during maturation of the immune system (46). This emerging concept is replacing the traditional beliefs that proteins with tissue-restricted or peripheral expression are not available for presentation in the thymus and that tolerance to such proteins can only be achieved through mechanisms of peripheral tolerance (47). Moreover, studies in transgenic mice and fetal organ thymic cultures have provided both *in vivo* and *in vitro* functional data showing that thymic expression of self-antigens and their levels of expression dramatically affect the development of self-tolerance (46,48-52). The importance, for immune tolerance, of thymic vs. pancreatic *INS* expression is underscored by studies showing that tolerance to a transgenic allogeneic or xenogeneic antigen expressed from the insulin promoter can be transferred by transplanting the transgenic thymus to non-transgenic syngeneic recipients (53,54).

Combined with evidence that negative selection of autoreactive thymocytes is dose-dependent (55), this led us to hypothesize that different *INS* VNTR alleles may modulate tolerance to insulin by differentially influencing the expression levels of insulin in the thymus. Consistent with this hypothesis, *INS* mRNA levels in the thymus were found to correlate with VNTR alleles in an opposite fashion to that observed in the pancreas. *INS* transcripts in *cis* with class III VNTR alleles are transcribed at much higher levels (on average 2-3 fold) than those in *cis* with class I VNTR alleles (Table 2) (36,37).

The increased transcription levels detected in thymus fit well with the dominant protective effect associated with class III VNTR alleles, as higher insulin levels in the thymus may more efficiently induce negative selection of insulin-specific T-lymphocytes. In contrast, homozygosity for diabetes-associated class I VNTR alleles results in lower insulin levels that may be associated with a less efficient deletion of insulin-specific autoreactive T-cells. Specific functional evidence for this interpretation has been recently provided by the finding that transgenic expression of increased levels of proinsulin in the thymus (in MHC class II-positive cells) of nonobese diabetic (NOD) mice is sufficient to prevent diabetes (56). Proinsulin expression may be sufficient to obtain tolerance to insulin since most of the known immunodominant epitopes identified as targets of the insulin autoimmune responses in type 1 diabetes are shared by both insulin and proinsulin (57-59). *INS* transcription in human thymus also correlates with protein production in

Table 2. Summary of in vivo expression in pancreas and thymus from chromosomes carrying class I vs. class III INS VNTR alleles.

Report	Relative Expression	Fold Increase	Tissue
Bennet *et al.*, Ref. 10, 12	I > III	~1.25	Adult pancreas
Vafiadis *et al.*, Ref. 20	I > III	~1.15	Fetal pancreas, 7 - 20 weeks
Vafiadis *et al.*, Ref. 36	III > I	2.7 ± 0.7	Fetal thymus, 7-20 weeks
Pugliese *et al.*, Ref. 37	III > I	2.4 ± 0.7	Fetal and post-natal thymus

the thymus (36,37), where proinsulin may be the main product of the insulin gene. This is not surprising since thymus cells expressing proinsulin are not likely to possess or need the refined machinery necessary to process proinsulin to mature insulin.

These findings also raise intriguing questions about the possibility of imprinted extra-pancreatic *INS* expression in the thymus, as is known to be the case in the yolk sack. Although most thymus samples studied express both *INS* alleles, 5 out of 22 heterozygous samples expressed only one allele (36,37). Of note, in all instances the silenced allele was the one in *cis* to a class III VNTR. If this represents imprinted expression, then the maternal (or conceivably paternal) *INS* copy can be silenced only in the presence of a specific class III allele. Differences in the frequency of these alleles in different populations might explain the discrepancies among different studies as to the presence or absence of a parental effect. Alternatively, certain specific alleles within class III may act as silencing (rather than enhancing) elements, regardless of parental origin. Unfortunately parental DNA was not available for any of these five samples, so we were unable to determine the parental origin of the silenced allele in order to distinguish between the two possibilities. In either case, the observation of silencing of thymic *INS* expression by specific class III alleles leads to the prediction that, in genetic studies, these alleles will behave as predisposing rather than protective. To test this hypothesis we have developed a PCR-based restriction fingerprinting method that uses *Msp*I, an endonuclease that cuts only rare variants of the consensus repeat unit. It generates a large number of possible band patterns, indicating the presence of a large number of class III alleles that are different even when they have the same overall size. Interestingly, three of the five "silencing" class III alleles have identical MspI fingerprints, and two of these are also identical in overall size (Polychronakos and Pugliese, unpublished observations). We are currently in the process of examining the transmission of these specific class III alleles to diabetic children from non-diabetic parents, to test the prediction that they will be over-transmitted and represent a predisposing rather than protective allele.

Overall, the functional studies described here strongly suggest that *IDDM2*-associated susceptibility and resistance may derive from the VNTR influence on *INS* transcription in the thymus, where production of self-antigens such as (pro)insulin may be key to the shaping of a self-tolerant T-cell repertoire. More recent studies have shown that proinsulin expression in the thymus is limited to a subset of antigen-presenting cells which appear to mediate a tolerogenic signal, both in mouse (46,54,60) and human thymus (Pugliese A, personal observation). Moreover, similar cells and *INS* transcription have also been demonstrated in peripheral lymphoid organs (Pugliese A, personal observation), suggesting that insulin expression in lymphoid organs may also play a role in maintaining peripheral self-tolerance throughout life. Based on the available evidence, the *IDDM2* locus appears to act as a quantitative trait affecting the probability of developing autoimmune responses to insulin. Allelic variation at this locus, as well as complex parental and epigenetic effects controlling insulin expression in the immune system, may affect this probability by determining the number of insulin-specific autoreactive T-cells in the peripheral pool, both via thymic selection and peripheral tolerance mechanisms.

REFERENCES

1. Risch, N. 1987. Assessing the role of HLA-linked and unlinked determinants of disease. *Am. J. Hum. Genet.* 40: 1-14.
2. Bennett, S.T and Todd JA. 1996. Human type 1 diabetes and the insulin gene: principles of mapping polygenes. *Ann. Rev. Genet.* 30:343-370.
3. Lander, E.S. and Schork NJ. 1994. Genetic dissection of complex traits *Science.* 265:2037-48.
4. Owerbach, D. and Aagaard, L. 1984. Analysis of a 1963-bp polymorphic region flanking the human insulin gene. *Gene* 32:475-479.
5. Rotwein, P., Yokoyama, S., Didier, D.K. and Chirgwin. J.M. 1986. Genetic analysis of the hypervariable region flanking the human insulin gene. *Am. J. Hum. Gene*t, 39:291-299.
6. Bell, G.I., Horita, S. and Karam. J.H. 1984. A polymorphic locus near the human insulin gene is associated with insulin-dependent diabetes mellitus *Diabetes* 33:176-83.
7. Julier, C., Hyer, R.N., Davies. J., Merlin, F., Soularue, P., Briant, L., Cathelineau, G., Deschamps, I., Rotter, J.I., Froguel, P., Boitrand, C., Bell, J.I. and Lathrop, G.M. 1991. Insulin-IGF2 region on chromosome 11p encodes a gene implicated in HLA-DR4-dependent diabetes susceptibility. *Nature* 354:155-159.
8. Bain, S.C, Prins, J.B, Hearne, C.M., Rodrigues, N.R., Rowe, B.R., Pritchard, L.E., Richie, R.J., Hall, J.R., Undlien, D.E., Ronningen, K.S., Dunger, D.B., Barnett, A.H. and Todd, J.A. 1992. Insulin gene region-encoded susceptibility to type 1 diabetes is not restricted to HLA-DR4-positive individuals. *Nat. Genet.* 2:212-215.

9. Owerbach, D. and Gabbay, K.H. 1993. Localization of a Type I diabetes susceptibility locus to the variable tandem repeat region flanking the insulin gene. *Diabetes* 42:1708-1714.
10. Bennett, S.T., A.J. Wilson, F. Cucca, J. Nerup, F. Pociot, P.A. McKinney, A.H. Barnett, S.C. Bain, and J.A. Todd. 1996. *IDDM2*-VNTR-encoded susceptibility to type 1 diabetes: dominant protection and parental transmission of alleles of the insulin gene-linked minisatellite locus. *J. Autoimmun.* 9:415-421.
11. Lucassen, A.M., Julier, C., Beressi, J..P, Boitard, C., Froguel, P., Lathrop, M. and Bell, J.I. 1993. Susceptibility to insulin dependent diabetes mellitus maps to a 4.1 kb segment of DNA spanning the insulin gene and associated VNTR. *Nat. Genet.* 4:305-310.
12. Bennett, S.T., Lucassen, A.M., Gough, S.C., Powell, E.E., Undlien, D.E., Pritchard, L.E., Merriman, M.E., Kawaguchi, Y,., Dronsfield, M.J., Pociot, F., Nerup, J., Bouzekri, N., Cambon-Thomsen, A., Ronningen, K.S., Barnett, A.H., Bain, S.C. and Todd, J.A. 1995. Susceptibility to human type 1 diabetes at IDDM2 is determined by tandem repeat variation at the insulin gene minisatellite locus. *Nat. Genet.* 9:284-292.
13. Undlien, D.E., Bennett, S.T., Todd, J.A., Akselsen, H.E., Ikaheimo, I., Reijonen, H., Knip, M., Thorsby, E. and Ronningen, K.S. 1995. Insulin gene region-encoded susceptibility to IDDM maps upstream of the insulin gene. *Diabetes* 44:620-625.
14. Doria, A., Lee, J., Warram, J.H. and Krolewski, A.S. 1996. Diabetes susceptibility at IDDM2 cannot be positively mapped to the VNTR locus of the insulin gene. *Diabetologia* 39:594-599.
15. Bennett, S.T. and Todd, J.A. 1996. Human type 1 diabetes and the insulin gene: principles of mapping polygenes. *Ann. Rev. Genet.* 30:343-370.
16. Hoffman, A.R. and T.H. Vu. 1996. Genomic Imprinting. *Scientific American* 1:52-61
17. Giannoukakis, N., C. Deal, J. Paquette, C.G. Goodyer, and C. Polychronakos. 1993. Parental genomic imprinting of the human IGF2 gene. *Nat. Genet.* 4:98-101.
18. Feinberg, A.P. 1999. Imprinting of a genomic domain of 11p15 and loss of imprinting in cancer: an introduction. *Cancer Research* 59(7 Suppl):1743s-1746s.
19. Giddings, S.J., C.D. King, K.W. Harman, J.F. Flood, and L.R. Carnaghi. 1994. Allele specific inactivation of insulin 1 and 2, in the mouse yolk, indicates imprinting. *Nat. Genet.* 6:310-313.
20. Vafiadis, P., Bennett, S.T., Colle, E., Grabs, R., Goodyear, C.G. and Polychronakos, C. 1996. Imprinted and genotype-specific expression of genes at the *IDDM2* locus in pancreas and leucocytes. *J. Autoimmun.* 9:397-403.
21. Deltour, L., Montagutelli, X., Guenet, J.L., Jami, J., and Paldi A. 1995. Tissue- and developmental stage-specific imprinting of the mouse proinsulin gene, *Ins2*. *Developmental Biology* 168:686-688.
22. Pugliese, A., Awdeh, Z.L., Alper, C.A., Jackson, R.A. and Eisenbarth, G.S. The paternally inherited insulin gene B allele (1,428 FokI site) confers protection from insulin-dependent diabetes in families. *J Autoimmun* 7:687-694, 1994.
23. Polychronakos, C., Kukuvitis, A., Giannoukakis, N. and Colle, E. 1995. Parental imprinting effect at the INS-IGF2 diabetes susceptibility locus. *Diabetologia* 38:715-9.
24. Bui, M.M., Luo, D.F., She, J.Y., Maclaren, N.K., Muir, A., Thomson, G. and She JX. 1996. Paternally transmitted IDDM2 influences diabetes susceptibility despite biallelic expression of the insulin gene in human pancreas. *J. Autoimmun.* 9:97-103
25. Bennett, S.T., A.J. Wilson, L. Esposito, N. Bouzekri, D.E. Undlien, F. Cucca, L. Nistico', R. Buzzetti, B.E. the IMDIAB Group, F. Pociot, J. Nerup, A. Cambon-Thomsen, A. Pugliese, J.P.H. Shield, P.A. McKinney, S.C. Bain, C. Polychronakos, and J.A. Todd . 1997. Insulin VNTR allele-specific effect in type 1 diabetes depends on identity of untrasmitted paternal allele. *Nat. Genet.* 17:350-352.
26. Hollick, J., Dorweiler, J. and Chandler, V. 1997. Paramutation and related allelic interactions. *Trends Genet.* 13: 302-308.
27. LaSalle, J.M. and Lalande, M. 1996. Homologous association of oppositely imprinted chromosomal domains. *Science* 272:725-728.

28. Duvillié, B., Bucchini, D., Tang, T., Jami, J., and Paldi, A. 1998. Imprinting at the mouse Ins2 locus: Evidence for *cis*- and trans-allelic interactions . *Genomics* 47:52-57.
29. Ahmed, S., Bennett, S.T., Huxtable S.J., Todd, J.A., Matthews, D.R. and Gough SC. 1999. *INS* VNTR allelic variation and dynamic insulin secretion in healthy adult non-diabetic Caucasian subjects. *Diabetic Medicine*. 16:910-7.
30. Christofori, G., Naik, P. and Hanahan, D. 1995. Deregulation of both imprinted and expressed alleles of IGF2 gene during β-cell tumorigenesis. *Nat. Genet.* ,10:196-201.
31. Hill, D.J. and, Hogg J. 1991. Growth factor control of pancreatic B cell hyperplasia. *Baillieres Clin Endocrinol Metab* 5:689-98.
32. Nyman, T. and Pekonen, F. 1993. The expression of IGFs and their binding proteins in normal human lymphocytes. *Acta Endocrinologica* 128:168-72.
33. Lucassen, A.M., Screaton, G.R. Julier, C., Elliott, T.J., Lathrop, M. and Bell, J.I.. 1995. Regulation of insulin gene expression by the IDDM associated, insulin locus haplotype. *Hum. Mol. Genet.* 4:501-506.
34. Catignani Kennedy, G., German, M.S., and Rutter W.J. 1995. The minisatellite in the diabetes susceptibility locus IDDM2 regulates insulin transcription. *Nat. Genet.* 9:293-298.
35. Paquette, J., Giannoukakis, N., Polychronakos, C., Vafiadis, P. and Deal, C. 1998. The INS 5' variable number of tandem repeats is associated with IGF2 expression in humans. *J. Biol. Chem.* 273:14158-14164.
36. Vafiadis, P., S.T. Bennett, J.A. Todd, J. Nadeau, R. Grabs, C.G. Goodyear, S. Wickramasinghe, E. Colle, and C. Polychronakos. 1997. Insulin expression in the thymus is modulated by *INS* VNTR alleles at the *IDDM2* locus. *Nat. Genet.* 15:289-292.
37. Pugliese, A., Zeller, M., Fernandez, A.Jr., Zalcberg, L.J., Bartlett, R.J., Ricordi, C., Pietropaolo, M., Eisenbarth, G.S., Bennett, S.T. and Patel D.D. 1997. The insulin gene is transcribed in the human thymus and transcription levels correlate with allelic variation at the *INS* VNTR-*IDDM2* susceptibility locus for type 1 diabetes. *Nat. Genet.* 15:293-297.
38. Polychronakos, C., Giannoukakis N., and Deal, C. 1995. *IGF2* imprinting, insulin-dependent diabetes, immune function, and apoptosis: A hypothesis. *Developmental Genetics* 17:253-262
39. Vafiadis. P., Grabs. R., Goodyer, C.G., Colle, E. and Polychronakos C. 1998. A functional analysis of the role of IGF2 in *IDDM2* encoded susceptibility to type 1 diabetes. *Diabetes* 47:831-836.
40. Cu, H., Horon, I.L., Ohlsson, R., Hamilton, S.R. and Feinberg, A.P. 1998. Loss of imprinting in normal tissue of colorectal cancer patients with microsatellite instability *Nat. Medicine*. 4:1276-80.
41. Vafiadis, P., Bennett, S.T., Todd, J.A. and Polychronakos C. 1998. Divergence between genetic determinants of IGF2 transcription levels in leukocytes and of *IDDM2*-encoded susceptibility to type 1 diabetes. *J. Clin. Endocrinol. Metab.* 83:2933-9.
42. Jolicouer, C., Hanahan, D. and Smith, K.M.. 1994. T-cell tolerance toward a transgenic beta-cell antigen and transcription of endogenous pancreatic genes in thymus. *Proc. Natl. Acad. Sci. USA* 91:6707-6711.
43. Heath, V.L., Moore, N.C., Parnell S.M. and Mason, D.W. 1998. Intrathymic expression of genes involved in organ specific autoimmune disease. *J. Autoimmun.* 11:309-318.
44. Sospedra, M., Ferrer-Francesch, X., Dominguez, O., Juan, M., Foz-Sala, M., and Pujol-Borrell, R. 1998. Transcription of a broad range of self-antigens in human thymus suggests a role for central mechanisms in tolerance toward peripheral antigens. *J.Immunol.* 161:5918-5929.
45. Werdelin, O., Cordes, U., and Jensen, T. 1998. Aberrant expression of tissue-specific proteins in the thymus: a hypothesis for the development of central tolerance. *Scand. J. Immunol.* 47:95-100.
46. Hanahan, D. 1998. Peripheral-antigen-expressing cells in thymic medulla: factors in self-tolerance and autoimmunity. *Curr. Opin. Immunol.* 10:656-662.

47. Mason, D. and F. Powrie. 1998. Control of immune pathology by regulatory T cells. *Curr. Opin. Immunol.* 10:649-655.
48. Salmon, A.M., C. Bruand, A. Cardona, J.P. Changeux, and S. Berrih-Aknin. 1998. An acetylcholine receptor alpha subunit promoter confers intrathymic expression in transgenic mice. Implications for tolerance of a transgenic self-antigen and for autoreactivity in myasthenia gravis. *J. Clin. Invest.* 101:2340-2350.
49. Sebzda, E., Wallace, V.A., Mayer, J., Yeung, R.S.M., Mak, T.W., and Ohashi, P.S. 1994. Positive and negative thymocyte selection induced by different concentrations of a single peptide. *Science* 263:1615-1618.
50. Sprent, J. and Webb, S.R. 1995. Intrathymic and extrathymic clonal deletion of T cells. *Curr. Opinion. Immunol.* 7:196-205. 17.
51. Oehen, S.U., Ohashi, P.S., Burki, K., Hengartner, H., Zinkernagel, R.M., and Aichele, P. 1994. Escape of thymocytes and mature T cells from clonal deletion due to limiting tolerogen expression levels. *Cellular Immunology* M. 158:342-352.
52. Liblau, R.S., Tisch, R., Shokat, K., Yang, X., Dumont, N., Goodnow, C.C. and McDevitt H.O. 1993. Intravenous injection of soluble antigen induces thymic and peripheral T-cell apoptosis. *Proc. Natl. Acad. Sci. USA* 93:3031-3036.
53. Heath, W.R., Allison, J., Hoffmann, M.W., Schonrich, G., Hammerling, G., Arnold, B., Miller, J.F. Autoimmune diabetes as a consequence of locally produced intereukin- 2. *Nature* 359:547-49, 1992.
54. Smith, K.M., Olson, D.C., Hirose, R., and Hanahan, D. 1997. Pancreatic gene expression in rare cells of thymic medulla: evidence for functional contribution to T cell tolerance. *Internat. Immunol.* 9:1655-1665.
55. Ashton-Rickardt, P.G., Bandeira, A., Delaney, J.R., van Kaer, L., Pircher, H.P., Zinkernagel, R.M. and Tonegawa. S. 1994. Evidence for a differential avidity model of T cell selection in the thymus. *Cell* 76:651-663.
56. French, M.B., Allison, J., Cram, A.S., Thomas, H.E., Dempsey-Collier, M., Silva, A., Georgiou, H.M., Kay, T.W., Harrison, L.C. and Lew, A.M. 1997. Transgenic expression of mouse proinsulin II prevents diabetes in nonobese diabetic mice. *Diabetes* 46:34-39.
57. Kuglin, B., Gries, F.A. and Kolb, H. 1988. Evidence for IgG autoantibodies against human proinsulin in patients with IDDM before insulin treatment. *Diabetes* 37:130-132.
58. Castano, L., Ziegler, A., Ziegler, R., Shoelson, S. and Eisenbarth G.S. 1993. Characterization of insulin autoantibodies in relatives of patients with insulin-dependent diabetes mellitus. *Diabetes* 42:1202-1209.
59. Keilacker, H., Rjasanowski, I. Besch, G.S. and Kohnert K.D. 1995. Autoantibodies to insulin and to proinsulin in type 1 diabetic patients and in at-risk probands differentiate only little between both antigens. *Hormone Metabolic Research* 27:90-94.
60. Throsby, M., Homo-Delarche, F., Chevenne, D., Goya, R., Dardenne, M. and Pleau, J. 1998. Pancreatic Hormone Expression in the Murine Thymus: Localization in Dendritic Cells and Macrophages. *Endocrinology* 139:2399-240
61. Owerbach, D. and Gabbay, K.H. 1996. The search for IDDM susceptibility genes: the next generation. *Diabetes.* 45: 544-551

5

MATURITY ONSET DIABETES OF THE YOUNG (MODY)

Philippe Froguel, M.D., PhD
Queen Mary and Westfield College Genomic Center, University of London, London, UK

Gilberto Velho, M.D., PhD
INSERM U342, Institut Cochin de Génétique Moléculaire, Paris, France

INTRODUCTION

Maturity Onset Diabetes of the Young (MODY) is a familial form of non-insulin dependent diabetes with autosomal dominant inheritance. Hyperglycemia in MODY subjects usually develops at childhood, adolescence or young adulthood, and is associated with primary insulin-secretion defects (1, 2). Early studies showed that subjects from different families with MODY could present with variable phenotypes (3), which suggested that the disorder was genetically heterogeneous. MODY is an attractive model for genetic studies because of its well-defined monogenic mode of inheritance with high penetrance and its early age of onset allowing the collection of pedigrees with several generations of affected subjects. For these reasons, the investigation of genetic determinants of MODY proceeded faster than that of polygenic forms of diabetes and it is now recognized that MODY is not a single entity, but presents genetic as well as metabolic and clinical heterogeneity. Mutations in six genes cause most of the MODY cases. These genes encode the enzyme glucokinase (MODY2/GCK) (4-6) and the transcription factors Hepatocyte Nuclear Factor 4 alpha (HNF-4α/MODY1) (7, 8), Hepatocyte Nuclear Factor 1 alpha (HNF-1α/MODY3) (9-11), Insulin Promoter Factor 1 (IPF-1/MODY4) (12, 13), Hepatocyte Nuclear Factor 1 beta (HNF-1β/MODY5) (14), and NeuroD1/Beta2 (15). Moreover, additional MODY genes probably exist, since there are families in which MODY does not co-segregate with markers tightly linked to the known MODY loci (16).

MODY seems to have a worldwide distribution, but its prevalence is still unknown. Although commonly thought to be a relatively rare form of diabetes, its frequency might have been underestimated, as the hyperglycemia can remain undiagnosed until adulthood. It has been estimated that 2-5% of patients with Type 2 Diabetes may in fact have MODY (17). Furthermore, it has been shown that as much as 10% of subjects originally classified as having type 1 diabetes but without carrying high-risk HLA-haplotypes might indeed have MODY (18). The relative prevalence of the different subtypes of MODY has been shown to vary greatly in studies of MODY families from different populations (16, 19-21). MODY2 represents from 8 to 63% of cases (the most prevalent form in French families) and MODY3 from 21 to 64% of cases (the most prevalent form in British families). The other MODY subtypes are rare disorders in all these populations, having been described only in a few families, while additional unknown MODY locus or loci (MODY-X) represent 16 to 45% of the cases of MODY (the most prevalent form in German and Spanish families). These contrasting results may be due to differences in the genetic background of these populations, or else, may reflect, at least partly, ascertainment bias in the recruitment of families.

GLUCOKINASE MUTATIONS AND MODY2

Glucokinase phosphorylates glucose to glucose-6-phosphate in pancreatic beta cells and hepatocytes, and plays a major role in the regulation and integration of glucose metabolism (22). More than 80 different GCK mutations associated with MODY have been observed to date (6, 23). Expression studies have shown that the enzymatic activity of the mutant proteins was impaired (24), resulting in decreased glycolytic flux in pancreatic beta-cells (25). This defect translates in vivo as a glucose-sensing defect leading to an increase in the blood glucose threshold that triggers insulin secretion (26), and a right shift in the dose response curve of glucose-induced insulin secretion (27). Comparison of insulin secretion rates at different glucose levels demonstrated that glucokinase-deficient MODY2 subjects present an average 60% reduction in insulin secretion for a given glucose level (27). The release of insulin in response to arginine is usually well preserved which suggests that this secretory defect is indeed related to glucose sensing (28). Decreased net accumulation of hepatic glycogen and increased hepatic gluconeogenesis following meals were observed in glucokinase-deficient subjects (29). In addition, these subjects have decreased hepatic glucose cycling and endogenous glucose production abnormally high in relation to their plasma glucose levels, with a blunted suppression after oral glucose administration (30). These results demonstrate that in addition to the altered beta cell function, abnormalities in liver glucose metabolism contribute to the pathogenesis of hyperglycemia in patients with MODY2.

Despite these multiple defects in the pancreas and the liver, the hyperglycemia associated with GCK mutations is often mild, with fewer than 50% of subjects presenting overt diabetes (6). There is a lower prevalence of diabetes microvascular complications (retinopathy and proteinuria) in MODY2 than in other subtypes of MODY and late-onset Type 2 Diabetes (6, 31). Interestingly, inheritance of a glucokinase mutation not only results in hyperglycemia after birth, but also reduced fetal growth and decreased birth weight (32, 33). This effect might be due to a reduction in fetal insulin secretion in response to maternal blood glucose level (34). Despite the reduced birth weight, no differences in height, weight or BMI are observed in pre-adolescent, adolescent and adult MODY2 subjects as compared to their unaffected sibs (33). This post-natal realignment of weight (catch-up) is in agreement with observations that MODY2 subjects maintain relatively normal insulin levels throughout the day at the expense of hyperglycemia (27, 29).

HNF-1α AND MODY3

Positional cloning of MODY loci and studies in candidate genes have led to the identification of mutations in six transcription factors: HNF-1α, HNF-1β, HNF-4α, IPF1 and NeuroD1/Beta2 (8, 10, 13-15). Gene targeting in animals demonstrated that many of these islet-expressed genes play a key role in the fetal development, beta-cell differentiation, proliferation and neogenesis (35-37). Mutations in HNF-1α account for most of the mutations associated with MODY identified in nuclear factors. More than 80 different mutations located in the coding regions or in the promoter were found in various populations (10, 11, 16, 19, 38-42). An insulin secretory defect in the absence of insulin resistance was observed in diabetic and non-diabetic carriers of MODY3 mutations (43, 44), suggesting that HNF-1α is indeed implicated in pancreatic beta-cell function. Decreased stimulation of glucose utilization, oxidation, and nonoxidative glucose disposal, as well as a blunted suppression of endogenous glucose production were also observed in MODY3 subjects (45). However, these phenomena were found to be essentially secondary to insulinopenia due to the beta-cell defect (45). In contrast to the usually mild hyperglycemia due to glucokinase deficiency, MODY3 is a severe form of diabetes, often evolving to insulin-requirement (11, 31). Microvascular complications of diabetes are observed as frequently in MODY3 subjects as in subjects with type 2 diabetes with late onset (31, 46). HNF-1α is also expressed in the kidney, and a defect in the renal resorption of glucose characterized by decreased glucose threshold for glucosuria is often found in MODY3 subjects (47, 48).

The genetic and metabolic mechanisms, as well as the target genes associated with the beta-cell defect of MODY3 remain mostly unknown.

Heterozygous knock-out mice lacking one copy HNF-1α have a normal phenotype, while MODY3 subjects are all heterozygous for their mutations and fully express the diabetes phenotype (49, 50). This observation suggests that these mutations might have a dominant negative effect. However, experimental data show that only the mutations located in the transactivation domain have a dominant negative effect on HNF-1α transactivation potential (51). Mutations located elsewhere in the protein might not interfere with the activity of the normal allele. Studies in beta-cells from knock-out mice show a defect in ATP production in response to glucose, related to failure to generate NADH from glycolytic substrates (52). Although the precise nature of the signal defect remains elusive, these studies suggest that a reduction in the expression of one or more of the enzymes of the glycolytic pathway proximal to the enolase step accounts for the defects observed in glucose-stimulated signal transduction observed in these animals (52). On the other hand, contrasting results were observed in studies of beta-cells from knock-out mice (50) and a beta-cell-derived insulinoma cell line (53) regarding a possible defect in the expression of the insulin gene.

OTHER TRANSCRIPTION FACTORS AND MODY

MODY1 is much less prevalent than MODY2 and MODY3, and only a few kindred other than the large American RW family were found to carry HNF-4α mutations (8, 54-56). MODY1 subjects usually present a severe form of diabetes, which is often associated with microvascular complications (57). A primary pancreatic beta-cell defect was observed in these subjects (58, 59). HNF-4α is a member of the steroid/thyroid hormone receptor superfamily. Interestingly, it was demonstrated that long-chain fatty acids directly modulates the transcriptional activity of HNF-4α by binding as acyl-CoA thioesters to the ligand binding domain of HNF-4α gene (60). This binding results in the activation or the inhibition of HNF-4α transcriptional activity as a function of chain length and the degree of saturation of the fatty acyl-CoA ligand (60). This observation contributes important data to the understanding of the role of dietary fats in the control of insulin secretion. Here again, the molecular mechanisms by which a reduction of HNF-4α activity results in beta-cell defects and diabetes are not clearly determined. Studies in embryonic stem cells demonstrated that loss of function of HNF-4α leads to impaired expression of genes involved in glucose transport (GLUT-2) and glycolysis (aldolase B, glyceraldehyde-3-phosphate dehydrogenase), as well as the gene encoding liver pyruvate kinase (61). HNF-4α is an upstream regulator of HNF-1α/MODY3 expression. Decrease of HNF-1α expression as a result of an HNF-4α mutation might thus contribute to the MODY1 phenotype. This hypothesis is supported by the observation that a mutation in the HNF-4α binding site in the promoter of HNF-1α gene results in MODY3 (40).

Mutations in HNF-1β were recently described in a few families with familial diabetes with early onset consistent with MODY (14, 62). In these pedigrees HNF-1β mutations were associated with diabetes and severe kidney disease, which may appear before the impairment of glucose tolerance. Polycystic renal disease and/or particular histological abnormalities showing meganephrons were present in some subjects, suggesting that this gene could play a major role in kidney development and nephron differentiation. It is noteworthy that HNF-1β functions as a homodimer or as a heterodimer with the structurally related HNF-1α to bind to DNA (63).

All of these genetic defects in transcription factors lead to abnormalities of glucose homeostasis, and thereby promote the development of chronic hyperglycemia, through alterations in insulin secretion and possibly, in the development of the pancreatic islets. In this regard, a deletion in the homeodomain transcription factor insulin promoter factor-1 (IPF-1 or IDX-1, STF-1, PDX-1), was found to co-segregate with MODY in a large kindred presenting a consanguineous link (13). This mutation results in a premature stop codon and a protein lacking a domain that is crucial for DNA-binding. The phenotype of the subjects who are heterozygous for the mutation ranges from normal to impaired glucose tolerance to overt non insulin-dependent diabetes. One child who is homozygous for the mutation was born with pancreatic agenesis, and suffers from diabetes as well as exocrine insufficiency (12). IPF-1 is critically required for the embryonic development of the pancreatic islets as well as for transcriptional regulation of endocrine pancreatic tissue-specific genes in adults, such as the insulin, glucose transporter-2 (GLUT2) and glucokinase genes in beta cells, and the somatostatin gene in d-cells. IPF-1 is normally expressed in all cells of the pancreatic bud, and its absence in mice arrests development at the bud stage leading to pancreatic agenesis (35).

The transcription factor NeuroD1 (also known as Beta 2) is involved in the regulation of endocrine pancreas development. In mice homozygous for a targeted disruption of the NeuroD1 gene, pancreatic islet morphogenesis is abnormal and hyperglycemia develops, due, in part, to inadequate expression of the insulin gene (36). Recently, mutations in NeuroD1 were shown to co-segregate in with Type 2 diabetes of early age of onset and autosomal dominant-like transmission in two Caucasian kindred (15). This observation suggests that NeuroD1 might also play an important role on endocrine pancreas development and/or insulin gene expression in humans.

MODY GENES AND LATE ONSET TYPE 2 DIABETES

The full expression of hyperglycemia in subjects with Type 2 diabetes with late onset requires defective or deficient beta-cell function. For obvious reasons the MODY genes were considered as strong candidate genes for this insulin secretory defect. Positive associations between Type 2 diabetes and particular glucokinase alleles were observed in African-American and Mauritian Creole subjects (64). Mutations in the coding regions of the glucokinase gene were not found in these subjects, nor in other cohorts and populations (65), suggesting that glucokinase is not a major susceptibility gene for Type 2 diabetes. However, it is possible that variants in the regulatory regions upstream the promoter might play a minor role in a polygenic context, at least in some families or populations. A polymorphism at position –30 bp in the pancreatic promoter region was found to co-segregate with Type 2 diabetes with late onset in one French family (65). Moreover, this variant was associated with reduced beta-cell function in Japanese-American subjects with normal or impaired glucose tolerance (66), although this effect was not observed in Danish subjects (67).

The role of MODY and other transcription factors in the development of Type 2 diabetes is still under investigation. Linkage analyses studies and screening for mutations have excluded a role as major susceptibility genes for the five known MODY genes encoding transcription factors. However, mutations in HNF-1α were identified in African-Americans and Japanese subjects with atypical non-autoimmune diabetes with acute onset (68, 69), and a common polymorphism in HNF-1α was found to be associated with mild insulin secretion defects (70). Moreover, mutations in HNF-4α (71) and IPF1 (72, 73) were recently identified in a few families with late-onset Type 2 diabetes. Several other transcription factors have been studied, and a mutation in Islet Brain 1 (IB1) was found to be associated with diabetes in one family (74). IB1 is a homologue of the c-jun amino-terminal kinase interacting protein 1 (JIP-1), which plays a role in the modulation of apoptosis. IB1 is also a transactivator of the islet glucose transporter GLUT2. The mutant IB1 was found to be unable to prevent apoptosis in vitro. It is thus possible that the abnormal function of this mutant IB1 may render beta cells more susceptible to apoptotic stimuli, thus decreasing beta-cell mass. As glucotoxicity and lipotoxicity are known to induce both apoptosis and transcription factor down regulation in pancreatic beta cells, inherited or acquired limitations in IB1 activity could have deleterious effects in beta-cell function.

Together, these data suggest that mutations in transcription factors may contribute to the genetic risk to Type 2 diabetes through various mechanisms: dysregulation of target genes involved in glucose or lipid metabolism (HNFs, IPF1, IB1), abnormal beta-cell development and differentiation (IPF1, NeuroD1/Beta2), and dysregulation of beta-cell apoptosis (IB1). Deleterious mutations that significantly impair the transactivational activity of these transcription factors can be responsible in some families for monogenic-like forms of diabetes with late age of onset, which may represent an intermediary phenotype between MODY and the most common forms of Type 2 diabetes.

CONCLUSIONS

The identification of glucokinase as a diabetes susceptibility gene has provided a major impulse for the reassessment of the physiological role as "glucose sensor" and the understanding of pathophysiological importance of this key enzyme of glucose homeostasis (22, 75). More recently, the recognition of the role of transcription factors in MODY opened entirely new perspectives in the understanding of the molecular basis not only of MODY, but also of other forms of diabetes (76). The identification of the remaining MODY genes will certainly further understanding of glucose homeostasis and pathophysiology of hyperglycemia and contribute to a more rational classification of diabetes based on etiology and pathophysiology.

REFERENCES

1. Velho, G., and Froguel, P. 1998. Genetic, metabolic and clinical characteristics of maturity onset diabetes of the young. *Eur. J. Endocrinol.* 138:233-239.
2. Froguel, P., and Velho, G. 1999. Molecular genetics of maturity onset diabetes of the young. *Trends Endocrinol. Metab.* 10:142-146.
3. Fajans, S.S. 1990. Scope and heterogeneous nature of MODY. *Diabetes Care.* 13:49-64.
4. Froguel, P., et al. 1992. The glucokinase locus on chromosome 7p is closely linked to early onset non insulin dependent diabetes mellitus. *Nature.* 356:162-164.
5. Froguel, P., et al. 1993. Familial hyperglycemia due to mutations in glucokinase: definition of a subtype of diabetes mellitus. *N. Engl. J. Med.* 328:697-702.
6. Velho, G., et al. 1997. Identification of 14 new glucokinase mutations and description of the clinical profile of 42 MODY-2 families. *Diabetologia.* 40:217-224.
7. Bell, G.I., Xiang, K.S., Newman, M.V., Wu, S.H., Wright, L.G., Fajans, S.S., and Cox, N.J. 1991. Gene for non insulin dependent diabetes mellitus (maturity onset diabetes of the young subtype) is linked to DNA polymorphism on chromosome 20q. *Proc. Natl. Acad. Sci. U.S.A.* 88:1484-1488.
8. Yamagata, K., Furuta, H., Oda, O., Kaisaki, P.J., Menzel, S., Cox, N.J., Fajans, S.S., Signorini, S., Stoffel, M., and Bell, G.I. 1996. Mutations in the hepatocyte nuclear factor 4 alpha gene in maturity-onset diabetes of the young (MODY1). *Nature.* 384:458-460.
9. Vaxillaire, M., Boccio, V., Philippi, A., Vigouroux, C., Terwilliger, J., Passa, P., Beckman, J.S., Velho, G., Lathrop, G.M., and Froguel, P. 1995. A gene for maturity onset diabetes of the young (MODY) maps to chromosome 12q. *Nature Genetics.* 9:418-423.
10. Yamagata, K., et al. 1996. Mutations in the hepatocyte nuclear factor 1 alpha gene in maturity-onset diabetes of the young (MODY3). *Nature.* 384:455-458.
11. Vaxillaire, M., et al. 1997. Identification of nine novel mutations in the hepatocyte nuclear factor 1 alpha gene associated with maturity-onset diabetes of the young (MODY3). *Hum. Mol. Genet.* 6:583-586.

12. Stoffers, D.A., Zinkin, N.T., Stanojevic, V., W.L., C., and Habener, J.F. 1997. Pancreatic agenesis attributable to a single nucleotide deletion in the human *IPF1* gene coding sequence. *Nature Genet.* 15:106-110.
13. Stoffers, D.A., Ferrer, J., Clarke, W.L., and Habener, J.F. 1997. Early-onset type 2 diabetes mellitus (MODY4) linked to IPF1. *Nature Genet.* 17:138-139.
14. Horikawa, Y., et al. 1997. Mutation in hepatocyte nuclear factor-1ß gene (TCF2) associated with MODY. *Nature Genet.* 17:384-385.
15. Malecki, M.T., Jhala, U.S., Antonellis, A., Fields, L., Doria, A., Orban, T., Saad, M., Warram, J.H., Montminy, M., and Krolewski, A.S. 1999. Mutations in NEUROD1 are associated with the development of type 2 diabetes mellitus. *Nature Genet.* 23:323-328.
16. Chèvre, J.C., et al. 1998. Mutation screening in 18 caucasian families suggests the existence of other MODY genes. *Diabetologia.* 41:1017-1023.
17. Ledermann, H.M. 1995. Is maturity onset diabetes at young age (MODY) more common in Europe than previously assumed? *Lancet.* 345:648.
18. Moller, A.M., Dalgaard, L.T., Pociot, F., Nerup, J., Hansen, T., and Pedersen, O. 1998. Mutations in the hepatocyte nuclear factor-1 alpha gene in Caucasian families originally classified as having Type I diabetes. *Diabetologia.* 41:1528-1531.
19. Frayling, T.M., et al. 1997. Mutations in the hepatocyte nuclear factor-1 alpha gene are a common cause of maturity-onset diabetes of the young in the U.K. *Diabetes.* 46:720-725.
20. Lindner, T.H., Cockburn, B.N., and Bell, G.I. 1999. Molecular genetics of MODY in Germany. *Diabetologia.* 42:121-123.
21. Costa, A., et al. 2000. Genetic and clinical characterisation of MODY in Spanish families. *Eur. J. Endocrinol.* 142:380-386.
22. Matschinsky, F.M. 1996. A lesson in metabolic regulation inspired by the glucokinase glucose sensor paradigm. *Diabetes.* 45:223-241.
23. Blanché, H., et al. 1997. Criblage moléculaire de la glucokinase: 37 nouvelles mutations. (Abstract). *Diab. Metab.* 23 (suppl.1):29.
24. Gidh-Jain, M., et al. 1993. Glucokinase mutations associated with non insulin dependent (type 2) diabetes mellitus have decreased enzymatic activity: implications for structure/function relationships. *Proc. Natl. Acad. Sci. U.S.A.* 90:1932-1936.
25. Sturis, J., Kurland, I.J., Byrne, M.M., Mosekilde, E., Froguel, P., Pilkis, S.J., Bell, G.I., and Polonsky, K.S. 1994. Compensation in pancreatic beta-cell function in subjects with glucokinase mutations. *Diabetes.* 43:718-723.
26. Velho, G., Froguel, P., Clément, K., Pueyo, M.E., Rakotoambinina, B., Zouali, H., Passa, P., Cohen, D., and Robert, J.J. 1992. Primary pancreatic beta-cell secretory defect caused by mutations in the glucokinase in kindreds of maturity onset diabetes of the young. *Lancet.* 340:444-448.
27. Byrne, M.M., et al. 1994. Insulin secretory abnormalities in subjects with hyperglycemia due to glucokinase mutations. *J. Clin. Invest.* 93:1120-1130.
28. Pueyo, M.E., Clement, K., Vaxillaire, M., Passa, P., Froguel, P., Robert, J.J., and Velho, G. 1994. Arginine-induced insulin release in glucokinase-deficient subjects. *Diabetes Care.* 17:1015-1021.
29. Velho, G., Petersen, K.F., Perseghin, G., Hwang, J.-H., Rothman, D.L., Pueyo, M.E., Cline, G.W., Froguel, P., and Shulman, G.I. 1996. Impaired hepatic glycogen synthesis in glucokinase-deficient (MODY-2) subjects. *J. Clin. Invest.* 98:1755-1761.
30. Tappy, L., Dussoix, P., Iynedjian, P., Henry, S., Schneiter, P., Zahnd, G., Jéquier, E., and Philippe, J. 1997. Abnormal regulation of hepatic glucose output in maturity onset diabetes of the young caused by a specific mutation of the glucokinase gene. *Diabetes.* 46:204-208.
31. Velho, G., Vaxillaire, M., Boccio, V., Charpentier, G., and Froguel, P. 1996. Diabetes complications in NIDDM kindreds linked to the MODY-3 locus on chromosome 12q. *Diabetes Care.* 19:915-919.

32. Hattersley, A.T., Beards, F., Ballantyne, E., Appleton, M., Harvey, R., and Ellard, S. 1998. Mutations in the glucokinase gene of the fetus result in reduced birth weight. *Nature Genet.* 19:268-270.
33. Velho, G., Hattersley, A.T., and Froguel, P. 2000. Maternal diabetes alters birth weight in glucokinase-deficient (MODY2) kindreds but has no influence on adult weight, height, insulin secretion or insulin sensitivity. *Diabetologia.* 43: (in press).
34. Hattersley, A.T., and Tooke, J.E. 1999. The fetal insulin hypothesis: an alternative explanation of the association of low birthweight with diabetes and vascular disease. *Lancet.* 353:1789-1792.
35. Jonsson, J., Carisson, L., Edlund, T., and Edlund, H. 1994. Insulin-promoter-factor 1 is required for pancreas development in mice. *Nature.* 371:606-609.
36. Naya, F.J., Huang, H.P., Qiu, Y.H., Mutoh, H., DeMayo, F.J., Leiter, A.B., and Tsai, M.J. 1997. Diabetes, defective pancreatic morphogenesis, and abnormal enteroendocrine differentiation in BETA2/NeuroD-deficient mice. *Gene. Develop.* 11:2323-2334.
37. Ahlgren, U., Jonsson, J., Jonsson, L., Simu, K., and Edlund, H. 1998. Beta-cell-specific inactivation of the mouse Ipf1/Pdx1 gene results in loss of the beta-cell phenotype and maturity onset diabetes. *Gene. Develop.* 12:1763-1768.
38. Boutin, P., Chèvre, J.C., Gomis, R., Pardini, V.C., Guillausseau, P.J., Velho, G., and Froguel, P. 1997. An automated fluorescent SSCP technique for screening for mutations the hepatocyte nuclear factor 1 alpha gene (MODY3). *Diabetes.* 46:2108-2109.
39. Glucksmann, M.A., et al. 1997. Novel mutations and a mutational hotspot in the MODY3 gene. *Diabetes.* 46:1081-1086.
40. Gragnoli, C., Lindner, T., Cockburn, B.N., Kaisaki, P.J., Gragnoli, F., Marozzi, G., and Bell, G.I. 1997. Maturity-onset diabetes of the young due to a mutation in the hepatocyte nuclear factor-4 alpha binding site in the promoter of the hepatocyte nuclear factor-1 alpha gene. *Diabetes.* 46:1648-1651.
41. Hansen, T., et al. 1997. Novel MODY3 mutations in the hepatocyte nuclear factor-1 alpha gene: Evidence for a hyperexcitability of pancreatic beta-cells to intravenous secretagogues in a glucose-tolerant carrier of a P447L mutation. *Diabetes.* 46:726-730.
42. Kaisaki, P.J., et al. 1997. Mutations in the hepatocyte nuclear factor-1 alpha gene in MODY and early-onset NIDDM: Evidence for a mutational hotspot in exon 4. *Diabetes.* 46:528-535.
43. Byrne, M.M., et al. 1996. Altered insulin secretory responses to glucose in diabetic and nondiabetic subjects with mutations in the diabetes mellitus susceptibility gene MODY on chromosome 12. *Diabetes.* 45:1503-1510.
44. Vaxillaire, M., Pueyo, M.E., Clément, K., Fiet, J., Timsit, J., Philippe, J., Robert, J.-J., Tappy, L., Froguel, P., and Velho, G. 1999. Insulin secretion and insulin sensitivity in diabetic and nondiabetic subjects with HNF-1α (MODY3) mutations. *Eur. J. Endocrinol.* 141:609-618.
45. Surmely, J.F., Guenat, E., Philippe, J., Dussoix, P., Schneiter, P., Temler, E., Vaxillaire, M., Froguel, P., Jequier, E., and Tappy, L. 1998. Glucose utilization and production in patients with maturity-onset diabetes of the young caused by a mutation of the hepatocyte nuclear factor-1 alpha gene. *Diabetes.* 47:1459-1463.
46. Isomaa, B., Henricsson, M., Lehto, M., Forsblom, C., Karanko, S., Sarelin, L., Haggblom, M., and Groop, L. 1998. Chronic diabetic complications in patients with MODY3 diabetes. *Diabetologia.* 41:467-473.
47. Menzel, R., Kaiasaki, P.J., Rjasanowski, I., Heinke, P., Kerner, W., and Menzel, S. 1998. A low renal threshold for glucose in diabetic patients with a mutation in the hepatocyte nuclear factor 1α (HNF-1α) gene. *Diabet. Med.* 15:816-820.
48. Velho, G., Benqué-Blanchet, F., Vaxillaire, M., Pontoglio, M., Froguel, P., Friedlander, G., and Prié, D. 1998. Renal proximal tubular defects associated to the MODY3 phenotype. (Abstract). *Diabetologia.* 41 (suppl.1):A108.

49. Pontoglio, M., Barra, J., Hadchouel, M., Doyen, A., Kress, C., Poggi Bach, J., Babinet, C., and Yaniv, M. 1996. Hepatocyte Nuclear Factor 1 inactivation results in hepatic dysfunction, phenylketonuria, and renal Fanconi syndrome. *Cell*. 84:572-585.
50. Pontoglio, M., et al. 1998. Defective insulin secretion in hepatocyte nuclear factor 1 alpha-deficient mice. *J. Clin. Invest.* 101:2215-2222.
51. Vaxillaire, M., Abderrahmani, A., Boutin, P., Bailleul, B., P., F., Yaniv, M., and Pontoglio, M. 1999. Anatomy of a homeoprotein revealed by the analysis of human MODY3 mutations. *J. Biol. Chem.* 274:35639-35646.
52. Dukes, I.D., et al. 1998. Defective pancreatic b-cell glycolytic signaling in Hepatocyte Nuclear Factor-1α-deficient mice. *J. Biol. Chem.* 273:24457-24464.
53. Wang, H., Maechier, P., Hagenfeldt, K.A., and Wollheim, C.B. 1998. Dominant-negative suppression of HNF-1α function results in defective insulin gene transcription and impaired metabolism-secretion coupling in a pancreatic β-cell line. *EMBO J.* 17:6701-6713.
54. Lindner, T., Gragnoli, C., Furuta, H., Cockburn, B.N., Petzold, C., Rietzsch, H., Weiss, U., Schulze, J., and Bell, G.I. 1997. Hepatic function in a family with a nonsense mutation (R154X) in the hepatocyte nuclear factor-4 alpha 1/MODY1 gene. *J. Clin. Invest.* 100:1400-1405.
55. Furuta, H., et al. 1997. Organization and partial sequence of the hepatocyte nuclear factor-4 alpha MODY1 gene and identification of a missense mutation, R127W, in a Japanese family with MODY. *Diabetes*. 46:1652-1657.
56. Bulman, M.P., Dronsfield, M.J., Frayling, T., Appleton, M., Bain, S.C., Ellard, S., and Hattersley, A.T. 1997. A missense mutation in the hepatocyte nuclear factor 4 alpha gene in a UK pedigree with maturity-onset diabetes of the young. *Diabetologia*. 40:859-862.
57. Fajans, S.S., Bell, G.I., Bowden, D.W., Halter, J.B., and Polonsky, K.S. 1994. Maturity-onset diabetes of the young. *Life Science*. 55:413-422.
58. Herman, W.H., Fajans, S.S., Ortiz, F.J., Smith, M.J., Sturis, J., Bell, G.I., Polonsky, K.S., and Halter, J.B. 1994. Abnormal insulin secretion, not insulin resistance, is the genetic or primary defect of MODY in the RW pedigree. *Diabetes*. 43:40-46.
59. Byrne, M.M., Sturis, J., Fajans, S.S., Ortiz, F.J., Stoltz, A., Stoffel, M., Smith, M.J., Bell, G.I., Halter, J.B., and Polonsky, K.S. 1995. Altered insulin secretory responses to glucose in subjects with a mutation in the MODY1 gene on chromosome 20. *Diabetes*. 44:699-704.
60. Hertz, R., Magenheim, J., Berman, I., and Bar-Tana, J. 1998. Fatty acyl-CoA thioesters are ligands of hepatic nuclear factor 4 alpha. *Nature*. 392:512-516.
61. Stoffel, M., and Duncan, S.A. 1997. The maturity-onset diabetes of the young (MODY1) transcription factor HNF4 alpha regulates expression of genes required for glucose transport and metabolism. *Proc. Natl. Acad. Sci. USA*. 94:13209-13214.
62. Nishigori, H., Yamada, S., Kohama, T., Tomura, H., Sho, K., Horikawa, Y., Bell, G.I., Takeuchi, T., and Takeda, J. 1998. Frameshift mutation, A263fsinsGG, in the hepatocyte nuclear factor-1 beta gene associated with diabetes and renal dysfunction. *Diabetes*. 47:1354-1355.
63. Tronche, F., and Yaniv, M. 1992. HNF1, a homeoprotein member of the hepatic transcription regulatory network. *Bioessays*. 14:579-587.
64. Permutt, M.A., Chiu, K.C., and Tanizawa, Y. 1992. Glucokinase and NIDDM: a candidate gene that paid off. *Diabetes*. 41:1367-1372.
65. Zouali, H., et al. 1993. Linkage analysis and molecular scanning of the glucokinase gene in NIDDM families. *Diabetes*. 42:1238-1245.
66. Stone, L.M., Kahn, S.E., Fujimoto, W.Y., Deeb, S.S., and Porte, D., Jr. 1996. A variant at position -30 of the ß-cell glucokinase gene promoter is associated with reduced ß-cell function in middle-aged Japanese-American men. *Diabetes*. 45:422-428.
67. Urhammer, S.A., Hansen, T., Clausen, J.O., Eiberg, H., and Pedersen, O. 1998. The g/a nucleotide variant at position -30 in the beta-cell-specific glucokinase gene promoter has no impact on the beta-cell function in Danish Caucasians. *Diabetes*. 47:1359-1361.

68. Boutin, P., Gresh, L., Cisse, A., Hara, M., Bell, G., Babu, S., Eisenbarth, G., and Froguel, P. 1999. Missense mutation Gly574Ser in the transcription factor HNF-1 alpha, is a marker of atypical diabetes mellitus in African-American children. *Diabetologia*. 42:380-381.
69. Iwasaki, N., et al. 1997. Mutations in the hepatocyte nuclear factor-1 alpha/MODY3 gene in Japanese subjects with early- and late-onset NIDDM. *Diabetes*. 46:1504-1508.
70. Urhammer, S.A., et al. 1997. Genetic variation in the hepatocyte nuclear factor-1 alpha gene in Danish Caucasians with late-onset NIDDM. *Diabetologia*. 40:473-475.
71. Hani, E.H., et al. 1998. A missense mutation in the Hepatocyte Nuclear Factor 4-Alpha, resulting in a reduced transactivational activity, in human late-onset non insulin-dependent diabetes mellitus. *J. Clin. Invest.* 101:521-526.
72. Hani, E.H., Stoffers, D.A., Chevre, J.C., Durand, E., Stanojevic, V., Dina, C., Habener, J.F., and Froguel, P. 1999. Defective mutations in the insulin promoter factor-1 (IPF-1) gene in late-onset type 2 diabetes mellitus. *J. Clin. Invest.* 104:R41-R48.
73. Macfarlane, W.M., et al. 1999. Missense mutations in the insulin promoter factor-1 gene predispose to type 2 diabetes. *J. Clin. Invest.* 104:R33-R39.
74. Waeber, G., et al. 2000. The gene MAPK8IP1, encoding islet-brain-1, is a candidate for type 2 diabetes. *Nature Genet.* 24:291-295.
75. Matschinsky, F.M., Glaser, B., and Magnuson, M.A. 1998. Pancreatic beta-cell glucokinase: Closing the gap between theoretical concepts and experimental realities. *Diabetes*. 47:307-315.
76. St-Onge, L., Wehr, P., and Gruss, P. 1999. Pancreas development and diabetes. *Curr. Opin. Genet. Develop.* 9:295-300.

6
GENETICS OF MITOCHONDRIA-RELATED FORMS OF SYNDROMIC DIABETES MELLITUS

Sabine Hofmann, Ph.D., Matthias F. Bauer, M.D.
and Klaus-Dieter Gerbitz, M.D.
Academic Hospital Munich-Schwabing, D-80804 Munich, Germany

INTRODUCTION

Mitochondria play a pivotal role in cellular metabolism and in energy production in particular. They generate cellular energy in the form of ATP by coupling the electron flux along the respiratory chain to the process of oxidative phosphorylation (OXPHOS). Depending on their energy demand, different cell types contain different amounts of mitochondria, ranging from only a few in the spermatozoon to several thousands in cells of skeletal muscle, heart and brain and, about 10^5 in oocytes. Defects in structures or functions of mitochondria, mainly affecting the OXPHOS system, have been shown to be involved in the pathogenesis of a variety of systemic or organ-specific manifestations (reviewed in (1)). In particular, organ systems with high energy requirements, such as the central nervous system, heart, skeletal muscle, kidney and the endocrine system are susceptible to mitochondrial dysfunction. Neurological defects such as psychomotor retardation, hypotonia or ataxia, myo- or cardiomyopathies, optic atrophy or sensorineural hearing loss are among the most frequent clinical symptoms observed in OXPHOS disorders. Because of their high metabolic activity, pancreatic β-cells are also highly sensitive to ATP-supply defects. Diabetes mellitus is, therefore, frequently observed as one symptom in patients with complex mitochondrial disorders, in particular in those carrying mitochondrial DNA (mtDNA) mutations.

Besides its role in energy production, the mitochondrial OXPHOS contributes two further aspects to the pathogenesis of diabetes mellitus. First, the generation of oxygen radicals along the mitochondrial respiratory chain has been suggested to contribute to the progression of neurodegenerative disorders and normal aging - a mechanism which is also used to explain selective damage of pancreatic β-cells in certain forms of diabetes (2). Secondly, apoptosis has been proposed as a mechanism of pancreatic β-cell death in autoimmune diabetes. As mitochondria play an important role in the initial steps of the programmed cell death, it was concluded that mitochondrial dysfunction is, at least, indirectly involved in β-cell loss (3).

In contrast to type 1 and type 2 diabetes mellitus, which are complex and polygenic disorders (see Chapter 1), syndromic forms of diabetes constitute a mixture of distinct, presumptively monogenic diseases. In most cases, the underlying genetic defect is unknown. One of the first diabetes syndromes which has been genetically characterized is so-called mitochondrial diabetes mellitus (MDM), which is caused by mutations of mitochondrial DNA (mtDNA). Since the first description of diabetes associated mtDNA alterations in 1992 (4-6), many reports have confirmed that mtDNA defects contribute significantly to the development of diabetes in different ethnic populations. In this review, we will summarize the current state of knowledge about mitochondrial diabetes mellitus and on the possible mechanisms leading to defective insulin secretion. We will also discuss some of the most recent findings in the field of nuclear-encoded forms of syndromic diabetes. The genetic and functional characterization of mitochondria-related syndromes such as Friedreich ataxia, Wolfram syndrome and Rogers syndrome has provided important insights into possible mechanisms contributing to the development of diabetes.

MITOCHONDRIAL GENETICS

Most cells contain hundreds to thousands of mitochondria. Mitochondria have a double membrane structure and possesses their own genome; both features are considered to reflect the endosymbiotic origin of this organelle. Although mitochondria encode their own translational apparatus, the mitochondria-specific transcription, translation and protein assembly systems are under control of the nucleus, as proteins such as mitochondrial DNA and RNA polymerases, ribosomal proteins, or transcription factors are encoded by the nuclear genome. The mitochondrial genome, fully sequenced in 1981 (7), is a circular and double stranded molecule, about 16.5 kb in length (Figure 1). The mammalian mtDNA retains only 13 polypeptide genes, all of which encode components of the OXPHOS cascade in the inner membrane. In addition, it also codes for two RNA species (12S and 16S rRNA) and the 22 tRNAs necessary for mitochondrial protein biosynthesis.

Mitochondria are transmitted through the oocyte's cytoplasm at fertilization. The mtDNA exhibits strict maternal inheritance as it is exclusively transmitted from a mother to her offspring (8). Due to its compact structure, its lack of histone protection, its insufficient repair mechanisms and its exposure to oxygen radicals generated along the respiratory chain, the mtDNA is vulnerable and demonstrates a high mutation rate which is about 10 to 20 that of nuclear DNA. When a mutation arises, the cell initially contains a mixture of normal and mutant mtDNA molecules, a state which is referred to as heteroplasmy. During meiotic or mitotic cytokinesis of a heteroplasmic cell, both normal and mutated types of mtDNA are divided unevenly into daughter cells. After repeated cell divisions, the cellular mtDNA population can shift toward predominantly mutant or wild-type (homoplasmy). This phenomenon is also named replicative segregation. As the percentage of mutant mtDNA increases, the energy output falls below a threshold level necessary for minimal cell function. Beyond this point, clinical symptoms appear.

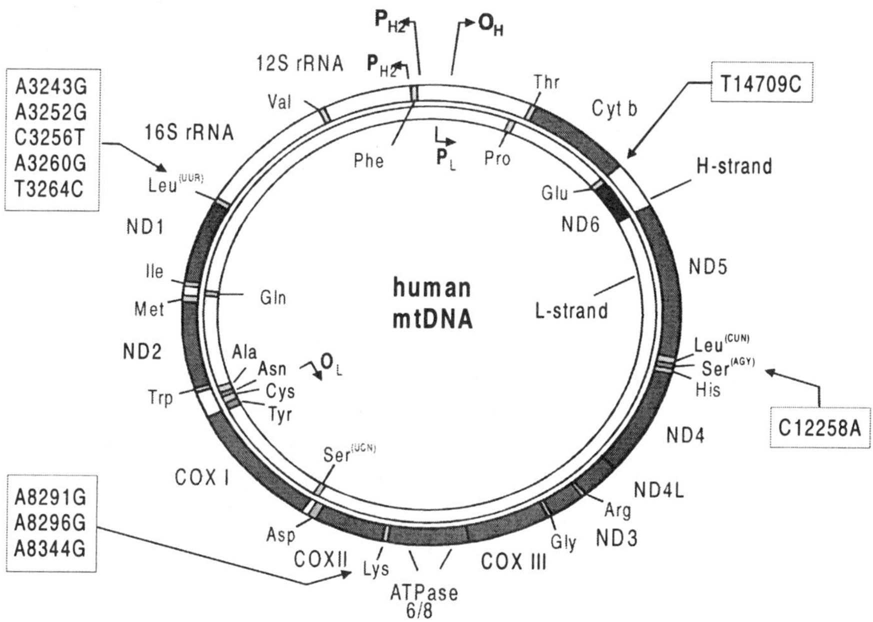

Figure 1. Map of human mitochondrial DNA. Positions of pathogenic point mutations that have been associated with diabetes mellitus are shown outside the circle. ND, NADH dehydrogenase genes; cytb, cytochrome b gene; COXI-III, cytochrome *c* oxidase subunits I-III genes; O_H and O_L, origin of replication of the heavy (H) and light (L) strand, respectively; P_{H1}, major promoter of the heavy strand; P_{H2}, minor promoter of the heavy strand; P_L, light strand promoter.

Maternally inherited mtDNA mutations range from neutral polymorphisms to severe or even lethal mutations (1). Neutral polymorphisms are often ancient and have accumulated along mtDNA lineages, therefore correlating with ethnic and geographic origins (9). Mildly deleterious mutations may not be expressed until late in life and are transmitted to the offspring. Thus, they may have arisen a long time ago and became fixed in the population as low-frequency polymorphisms. In contrast, severe mutations usually do not persist in the maternal lineage and will not be transmitted to the next generation. It is, therefore, widely accepted that deleterious mutations have evolved more recently.

To date, more than 50 point mutations in protein coding regions, tRNA or rRNA genes and over 100 length mutations including deletions, insertions or rearrangements of the mitochondrial genome have been associated with a mitochondrial disease phenotype (see updated version of MITOMAP, *www.gen.emory.edu/mitomap.html*). Not all of these mtDNA mutations will be inherited to the next generation. Somatic mutations which occur sporadically during the life-time of a single individual are not inheritable. Most of the somatic mutations of mtDNA are length mutations flanked by identical repeats. It seems likely that free radical damage is important for the occurrence of these mutations (10). There is an ongoing debate as to whether accumulation of somatic mutations during one's lifetime contributes to various degenerative disorders and to aging itself (11).

MITOCHONDRIAL FUNCTIONS

Energy production

In the mitochondrion, various metabolic pathways are bundled. These processes are, in particular, the carnitine-dependent transport of fatty acids and their β-oxidation, pyruvate carboxylation and decarboxylation, the Krebs-cycle, iron metabolism, the urea cycle, or parts of steroid and nitric oxide synthesis. Most of the catabolic pathways are interwoven and coupled to the energy-generating OXPHOS system. Reduction equivalents sequentially released during oxidation of carbon hydrates and fatty or amino acids are shuttled into the redox system of the respiratory chain (RC) thereby coupling substrate oxidation with the generation of a transmembrane proton motif force able to drive synthesis of ATP from ADP and inorganic phosphate (oxidative phosphorylation) (Figure 2).

The RC-OXPHOS system is located within the inner mitochondrial membrane and consists of five multisubunit enzyme complexes. Within the electron-conducting cascade of the respiratory chain, two complexes act as electron acceptors: (i) Complex I (NADH dehydrogenase) serves as an electron acceptor for several NADH producing reactions, and (ii) Complex II (succinate dehydrogenase) acquires electrons from succinate via $FADH_2$.

From both complexes, electrons are transferred to ubiquinone (Coenzyme Q, CoQ). In addition to Complex I and Complex II, two other redox pathways directly feed electrons to ubiquinone: flavoprotein (ETF), supplying electrons from the flavoprotein-linked step of fatty acid β-oxidation, and mitochondrial glycerophosphate dehydrogenase. Electrons are then transferred to cytochrome *c* via Complex III (cyt bc_1 complex) and, finally, to molecular oxygen by Complex IV (cytochrome *c* oxidase) to form H_2O. In Complex I, Complex III and IV electron transfer drives the translocation of protons from the matrix to the intermembrane space thereby generating an electrochemical gradient across the inner membrane (Figure 2). This gradient provides a proton-motif force which is used by the F_1F_0-ATP synthase (Complex V) to synthesize ATP. ATP constitutes the universally usable form of energy in all cellular compartments and is released from the mitochondrion via specialized carrier proteins, the so-called ATP/ADP translocators (ANT).

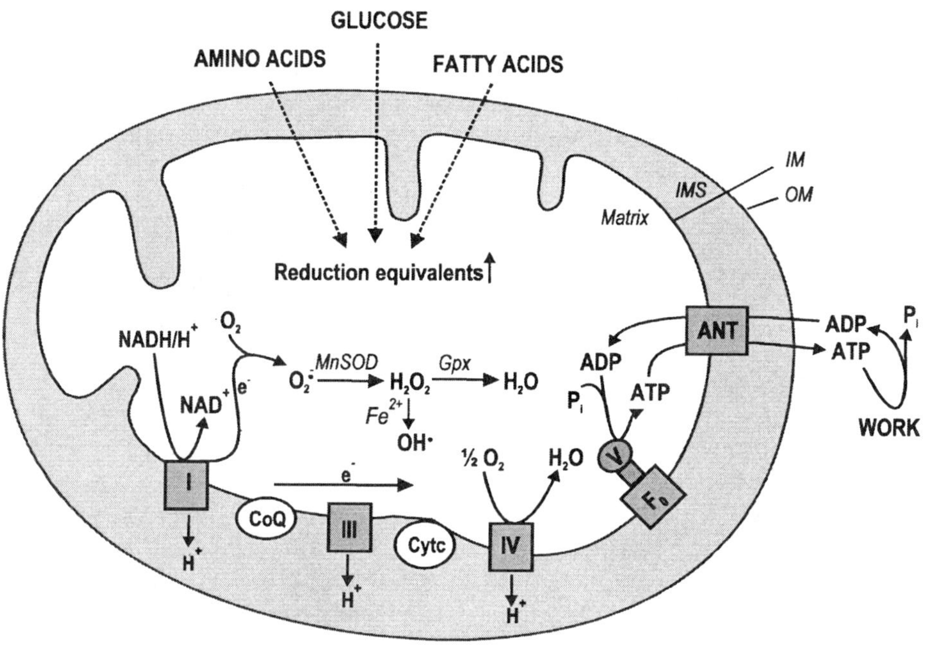

Figure 2. Diagram of a mitochondrion, showing the relationships between mitochondrial OXPHOS, ATP production and usage, and generation of reactive oxygen species (see text). OM, mitochondrial outer membrane; IM, mitochondrial inner membrane; IMS, intermembrane space.

Generation of reactive oxygen species

OXPHOS is the major endogeneous source of reactive oxygen species (ROS) (Figure 2). When electron transfer along the respiratory chain is inhibited, the excess electrons are donated directly to molecular oxygen to produce superoxide anion (O_2^{-}•). Most superoxide anions are detoxified by reduction to hydrogen peroxide (H_2O_2) inside and outside the mitochondria by the action of three different superoxide dismutases (SOD1, -2, -3). The detoxification product, H_2O_2, is reduced to water by the glutathione peroxidase (GPx), present in the cytosol and the mitochondrial matrix, as well as by the peroxisomal enzyme catalase. In the presence of transition metals like Cu^{2+} and Fe^{2+}, H_2O_2 can be converted via the *Fenton* reaction to the highly reactive and toxic hydroxyl radical OH•. Exposure to all three of the ROS species (O_2^-•, H_2O_2 and OH•) is known to affect the integrity of the mitochondrial genome and inhibits multiple cellular functions. While chronic exposure to ROS leads to damage of DNA (in particular mtDNA) (12), protein and lipids (13), the acute increase of ROS can inactivate the iron-sulfur (Fe-S) centers of RC-complexes I, II, and III, and the Krebs cycle aconitase, leading ultimately to breakdown of mitochondrial energy production (14). The imbalance between pro-oxidants and antioxidants would reduce the energy output from mitochondrial OXPHOS, thereby presumably impairing multiple cellular processes on the one hand and leading to increased oxidative stress on the other. As a consequence, these two processes - increased oxidative stress and decreased energy levels - might initiate endogenous mechanisms that induce activation of the mitochondrial permeability transition state as the initial step of apoptosis.

DIABETES MELLITUS CAUSED BY ALTERATIONS OF MtDNA

MtDNA mutations in diabetes mellitus

During the last decade, a large number of studies in different ethnic populations have emphasized the role of mtDNA mutations in the etiology of diabetes mellitus. The most commonly reported mtDNA point mutation associated with diabetes is an A/G exchange at nucleotide position (np) 3243 in the $tRNA^{Leu(UUR)}$ (Figure 1). This mutation was first identified as cause of the MELAS syndrome (mitochondrial encephalopathy with lactic acidosis and stroke like episodes) (15). In 1992, two independent publications found the np 3243 mutation in a large Dutch (5) and a British (4) family with diabetes and deafness. During the following years, an increasing number of reports confirmed the causative function of the np 3243 mutation in the development of diabetes mellitus (16-20). In nearly 70% of MDM, diabetes is found in combination with deafness (21), whereas the association with other neurological symptoms is less common. This subform of diabetes is, therefore, also referred to as "maternally inherited diabetes and deafness" (MIDD) (19).

In addition, less frequent independent mutations also have been described in association with diabetes (Figure 1). In particular, the $tRNA^{Leu(UUR)}$ gene seems to be an etiological hot spot. At least 11 disease-related $tRNA^{Leu(UUR)}$ mutations have been described (22), five of which were found to be associated with syndromic diabetes. A mutation at np 3260 was found in a patient with maternally inherited myopathy, cardiomyopathy and diabetes (23); a C/T exchange at np 3256 in a patient with a MERRF-like disease (myoclonic-epilepsy and ragged red fibers) plus diabetes (24); an A/G transition at np 3252 in a patient suffering from mitochondrial encephalomyopathy, pigmentary retinopathy, dementia, diabetes and hypothyroidism (25), a T/C exchange at np 3264 in a patient with diabetes, cerebellar ataxia, hearing loss and ophthalmoplegia (26) and the np 3243 mutation. Diabetes is rarely found in association with the so-called MERRF mutations at np 8344 (27), np 8291 (28) and at np 8296 (29) in the mitochondrial $tRNA^{Lys}$ gene. In Japanese populations, this latter mutation was found to account for 1% of diabetes cases. Recently, two new tRNA exchanges have been described, a T/C transition at np 14709 in the $tRNA^{Glu}$ gene in patients with diabetes and myopathy (30) and a C/A exchange in the $tRNA^{Ser}$ gene at np 12258 in association with diabetes, cerebellar ataxia, deafness and cataracts (31).

Length mutations of the mtDNA were first described in 1988 in patients suffering from mitochondrial myopathies, such as "chronic progressive external ophthalmoplegia" (CPEO) or the complete Kearns-Sayre syndrome (KSS) (32, 33). Endocrine dysfunction, for example diabetes mellitus, hypogonadism, or hypothyroidism, is found in a high degree of KSS or CPEO patients (34, 35). In 1992, Ballinger et al. (6) described a large pedigree with a maternally inherited syndrome of diabetes and deafness carrying a 10.4 kb mtDNA deletion. Further study of this family revealed the presence of more complex mtDNA rearrangements, namely duplications and deletion dimers, rather than single deletions (36, 37). The proportion of each type of rearranged mtDNA molecule seems to vary between different tissues, and there is evidence that the balance of mtDNA rearrangements may be crucial to this form of mitochondrial diabetes.

How common is MDM? We have recently summarized reported prevalence rates from different countries (38). The np 3243 mutation accounts for 0.5-1.5% of unselected diabetic patients, independently of whether they are classified as having type 1 or type 2 diabetes. In diabetic patients with a family history, the percentage of np 3243 carriers increases to 10%, and in a population with diabetes and deafness up to 60 %. The prevalence of MDM seems not to vary substantially among various countries and populations (39, 40). Taking into account a prevalence of diabetes of about 5% in the whole Western European or North American population, the frequency of MDM is, therefore, about 0.06 % in the general population.

The most intriguing question is, of course, the molecular mechanisms by which mtDNA mutations, in particular the tRNA mutation at np 3243, cause cellular dysfunction and disease? The current opinion is that mutations in tRNA genes cause mitochondrial dysfunction by affecting mitochondrial protein synthesis in a quantitative and/or qualitative way and, as a consequence, reduce the amount and/or quality of mtDNA encoded RC subunits. Most molecular analyses of the np 3243 mutation have been performed on cybrid cells, where the properties of wild-type versus mutant mtDNA can be compared on a nuclear "control background". Results from these studies show that the mutant tRNAs are functionally deficient due to a reduced amount and degree of aminoacylation (41). This "loss-of-function" hypothesis is supported by our recent *in vivo* study (42). In muscle biopsies from np 3243-carriers, an under-representation of the mutant $tRNA^{Leu(UUR)}$ relative to the wild-type $tRNA^{Leu(UUR)}$ among aminoacylated tRNAs was demonstrated, indicating a specific defect of the mutant molecule in stability and/or aminoacylation. In contrast, in studies in HeLa-cell cybrids or patient-derived tumor cell lines, aminoacylation of the mutant tRNA appears normal (43), as is the expression level of the mutant tRNA and the overall amount of mitochondrial protein biosynthesis (44). However, the mutant tRNA lacks the wobble-base U hypermodification that discriminates leucine UUR (R, purine) from phenylalanine UUY (Y, pyrimidine) codons (43). As a consequence, the np 3243 mutation may lead to a frequent misreading of phenylalanine and perhaps some other codons, thereby impairing mitochondrial biosynthesis via a "gain-of-function". Taken together, the specific primary effect of the np 3243 mutation on tRNA function and on mitochondrial biosynthesis is less than clear. As recently discussed (45), the different pictures emerging from cell culture and *in vivo* studies might reflect the diversity of molecular consequences of the np 3243 mutation in the human organism.

Phenotypic variability of MDM

The clinical phenotype of diabetic subjects harboring the np 3243 mutation is extremely heterogeneous ranging from diabetes only, both diabetes and deafness, to more complex multisystemic manifestations including the devastating MELAS syndrome. We recently summarized the clinical symptoms in 199 affected members of 45 families with diabetes and the np 3243 mutation (38): nearly 50% suffered from diabetes and deafness, 21% had only diabetes, 13% had diabetes combined with deafness and neurological symptoms (including MELAS) and 15% had deafness alone or in combination with neurological abnormalities. As the degree of heteroplasmy is known to differ considerably between different cell types, the severity and the type of the clinical outcome might be related to the proportion of mutant mtDNA in the respective tissues and organs (1). This is supported by a study of Otabe and co-workers (46) who found an enrichment of mutated mtDNA in pancreatic specimens from MDM patients compared to lymphoblast cells. The phenotypic heterogeneity, however, can not be simply explained by differences in dosage and tissue distribution of the mutant mtDNA. Thus, additional factors must be involved. As mentioned above, these could include the nuclear-genetic background, the mitochondrial haplotype or other epigenetic processes, all of which might modify the compensatory or secondary effects in a cell or an organism in response to a pathogenic tRNA mutation (45).

Possible pathophysiological mechanisms in MDM

MDM is a distinct disease entity that can be clearly distinguished from the idiopathic forms of diabetes by several characteristic features (38): MDM patients, compared to type 2 diabetes patients, have an earlier onset of disease (<40 years), are non-obese, are generally insulin-dependent, and not insulin resistant. Compared to type 1 diabetes, MDM patients do not develop ketosis, and show no signs of β-cell auto-antibodies.

Several pathophysiological mechanisms might contribute to hyperglycemia in MDM. An intact OXPHOS system is required for normal β-cell function as mitochondrial ATP production is an essential step in glucose signaling (47). Elevated glycolytic flux rates in response to a postprandial glucose load are indirectly coupled to mitochondrial oxidative metabolism and mitochondrial ATP production. When the ATP/ADP ratio increases, ATP-sensitive K^+ channels are closed and the subsequent membrane depolarization leads to an influx of Ca^{2+}, thereby inducing insulin release. The dependency of nutrient-stimulated insulin secretion on mitochondrial OXPHOS is supported by several lines of evidence (48): insulin secretion is inhibited by (i) blocking the respiration with cyanide, (ii) uncoupling of respiration from oxidative phosphorylation, (iii) inhibiting the ATP/ADP translocator, (iv) lowering mtDNA transcription, or (v) removing the mtDNA (ρ^0 cells). Whereas ρ^0 cells completely fail to secrete insulin in response to a glucose load, the effect of KCl on membrane depolarization and insulin exocytosis remains preserved (49). Thus, the loss of a functional respiratory chain in mtDNA-less ρ^0 cells specifically inhibits glucose-signaling steps but does not affect other β-cell functions such as insulin production or exocytosis. Consistent with these findings, measurements of the insulin secretory capacity of β-cells in np 3243 mutation carriers revealed a delayed and insufficient insulin and C-peptide response to a glucose-load (38, 50). In contrast, a normal secretory response was obtained with arginine (50). The insulinotrophic action of arginine is thought to be mediated by the intracellular accumulation of positively charged arginine and subsequent depolarization of the plasma membrane. Therefore, the arginine test is considered to discriminate glucose-sensing defects from insulin-production defect. Based on these results, Velho *et al.* (50) suggested a defect in metabolic coupling caused by the progressive reduction of OXPHOS capacity as a primary event in development of hyperglycemia in MDM.

Several studies suggested that the decreased insulin secretory capacity results from a selective and progressive β-cell loss (46, 51), rather than from a functional defect as suggested by Velho *et al.* (50). The most striking finding in autopsy pancreata from np 3243 carriers who had suffered from MELAS with or without diabetes (46) or from insulin-dependent diabetes alone (51) is the markedly reduced number of insulin-positive islet cells and, to a lesser extent, α-cells. No evidence for insulitis or for apoptotic processes could be detected. The molecular analysis revealed an enrichment in mutated mtDNA in islets compared to peripheral blood cells (46). As there was no clear-cut correlation between the amount of mutated mtDNA in pancreatic specimens and the clinical outcome or degree of islet cell reduction, other mechanisms might contribute to the phenotypic expression of the np 3243 mutation. Oxidative stress induced by prolonged exposure to hyperglycemia and increased ROS production as a result of impaired OXPHOS in MDM patients may accelerate the progression of diabetes (52). As mtDNA and mitochondrial enyzmes are sensitive targets for oxidative damage, there would be a further decline in mitochondrial functionality and, finally, destruction of the β-cell.

CONTRIBUTION OF MITOCHONDRIAL DYSFUNCTION TO NUCLEAR-ENCODED DIABETES SYNDROMES

Diabetes mellitus is a common phenotype found in a large number of syndromic diseases - the Online Mendelian Inheritance of Man (OMIM) lists over 40 disease entries when queried with "diabetes" and "syndrome". Each of these diabetic syndromes is likely to be caused by a distinct gene defect. Some show the characteristic clinical features typical for mitochondrial diseases and may, therefore, be caused by defects in mitochondrial proteins or at least in cellular factors influencing mitochondrial function. The disease gene identification in diabetes syndromes such as Wolfram syndrome, Friedreich ataxia and Rogers syndrome - all of them former "candidates" for mitochondria-related disorders - has now shed some light on the possible mechanisms resulting in neurodegeneration and diabetes. With the identification and characterization of the defective protein in Friedreich ataxia, it is now recognized to be a mitochondrial disorder. In Wolfram or Rogers syndrome, the defective protein appears not to be located in mitochondria but may influence mitochondrial functions.

Wolfram syndrome

Wolfram syndrome is a rare progressive neurodegenerative disorder described more than 60 years ago by Wolfram and Wagener (53). The acronym "DIDMOAD" summarizes the most frequent clinical findings: diabetes insipidus, diabetes mellitus, optic atrophy and deafness whereby diabetes mellitus and optic atrophy have been taken as the essential features. Additional but less frequent clinical phenotypes are renal tract and neurological abnormalities, disturbances of neuroendocrine systems and a relatively high incidence of depression and psychotic behavior. An insulin-dependent, non-autoimmune diabetes is usually the first symptom with a mean onset at the age of 6, followed by optic atrophy at the age of about 11 years (54). As most of the clinical phenotypes resemble those observed in other respiratory chain diseases, Wolfram syndrome was proposed to be a mitochondrial disorder (55). Consistent with this hypothesis, deletions in mtDNA and morphological mitochondrial abnormalities were reported in some sporadic and familial cases (56, 57).

In 1994, the Wolfram disease gene was mapped to the short arm of chromosome 4 (58). Using a candidate gene approach, we identified the nuclear gene defect in Wolfram syndrome (59). Eight out of twelve Wolfram patients revealed mutations on both alleles in a novel gene on chromosome 4p16, named wolframin (59) or WFR1 (60). The mutations included stop, frameshift and splice site mutations, suggesting loss-of-function mutations in this gene as the cause of Wolfram syndrome. The wolframin gene appears to be ubiquitously expressed in human tissues with highest steady-state levels in brain and pancreas (59). As wolframin mutations lead to degeneration of neuronal and neuroendocrine cells, wolframin might be involved in development or maintenance of neuroectoderm-derived tissues (60, 61). The polypeptide contains 890 amino acids and is predicted to be a transmembrane protein. The function of the novel protein remains to be elucidated. So far, no significant homology to published protein sequences has been found. In particular, no wolframin homologue has been identified in model organisms such as *S.cerevisiae* or *C.elegans*. It is unclear whether wolframin is a mitochondrial protein or whether absence of wolframin results in mitochondrial dysfunction. In Spanish families with Wolfram syndrome, mtDNA deletions were found to co-segregate with wolframin gene defects (62). It is unlikely that the wolframin protein interacts directly with the mitochondrial genome. Rather, the observed mtDNA fragmentation might be secondary to increased oxidative stress or increased sensitivity to oxidative stress, ultimately leading to death of neuronal and neuroendocrine cells.

Rogers syndrome

Rogers syndrome is an early-onset, autosomal-recessive disorder defined by the occurrence of diabetes mellitus, deafness and thiamine-responsive megaloblastic anemia (63) and is, therefore, also named TRMA. The disorder represents a novel form of childhood non-type 1 diabetes mellitus. No anti-insulin or anti-islet antibodies could be detected in Rogers Syndrome patients. The treatment with pharmacological doses of thiamine improves hematological and endocrine dysfunction and, at least, prevents further progression of neurological symptoms. These data suggested an involvement of the TRMA disease gene in thiamine metabolism. Upon uptake of thiamine from the gut and transport into tissues and cells, thiamine is normally converted to thiamine pyrophosphate (TPP) by thiamine pyrophosphokinase (TPK). TPP then binds in the form of a cofactor to four enzymes: transketolase, pyruvate dehydrogenase, α-ketoglutarate dehydrogenase and branched-chain keto-acid dehydrogenase, the latter three are located in mitochondria. It is therefore possible that the mitochondrial disease-like phenotype of TRMA is associated with secondary abnormalities in thiamine-dependent mitochondrial enzyme complexes. The TRMA locus has been mapped to chromosome 1q23.3 (64). Observations made in patient-derived fibroblasts suggested that a defective high-affinity thiamine transporter is responsible for the clinical features in TRMA (65). Three independent studies identified loss-of-functions mutations in a novel gene (SLC19A2) encoding a functional thiamine transporter (66-68). Considering the predicted absence of SLC19A2 in TRMA patients, Fleming et al. (66) speculated that a secondary thiamine transport process allows sufficient thiamine uptake to prevent the metabolic condition of severe thiamine deficiency, beriberi.

Friedreich Ataxia

Friedreich ataxia (FA) is an autosomal recessive disorder with an estimated prevalence of 1:50,000 and a deduced carrier frequency of 1:120 in European populations, making it the most commonly inherited form of ataxia. Clinically, FA is a complex neurological disorder characterized by unsteady gait, limp areflexia, muscle weakness and hypertrophic cardiomyopathy (69). Patients suffering from FA often develop blindness, deafness and/or diabetes; glucose intolerance or diabetes mellitus is diagnosed in about 20% of cases. Genetically, FA belongs to a class of neurodegenerative disorders caused by unstable trinucleotide-repeats. In FA, hyper-expansive GAA repeats occur in the first intron of the disease gene, FRDA1 (70). In healthy subjects, the number of GAA repeats is less than 39. If the GAA expansion exceeds a critical threshold length (>66 repeats), FRDA expression is inhibited at the level of gene transcription resulting in decreased protein levels. The severity of the disease correlates with the length of the expanded GAA repeat. In some FA cases, elongation of up to 1700 repeat units has been found. The vast majority of FA patients (about 95%) are homozygous for the GAA repeat expansion and the remaining 5% are compound heterozygotes for the expansion and an additional point mutation in the FRDA1 gene.

The function of the encoded 210 amino acid protein, named frataxin, is not completely resolved. Based on its homology to a protein characterized in the model organism *S.cerevisiae*, a putative function of frataxin in cellular iron metabolism has been proposed (reviewed in (71)). The yeast frataxin homologue encoded by the *YFH1* gene is a mitochondrial protein. *YFH1* deletion strains exhibit a "petite" phenotype, i.e. they are unable to grow on nonfermentable carbon sources, grow poorly on fermentable carbon sources and are respiration deficient (72, 73). Furthermore, cells lacking the *YFH1* gene exhibit constitutive activity of the high affinity iron-uptake system, resulting in diminished levels of iron in cytosol and an ~10-fold increase in intramitochondrial iron levels (74). *YFH1* deletion strains are highly sensitive to oxidative stress, indicating that the accumulation of iron within mitochondria leads to formation of reactive oxygen radicals (ROS) via the iron-catalyzed *Fenton* reaction and subsequently to mitochondrial DNA damage, thus further impairing mitochondrial OXPHOS (74). The exact mechanism leading to mitochondrial iron accumulation is not clear; however, a role of YFH1P in efflux of iron from the mitochondria has been suggested (75).

Analogously to what is known from yeast studies, the human frataxin might be required for mitochondrial iron homeostasis, and FA might result from oxidative damage secondary to mitochondrial iron overload (Figure 3). Indeed, accumulation of iron has been observed in cardiac muscles from FA

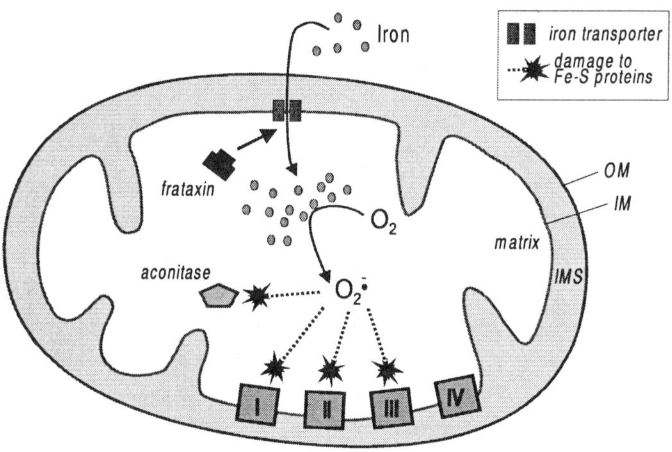

Figure 3. Model of mitochondrial dysfunction in FA patients as proposed by Rötig *et al.* (76). Frataxin regulates the mitochondrial iron transport system. Deficiency of frataxin in FA patients results in accumulation of iron within the mitochondrion. Iron-induced oxidative stress primarily destroys Fe-S clusters of mitochondrial respiratory chain enzyme complexes I, II and III and of the Krebs cycle enzyme aconitase thereby leading to a decline in mitochondrial energy output.

patients indicating similar functions of yeast YFH1P and human frataxin. Moreover, FA patients have a deficiency of iron-sulphur (Fe-S) cluster-containing subunits of the mitochondrial respiratory chain complexes I, II and III and of the Krebs cycle enzyme aconitase (76). The specific deficiency of iron proteins is thought to be related to mitochondrial iron accumulation (Figure 3), since Fe-S enzymes are known to be extremely sensitive to superoxide which is capable of attacking and destroying Fe-S clusters (71). As mutations in two other yeast proteins, the heat shock protein, Ssq1, and the cysteine desulphurase, Nfs1p, also result in massive intramitochondrial iron accumulation (personal communication, G. Kispal), the discovery of further neurodegenerative diseases with abnormal mitochondrial iron balance seems likely in the near future.

REFERENCES

1. Wallace, D.C. 1994. Mitochondrial DNA sequence variation in human evolution and disease. *Proc Natl Acad Sci U S A*. 91:8739-46.
2. Esposito, L.A., S. Melov, A. Panov, B.A. Cottrell, and D.C. Wallace. 1999. Mitochondrial disease in mouse results in increased oxidative stress. *Proc Natl Acad Sci U S A*. 96:4820-5.
3. Rabinovitch, A., W. Suarez-Pinzon, K. Strynadka, Q. Ju, D. Edelstein, M. Brownlee, G.S. Korbutt, and R.V. Rajotte. 1999. Transfection of human pancreatic islets with an anti-apoptotic gene (bcl-2) protects beta-cells from cytokine-induced destruction. *Diabetes*. 48:1223-9.
4. Reardon, W., R.J. Ross, M.G. Sweeney, L.M. Luxon, M.E. Pembrey, A.E. Harding, and R.C. Trembath. 1992. Diabetes mellitus associated with a pathogenic point mutation in mitochondrial DNA. *Lancet*. 340:1376-9.
5. van den Ouweland, J.M., H.H. Lemkes, W. Ruitenbeek, L.A. Sandkuijl, M.F. de Vijlder, P.A. Struyvenberg, J.J. van de Kamp, and J.A. Maassen. 1992. Mutation in mitochondrial tRNA(Leu)(UUR) gene in a large pedigree with maternally transmitted type II diabetes mellitus and deafness. *Nat Genet*. 1:368-71.
6. Ballinger, S.W., J.M. Shoffner, E.V. Hedaya, I. Trounce, M.A. Polak, D.A. Koontz, and D.C. Wallace. 1992. Maternally transmitted diabetes and deafness associated with a 10.4 kb mitochondrial DNA deletion. *Nat Genet*. 1:11-5.
7. Anderson, S., A.T. Bankier, B.G. Barrell, M.H. de Bruijn, A.R. Coulson, J. Drouin, I.C. Eperon, D.P. Nierlich, B.A. Roe, F. Sanger, P.H. Schreier, A.J. Smith, R. Staden, and I.G. Young. 1981. Sequence and organization of the human mitochondrial genome. *Nature*. 290:457-65.
8. Giles, R.E., H. Blanc, H.M. Cann, and D.C. Wallace. 1980. Maternal inheritance of human mitochondrial DNA. *Proc Natl Acad Sci U S A*. 77:6715-9.
9. Hofmann, S., M. Jaksch, R. Bezold, S. Mertens, S. Aholt, A. Paprotta, and K.D. Gerbitz. 1997. Population genetics and disease susceptibility: characterization of central European haplogroups by mtDNA gene mutations, correlation with D loop variants and association with disease. *Hum Mol Genet*. 6:1835-46.
10. Ames, B.N., M.K. Shigenaga, and T.M. Hagen. 1993. Oxidants, antioxidants, and the degenerative diseases of aging. *Proc Natl Acad Sci U S A*. 90:7915-22.
11. Lightowlers, R.N., H.T. Jacobs, and O.A. Kajander. 1999. Mitochondrial DNA--all things bad? *Trends Genet*. 15:91-3.
12. Ozawa, T. 1997. Oxidative damage and fragmentation of mitochondrial DNA in cellular apoptosis. *Biosci Rep*. 17:237-50.
13. Papa, S., and V.P. Skulachev. 1997. Reactive oxygen species, mitochondria, apoptosis and aging. *Mol Cell Biochem*. 174:305-19.
14. Wallace, D.C. 1999. Mitochondrial Diseases in Man and Mouse. *Science*. 283:1482-1488.
15. Goto, Y., I. Nonaka, and S. Horai. 1990. A mutation in the tRNA(Leu)(UUR) gene associated with the MELAS subgroup of mitochondrial encephalomyopathies. *Nature*. 348:651-3.
16. Gerbitz, K.D., A. Paprotta, M. Jaksch, S. Zierz, and J. Drechsel. 1993. Diabetes mellitus is one of the heterogeneous phenotypic features of a mitochondrial DNA point mutation within the tRNALeu(UUR) gene. *FEBS Lett*. 321:194-6.
17. Alcolado, J.C. 1993. Mitochondrial DNA defects in diabetes mellitus. *Diabetologia*. 36:578-9.

18. Vionnet, N., P. Passa, and P. Froguel. 1993. Prevalence of mitochondrial gene mutations in families with diabetes mellitus. *Lancet*. 342:1429-30.

19. van den Ouweland, J.M., H.H. Lemkes, R.C. Trembath, R. Ross, G. Velho, D. Cohen, P. Froguel, and J.A. Maassen. 1994. Maternally inherited diabetes and deafness is a distinct subtype of diabetes and associates with a single point mutation in the mitochondrial tRNA(Leu(UUR)) gene. *Diabetes*. 43:746-51.

20. Kadowaki, T., H. Kadowaki, Y. Mori, K. Tobe, R. Sakuta, Y. Suzuki, Y. Tanabe, H. Sakura, T. Awata, Y. Goto, and et al. 1994. A subtype of diabetes mellitus associated with a mutation of mitochondrial DNA. *N Engl J Med*. 330:962-8.

21. van den Ouweland, J.M., H.H. Lemkes, K.D. Gerbitz, and J.A. Maassen. 1995. Maternally inherited diabetes and deafness (MIDD): a distinct subtype of diabetes associated with a mitochondrial tRNA(Leu)(UUR) gene point mutation. *Muscle Nerve*. 3:S124-30.

22. Moraes, C.T., F. Ciacci, E. Bonilla, C. Jansen, M. Hirano, N. Rao, R.E. Lovelace, L.P. Rowland, E.A. Schon, and S. DiMauro. 1993. Two novel pathogenic mitochondrial DNA mutations affecting organelle number and protein synthesis. Is the tRNA(Leu(UUR)) gene an etiologic hot spot? *J Clin Invest*. 92:2906-15.

23. Zeviani, M., C. Gellera, C. Antozzi, M. Rimoldi, L. Morandi, F. Villani, V. Tiranti, and S. DiDonato. 1991. Maternally inherited myopathy and cardiomyopathy: association with mutation in mitochondrial DNA tRNA(Leu)(UUR). *Lancet*. 338:143-7.

24. Sano, M., M. Ozawa, S. Shiota, Y. Momose, M. Uchigata, and Y. Goto. 1996. The T-C(8356) mitochondrial DNA mutation in a Japanese family. *J Neurol*. 243:441-4.

25. Morten, K.J., J.M. Cooper, G.K. Brown, B.D. Lake, D. Pike, and J. Poulton. 1993. A new point mutation associated with mitochondrial encephalomyopathy. *Hum Mol Genet*. 2:2081-7.

26. Suzuki, Y., S. Suzuki, Y. Hinokio, M. Chiba, Y. Atsumi, K. Hosokawa, A. Shimada, T. Asahina, and K. Matsuoka. 1997. Diabetes associated with a novel 3264 mitochondrial tRNA(Leu)(UUR) mutation. *Diabetes Care*. 20:1138-40.

27. Shoffner, J.M., M.T. Lott, A.M. Lezza, P. Seibel, S.W. Ballinger, and D.C. Wallace. 1990. Myoclonic epilepsy and ragged-red fiber disease (MERRF) is associated with a mitochondrial DNA tRNA(Lys) mutation. *Cell*. 61:931-7.

28. Hirata, K., M. Nakagawa, I. Higuchi, K. Hashimoto, K. Hanada, K. Takahashi, T. Niiyama, K. Izumi, S. Sakoda, H. Yamada, and M. Osame. 1999. Adult onset limb-girdle type mitochondrial myopathy with a mitochondrial DNA np8291 A-to-G substitution. *J Hum Genet*. 44:210-4.

29. Kameoka, K., H. Isotani, K. Tanaka, K. Azukari, Y. Fujimura, Y. Shiota, E. Sasaki, M. Majima, K. Furukawa, S. Haginomori, H. Kitaoka, and N. Ohsawa. 1998. Novel mitochondrial DNA mutation in tRNA(Lys) (8296A-->G) associated with diabetes. *Biochem Biophys Res Commun*. 245:523-7.

30. Hao, H., E. Bonilla, G. Manfredi, S. DiMauro, and C.T. Moraes. 1995. Segregation patterns of a novel mutation in the mitochondrial tRNA glutamic acid gene associated with myopathy and diabetes mellitus. *Am J Hum Genet*. 56:1017-25.

31. Lynn, S., T. Wardell, M.A. Johnson, P.F. Chinnery, M.E. Daly, M. Walker, and D.M. Turnbull. 1998. Mitochondrial diabetes: investigation and identification of a novel mutation. *Diabetes*. 47:1800-2.

32. Holt, I.J., J.M. Cooper, J.A. Morgan-Hughes, and A.E. Harding. 1988. Deletions of muscle mitochondrial DNA [letter]. *Lancet*. 1:1462.

33. Lestienne, P., and G. Ponsot. 1988. Kearns-Sayre syndrome with muscle mitochondrial DNA deletion. *Lancet*. 1:885.

34. Tanabe, Y., S. Miyamoto, Y. Kinoshita, K. Yamada, N. Sasaki, E. Makino, and H. Nakajima. 1988. Diabetes mellitus in Kearns-Sayre syndrome. *Eur Neurol*. 28:34-8.

35. Quade, A., S. Zierz, and D. Klingmuller. 1992. Endocrine abnormalities in mitochondrial myopathy with external ophthalmoplegia. *Clin Investig*. 70:396-402.

36. Dunbar, D.R., P.A. Moonie, R.J. Swingler, D. Davidson, R. Roberts, and I.J. Holt. 1993. Maternally transmitted partial direct tandem duplication of mitochondrial DNA associated with diabetes mellitus. *Hum Mol Genet*. 2:1619-24.

37. Poulton, J., and I.J. Holt. 1994. Mitochondrial DNA: does more lead to less? *Nat Genet*. 8:313-5.

38. Gerbitz, K.D., J.M. van den Ouweland, J.A. Maassen, and M. Jaksch. 1995. Mitochondrial diabetes mellitus: a review. *Biochim Biophys Acta*. 1271:253-60.

39. Maassen, J.A., and T. Kadowaki. 1996. Maternally inherited diabetes and deafness: a new diabetes subtype. *Diabetologia*. 39:375-82.

40. Tsukuda, K., Y. Suzuki, K. Kameoka, N. Osawa, Y. Goto, H. Katagiri, T. Asano, Y. Yazaki, and Y. Oka. 1997. Screening of patients with maternally transmitted diabetes for mitochondrial gene mutations in the tRNA[Leu(UUR)] region. *Diabet Med*. 14:1032-7.

41. Janssen, G.M., J.A. Maassen, and J.M. van Den Ouweland. 1999. The diabetes-associated 3243 mutation in the mitochondrial tRNA(Leu(UUR)) gene causes severe mitochondrial dysfunction without a strong decrease in protein synthesis rate. *J Biol Chem*. 274:29744-8.

42. Borner, G.V., M. Zeviani, V. Tiranti, F. Carrara, S. Hoffmann, K.D. Gerbitz, H. Lochmuller, D. Pongratz, T. Klopstock, A. Melberg, E. Holme, and S. Paabo. 2000. Decreased aminoacylation of mutant tRNAs in MELAS but not in MERRF patients. *Hum Mol Genet*. 9:467-75.

43. Yasukawa, T., T. Suzuki, T. Ueda, S. Ohta, and K. Watanabe. 2000. Modification defect at anticodon wobble nucleotide of mitochondrial tRNAs(Leu)(UUR) with pathogenic mutations of mitochondrial myopathy, encephalopathy, lactic acidosis, and stroke-like episodes. *J Biol Chem*. 275:4251-7.

44. Flierl, A., H. Reichmann, and P. Seibel. 1997. Pathophysiology of the MELAS 3243 transition mutation. *J Biol Chem*. 272:27189-96.

45. Jacobs, H.T., and I.J. Holt. 2000. The np 3243 MELAS mutation: damned if you aminoacylate, damned if you don't. *Hum Mol Genet*. 9:463-5.

46. Otabe, S., K. Yasuda, Y. Mori, K. Shimokawa, H. Kadowaki, A. Jimi, K. Nonaka, Y. Akanuma, Y. Yazaki, and T. Kadowaki. 1999. Molecular and histological evaluation of pancreata from patients with a mitochondrial gene mutation associated with impaired insulin secretion. *Biochem Biophys Res Commun*. 259:149-156.

47. Wollheim, C.B. 2000. Beta-cell mitochondria in the regulation of insulin secretion: a new culprit in Type II diabetes. *Diabetologia*. 43:265-277.

48. Kagawa, Y., S.H. Cha, K. Hasegawa, T. Hamamoto, and H. Endo. 1999. Regulation of energy metabolism in human cells in aging and diabetes: FoF(1), mtDNA, UCP, and ROS. *Biochem Biophys Res Commun*. 266:662-76.

49. Kennedy, E.D., P. Maechler, and C.B. Wollheim. 1998. Effects of depletion of mitochondrial DNA in metabolism secretion coupling in INS-1 cells. *Diabetes*. 47:374-80.

50. Velho, G., M.M. Byrne, K. Clement, J. Sturis, M.E. Pueyo, H. Blanche, N. Vionnet, J. Fiet, P. Passa, J.J. Robert, K.S. Polonsky, and P. Froguel. 1996. Clinical phenotypes, insulin secretion, and insulin sensitivity in kindreds with maternally inherited diabetes and deafness due to mitochondrial tRNALeu(UUR) gene mutation. *Diabetes*. 45:478-87.

51. Kobayashi, T., K. Nakanishi, H. Nakase, H. Kajio, M. Okubo, T. Murase, and K. Kosaka. 1997. In situ characterization of islets in diabetes with a mitochondrial DNA mutation at nucleotide position 3243. *Diabetes*. 46:1567-71.

52. Gerbitz, K.D. 1992. Does the mitochondrial DNA play a role in the pathogenesis of diabetes? [see comments]. *Diabetologia*. 35:1181-6.

53. Wolfram, D.J., and H.P. Wagener. 1938. Diabetes mellitus and simple optic atrophy among siblings: report of four cases. *Mayo Clin. Proc.* 13:715-718.

54. Barrett, T.G., S.E. Bundey, and A.F. Macleod. 1995. Neurodegeneration and diabetes: UK nationwide study of Wolfram (DIDMOAD) syndrome. *Lancet*. 346:1458-63.
55. Bu, X., and J.I. Rotter. 1993. Wolfram syndrome: a mitochondrial-mediated disorder? *Lancet*. 342:598-600.
56. Rotig, A., V. Cormier, P. Chatelain, R. Francois, J.M. Saudubray, P. Rustin, and A. Munnich. 1993. Deletion of mitochondrial DNA in a case of early-onset diabetes mellitus, optic atrophy and deafness (DIDMOAD, Wolfram syndrome). *J Inherit Metab Dis*. 16:527-30.
57. Bundey, S., K. Poulton, H. Whitwell, E. Curtis, I.A. Brown, and A.R. Fielder. 1992. Mitochondrial abnormalities in the DIDMOAD syndrome. *J Inherit Metab Dis*. 15:315-9.
58. Polymeropoulos, M.H., R.G. Swift, and M. Swift. 1994. Linkage of the gene for Wolfram syndrome to markers on the short arm of chromosome 4. *Nat Genet*. 8:95-7.
59. Strom, T.M., K. Hortnagel, S. Hofmann, F. Gekeler, C. Scharfe, W. Rabl, K.D. Gerbitz, and T. Meitinger. 1998. Diabetes insipidus, diabetes mellitus, optic atrophy and deafness (DIDMOAD) caused by mutations in a novel gene (wolframin) coding for a predicted transmembrane protein. *Hum Mol Genet*. 7:2021-8.
60. Inoue, H., Y. Tanizawa, J. Wasson, P. Behn, K. Kalidas, E. Bernal-Mizrachi, M. Mueckler, H. Marshall, H. Donis-Keller, P. Crock, D. Rogers, M. Mikuni, H. Kumashiro, K. Higashi, G. Sobue, Y. Oka, and M.A. Permutt. 1998. A gene encoding a transmembrane protein is mutated in patients with diabetes mellitus and optic atrophy (Wolfram syndrome). *Nat Genet*. 20:143-8.
61. Garcia-Luna, P.P., E. Villechenous, A. Leal-Cerro, S. Duran, S. Jorge, I. Wichmann, A. Nunez-Roldan, and R. Astorga. 1988. Contrasting features of insulin dependent diabetes mellitus associated with neuroectodermal defects and classical insulin dependent diabetes mellitus. *Acta Paediatr Scand*. 77:413-8.
62. Barrientos, A., V. Volpini, J. Casademont, D. Genis, J.M. Manzanares, I. Ferrer, J. Corral, F. Cardellach, A. Urbano-Marquez, X. Estivill, and V. Nunes. 1996. A nuclear defect in the 4p16 region predisposes to multiple mitochondrial DNA deletions in families with Wolfram syndrome. *J Clin Invest*. 97:1570-6.
63. Rogers, L.E., F.S. Porter, and J.B. Sidbury. 1969. Thiamine-responsive megaloblastic anemia. *J. Pediatr*. 74:494-504.
64. Neufeld, E.J., H. Mandel, T. Raz, R. Szargel, C.N. Yandava, A. Stagg, S. Faure, T. Barrett, N. Buist, and N. Cohen. 1997. Localization of the gene for thiamine-responsive megaloblastic anemia syndrome, on the long arm of chromosome 1, by homozygosity mapping. *Am J Hum Genet*. 61:1335-41.
65. Stagg, A.R., J.C. Fleming, M.A. Baker, M. Sakamoto, N. Cohen, and E.J. Neufeld. 1999. Defective high-affinity thiamine transporter leads to cell death in thiamine-responsive megaloblastic anemia syndrome fibroblasts. *J Clin Invest*. 103:723-9.
66. Fleming, J.C., E. Tartaglini, M.P. Steinkamp, D.F. Schorderet, N. Cohen, and E.J. Neufeld. 1999. The gene mutated in thiamine-responsive anaemia with diabetes and deafness (TRMA) encodes a functional thiamine transporter. *Nat Genet*. 22:305-8.
67. Labay, V., T. Raz, D. Baron, H. Mandel, H. Williams, T. Barrett, R. Szargel, L. McDonald, A. Shalata, K. Nosaka, S. Gregory, and N. Cohen. 1999. Mutations in SLC19A2 cause thiamine-responsive megaloblastic anaemia associated with diabetes mellitus and deafness. *Nat Genet*. 22:300-4.
68. Diaz, G.A., M. Banikazemi, K. Oishi, R.J. Desnick, and B.D. Gelb. 1999. Mutations in a new gene encoding a thiamine transporter cause thiamine-responsive megaloblastic anaemia syndrome. *Nat Genet*. 22:309-12.
69. Durr, A., M. Cossee, Y. Agid, V. Campuzano, C. Mignard, C. Penet, J.L. Mandel, A. Brice, and M. Koenig. 1996. Clinical and genetic abnormalities in patients with Friedreich's ataxia. *N Engl J Med*. 335:1169-75.

70. Campuzano, V., L. Montermini, M.D. Molto, L. Pianese, M. Cossee, F. Cavalcanti, E. Monros, F. Rodius, F. Duclos, A. Monticelli, and et al. 1996. Friedreich's ataxia: autosomal recessive disease caused by an intronic GAA triplet repeat expansion. *Science*. 271:1423-7.

71. Knight, S.A., R. Kim, D. Pain, and A. Dancis. 1999. The yeast connection to Friedreich ataxia. *Am J Hum Genet*. 64:365-71.

72. Koutnikova, H., V. Campuzano, F. Foury, P. Dolle, O. Cazzalini, and M. Koenig. 1997. Studies of human, mouse and yeast homologues indicate a mitochondrial function for frataxin. *Nat Genet*. 16:345-51.

73. Wilson, R.B., and D.M. Roof. 1997. Respiratory deficiency due to loss of mitochondrial DNA in yeast lacking the frataxin homologue. *Nat Genet*. 16:352-7.

74. Babcock, M., D. de Silva, R. Oaks, S. Davis-Kaplan, S. Jiralerspong, L. Montermini, M. Pandolfo, and J. Kaplan. 1997. Regulation of mitochondrial iron accumulation by Yfh1p, a putative homolog of frataxin. *Science*. 276:1709-12.

relevance to human disease. *Trends Biochem Sci*. 23:135-8.

76. Rotig, A., P. de Lonlay, D. Chretien, F. Foury, M. Koenig, D. Sidi, A. Munnich, and P. Rustin. 1997. Aconitase and mitochondrial iron-sulphur protein deficiency in Friedreich ataxia. *Nat Genet*. 17:215-7.

7
REGULATION OF INSULIN SECRETION IN VIVO

Josep Vidal and Steven E. Kahn
University of Washington and VA Puget Sound Health Care System, Seattle, WA 98108 USA

INTRODUCTION

Disruption of the normal relationship between ß-cell function and insulin sensitivity is central to the pathogenesis of hyperglycemia in type 2 diabetes. Normal glucose regulation is dependent on a closed feedback loop relationship among the liver, peripheral tissues (primarily muscle) and pancreatic islet cells (1). In individuals with normal islet function, the pancreatic islet ß-cell adapts to reductions in insulin sensitivity in the hepatic and peripheral tissues by increasing insulin secretion and thereby prevents the development of fasting hyperglycemia. However, in type 2 diabetes, fasting hyperglycemia occurs when impaired islet ß-cell function results in an underproduction of insulin relative to the prevailing insulin sensitivity (1). This chapter aims to provide the basis for the understanding of ß-cell function measurements *in vivo* in as much as this can be useful in unraveling the genetic basis of type 2 diabetes.

BASIS OF SYNTHESIS AND RELEASE OF ß-CELL SECRETORY PRODUCTS

The pancreatic islet comprises a group of cells that synthesize and release a number of different hormones. The classical ones are insulin from the ß-cell, glucagon from the α-cell, somatostatin from the ∂-cell, and the more recently recognized islet amyloid polypeptide (IAPP, also known as amylin), which is also a secretory product of the ß-cell. The hormonal secretory activity of the islet is the net result of a complex interaction among the different cell types, with insulin secretion having been most extensively studied as a marker of islet function. In order to understand the basis for normal and abnormal islet function, it is important to briefly review the normal physiology of the biosynthetic and secretory systems operating in the ß-cell.

Glucose Metabolism in the ß-cell

ß-cell regulation of plasma glucose in a narrow range is dependent in large part on the ability of the ß-cell to take up and metabolize glucose (Figure 1) (2, 3). Glucose is transported into the ß-cell via the GLUT-2 glucose transporter and is then phosphorylated by the enzyme glucokinase. By virtue of glucokinase's unique properties, phosphorylation is considered to be a crucial step in ß-cell glucose metabolism, with glucokinase being considered as the ß-cell glucosensor (3). Following its phosphorylation, the ß-cell enzymatic machinery metabolizes glucose in the oxidative pathway, resulting in the net generation of ATP in the mitochondria (4). An increase in the ATP/ADP ratio results in closure of the ATP-dependent potassium channel (K_{ATP}), a complex composed by a pore-forming protein (Kir6.2) and a sulfonylurea receptor protein (SUR1) (5). Closure of the K_{ATP} channel complex results in plasma membrane depolarization and opening of the voltage-dependent-L-type calcium channels, which allows extracellular calcium to enter the intracellular pool of free calcium.

Glucose metabolism derived signals and intracellular calcium concentration changes secondary to the metabolism of the hexose are crucial to regulate insulin gene transcription and insulin processing, to stimulate insulin secretion, and also to modulate the secretory response to a variety of other ß-cell stimuli.

Insulin Transcription and Processing

Insulin gene transcription is regulated by multiple *cis*-acting elements located within a relatively short region upstream of the transcription start site (6). DNA-binding activity of a number of ß-cell transcription factors that recognize discrete elements in the promoter region of the insulin gene, among which the homeodomain transcription factor insulin promoter factor-1 (IPF-1) plays a particularly important role, is modulated by glucose metabolism and intracellular calcium. Translation of insulin mRNA in the rough endoplasmic reticulum results in the production of preproinsulin, which is immediately cleaved to proinsulin and then transported from the endoplasmic reticulum to the Golgi apparatus, where it is packaged into secretory granules. As the secretory granule matures, proinsulin is processed to insulin and C-peptide, resulting in the production of equimolar quantities of these two peptides. The production of insulin from its precursor proinsulin is an energy-requiring process dependent on ATP and the action of specific processing enzymes (PC1/3 and PC2) located within the secretory granule (7, 8). The activity of these proteases is both pH and calcium dependent. In healthy human subjects, the majority of, but not all, proinsulin is fully processed so that normal subjects release small (1-2% relative to the processed insulin) quantities of proinsulin in response to ß-cell stimulation (9, 10).

Noteworthy is the fact that in addition to the regulated secretory pathway, the ß-cell also secretes its products through a constitutive pathway. This pathway is characteristic of cell types that do not release products in response to secretagogues. Under normal conditions, the constitutive secretory pathway in the pancreatic ß-cell is quantitatively less important than the regulated pathway. The two pathways differ in that in the constitutive pathway the rate of hormone release is dependent on the rate of new protein synthesis and does not require secretagogue presentation and the presence of calcium. Moreover, the two specific proteases responsible for proinsulin processing in the regulated pathway are not present in the constitutive pathway so that proinsulin goes essentially unprocessed during its transit in this pathway and little to no insulin and C-peptide are released from it (11).

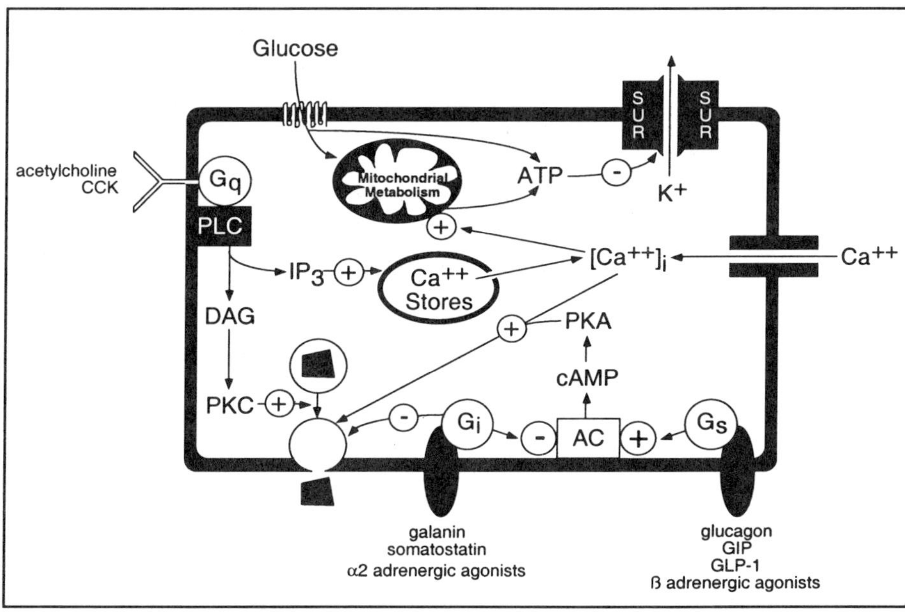

Figure 1: Intracellular signal transduction pathways in the pancreatic ß-cell thought to be most important in ß-cell secretory granule exocytosis. Glucose is transported into the cell via the GLUT2 glucose transporter and stimulates oxidative metabolism. Other modulators (neurotransmitters and hormones) act via either adenylate cyclase (AC) or phospholipase C (PLC). Gi, Gs and Gq are heterotrimeric GTPases that couple the action of receptor agonists to AC and PLC. Inhibitors of exocytosis through Gi interfere with cyclic adenosine monophosphate (cAMP) generation, channel activity and exocytosis itself. Closure of the potassium channel occurs by an increase in the ATP/ADP ratio or following sulfonylurea binding to the sulfonylurea receptor (SUR), which is then followed by calcium influx through the voltage-sensitive L-type calcium channel. Adapted from (12).

Insulin Secretion

Glucose-induced insulin secretion is tightly linked to changes in the adenosine compounds in the ß-cell resulting from the metabolism of the hexose (2). As described above, the net increase in the ATP/ADP ratio secondary to glucose metabolism is followed by a cascade of events that result in an increase in the intracellular calcium concentration. Adenosine compounds and calcium are the main modulators of the interaction and activators of the complex network of proteins involved in insulin granule exocytosis (Figure 1) (12).

Glucose is also important in regulating insulin secretory mechanisms that are not dependent on glycolysis. By providing additional phospholipid substrate or by activating membrane phosphodiesterases, glucose increases diacylglycerol (DAG) and inositol trisphosphate (IP3) concentrations. IP3 is soluble and released from the cytoplasm where it interacts with the endoplasmic reticulum to release stored calcium. With increases in cytosolic calcium, DAG activates protein kinase C that in turn can phosphorylate ß-cell proteins resulting in insulin secretion (Figure 1).

Finally, it is important to emphasize that although glucose regulation of proinsulin biosynthesis and insulin secretion share common metabolic requirements, there must be a point of divergence of these stimulus-response coupling pathways (13). The distal targets of the ß-cell's insulin exocytotic apparatus and protein synthesis machinery are distinctly different cellular mechanisms. The point of divergence of these two fundamental processes in the pancreatic ß-cell and its potential implications have not yet been clearly defined.

DYNAMICS OF INSULIN SECRETION *IN VIVO*

Insulin secretion under basal conditions is phasic, being secreted in a continuous pulsatile manner. The periodicity of insulin release appears to be of two types, with distinct pulses every 10 to 14 minutes superimposed on a longer rhythm of insulin secretion that has a periodicity of 105 to 120 minutes (14). While it is not entirely clear whether either or both of these pulsatile rhythms result from an intrinsic ß-cell pacemaker or are modulated by other factors, studies performed *in vitro* using islets (15) and *in vivo* in vagotomized humans (16) suggest that the shorter oscillations result at least in part from an intra-islet pacemaker which is influenced by vagal tone. Control of the slower ultradian oscillations may be linked to an oscillating peripheral metabolic signal or an interaction between the insulin response system and insulin's effects on circulating secretagogues, especially glucose.

Glucose Stimulated Insulin Secretion

The importance of glucose as a ß-cell stimulant following oral ingestion (17) and intravenous administration (18) has been recognized for many years. However, glucose-induced insulin secretion is not a linear function of the glucose concentration and comprises at least two phases (19). Both phases commence immediately following glucose administration but the second phase is only detectable once the rapid first phase response has diminished. As detailed subsequently, the glucose-stimulated insulin response is not only related to the magnitude of the glucose stimulus (20), but also varies based on tissue sensitivity to insulin (21), with obesity being a major contributor to differences in insulin sensitivity (18).

Glucose Modulation of Insulin Secretion

A number of other secretagogues, including hormones, gut peptides and amino acids, are also potent ß-cell secretagogues (Figure 1) (22). However, glucose is an important modulator of the magnitude of the ß-cell's response to these non-glucose secretagogues. It does so through two different mechanisms: potentiation and priming (23).

The relationship between glucose level and the degree of potentiation follows Michaelis-Menten type of kinetics, being non-linear in nature and reaching a maximum at a glucose level greater than 25 mM (24). One can analyze this curve and characterize its components into the maximal capacity of glucose to potentiate the ß-cell response to a non-glucose stimulus (AIRmax) and the plasma glucose concentration at which half-maximal potentiation of the insulin response occurs (PG50), representing the sensitivity of the system to glucose. Studies examining these two measures under a variety of different natural and experimental conditions have demonstrated that they can vary independently in different physiological and pathological conditions (25-29).

The priming of glucose is its ability to modulate the ß-cell's response to a subsequent glucose or non-glucose secretagogue administered shortly after the glucose level has returned back to basal (23). This ability of glucose to impact subsequent ß-cell responses has been used as another test of ß-cell integrity (30).

Insulin Sensitivity as a Modulator of Insulin Secretion

Regulation of insulin secretion is not limited to glucose and other secretagogues but is also determined by more indirect influences. For instance, it has long been recognized that insulin release is enhanced in obesity (18, 31), and that this obesity-associated enhancement of insulin secretion affects both the magnitude of the oscillatory insulin release and the acute responses to glucose and non-glucose secretagogues (14, 32). With application of measures of insulin sensitivity, it appears that this phenomenon is not accounted for by obesity *per se*, but rather that variations in insulin sensitivity are responsible for modulating ß-cell function.

We examined the nature of the interaction between measures of ß-cell function and insulin sensitivity by assessing these two variables in a large cohort of young, apparently healthy subjects (Figure 2) (21). In this population with normal glucose tolerance and varying degrees of obesity, the acute insulin response to an intravenous secretory challenge was immediate and profound. However, individual values for insulin sensitivity showed wide variation, and ß-cell function varied quantitatively with these differences in insulin sensitivity. As predicted by Bergman et al (33), when insulin secretion and sensitivity were plotted together, the relationship between these parameters was non-linear in nature and best described by a hyperbolic function. Thus, insulin sensitivity times ß-cell function is a constant for a given degree of glucose tolerance. This product is now commonly referred to as the disposition index. In order for glucose tolerance to remain constant when insulin sensitivity changes, a proportionate reciprocal alteration in insulin output has to occur so that the disposition index does not change. If insulin secretion does not change appropriately, glucose tolerance will differ.

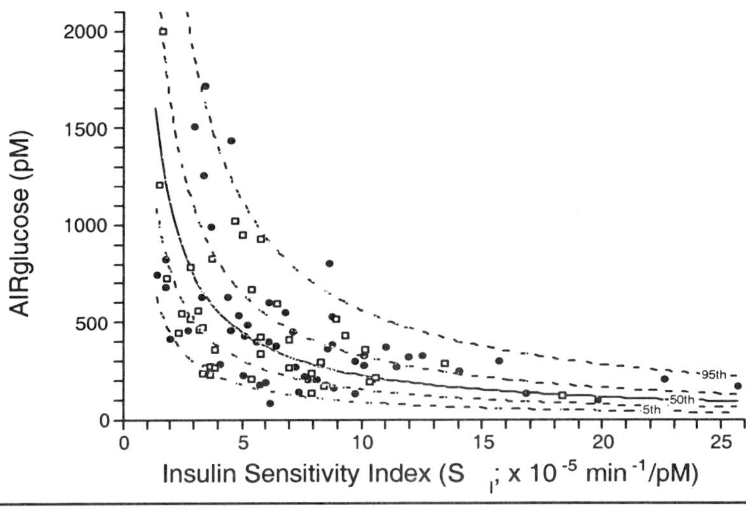

Figure 2: Relationship between insulin sensitivity and ß-cell function quantified as the first-phase insulin response (AIRglucose) in 93 apparently healthy, non-diabetic subjects under the age of 45 years. The cohort demonstrates a broad range of insulin sensitivity and ß-cell function. The solid line depicts the best-fit relationship (50th percentile), while the broken lines represent the 5th, 25th, 75th and 95th percentiles. The relationship is best described by a hyperbolic function so that any change in insulin sensitivity is balanced by a reciprocal and proportionate change in ß-cell function. Reproduced from (21).

This hyperbolic relationship implies that a feedback loop governs the interaction between the ß-cell and the peripheral tissues. Whether this regulation is governed by central neural control or is the result of a humoral metabolic signal arising in the peripheral tissues is unclear (34). However, what is certain is that an adaptive increase in insulin secretion in response to the development of insulin resistance can occur relatively quickly as demonstrated by an enhancement of insulin release following only two weeks of nicotinic acid-induced experimental insulin resistance in young healthy subjects (25). That complete adaptation is possible was demonstrated in a study of a group of older subjects who participated in a 6 month intensive exercise training program which resulted in a 36% increase in insulin sensitivity and a reciprocal 30% reduction in the insulin response (26). Thus, even though older individuals have reduced insulin responses to glucose and non-glucose secretagogues in relation to insulin sensitivity (35), their ß-cells appeared to adapt perfectly to the increase in insulin sensitivity from exercise such that glucose tolerance was not affected (26). On the other hand, that complete adaptation to an environmentally associated change in insulin sensitivity does not always occur was recently demonstrated in dogs fed a high-fat diet for 7 weeks. This intervention was associated with a 57% decrease in insulin sensitivity but no change in the acute insulin response, so that glucose tolerance consequently deteriorated (36).

IMPAIRED ß-CELL FUNCTION IN TYPE 2 DIABETES

The development of the insulin radioimmunoassay sparked considerable debate as to the pathogenesis of type 2 diabetes. The seminal work of Banting and Best conclusively demonstrated that a lack of insulin was vital to the development of hyperglycemia. Thus, it was somewhat of a surprise that the development of the insulin radioimmunoassay highlighted the fact that type 2 diabetes was not associated with an absolute deficiency of circulating insulin. Using insulin immunoassays as well as assays of proinsulin, C-peptide and IAPP, the importance of alterations in ß-cell function to the development of the hyperglycemia of type 2 diabetes has become apparent. Abnormalities in both glucose- and non-glucose-stimulated insulin secretion have been demonstrated. In the fasting state, disturbed oscillatory insulin release has been shown, involving both the rapid (37) and the more prolonged (38) pulses. This lack of pulsatility may contribute to the pathogenesis of the hyperglycemia since insulin may be more biologically effective when delivered in pulses (39).

Type 2 diabetes is also characterized by the loss of the first-phase insulin response to glucose, a defect which is observed in all individuals with fasting plasma glucose concentrations greater than 7.8 mM, and in most individuals whose basal glucose concentration is above 6.4 mM (40, 41).

While there is an absolute deficiency of first-phase secretion in type 2 diabetes, the presence of higher glucose levels in type 2 diabetes may make the second-phase response appear relatively intact. However, when ß-cell function is assessed after glucose levels are matched in healthy and type 2 diabetic subjects, it is apparent that a second-phase secretory defect is also characteristic of the disease (24).

The ability of glucose to potentiate the insulin response to non-glucose secretagogues is also reduced in type 2 diabetes (24, 42). By examination of the glucose-dose response curve of the relationship between glucose level and insulin response to a non-glucose stimulant, it is apparent that the decrease in glucose potentiation is the result of a reduction in ß-cell secretory capacity (reduced AIRmax) without an apparent change in sensitivity of the cell to glucose (unchanged PG50) (24). Since the reduction in AIRmax is curvilinearly proportionate to the degree of fasting hyperglycemia (42, 43), a large decline in AIRmax (about 75%) is already present at the diagnostic fasting glucose level for type 2 diabetes.

Not only have the classic defects in insulin secretory responses been well characterized as measures of ß-cell dysfunction in type 2 diabetes, but a disproportionate increase in the ß-cell release of proinsulin has also been demonstrated. Plasma proinsulin levels in healthy subjects in the basal state average approximately 15% of the circulating fasting immunoreactive insulin concentration (44-47). It should be emphasized that, because the clearance rate of circulating proinsulin is slower than that of insulin (48), the proportion of proinsulin in plasma is greater than that present in the mature secretory granule, which is around 2% (49). In subjects with type 2 diabetes, there is a disproportionate increase in the amount of proinsulin-like molecules circulating in plasma amounting to an average of 25-30% of immunoreactive insulin in the basal state (44-47).

Pathogenesis of the Impaired ß-cell Function of Type 2 Diabetes

Reduced pancreatic ß-cell mass appears to be a common anatomic finding in type 2 diabetic subjects (50-52). This reduction may be due at least in part to amyloid deposits localized in pancreatic islets that are observed in some 90% of individuals with type 2 diabetes (53), as first described by Opie in 1901 (54). However, based in part on studies performed in humans, dogs and rats, even a relative reduction of ß-cell mass of about 50% alone does not appear sufficient to explain the observed abnormalities (27, 55, 56). In none of these studies was fasting hyperglycemia observed. Persistent hyperglycemia has only been found in two studies. In one of the studies, glucose needed to be infused for weeks in partially pancreatectomized (50-65%) dogs in order to produce continuous hyperglycemia while dogs without pancreatic mass reduction did not develop hyperglycemia (57). In the other study, more than 90% of the pancreas had to be removed in rats in order for fasting hyperglycemia to develop (58). Thus, pancreatic resection producing a similar degree of ß-cell loss as observed in type 2 diabetes does not produce either the characteristic islet dysfunction seen in type 2 diabetes or persistent hyperglycemia. Therefore, it appears that functional factor(s) have to be involved in pathogenesis of the impaired ß-cell function of type 2 diabetes. It should be emphasized that the understanding of such functional factor(s) has not yet been well established.

The explanation for the disproportionate proinsulinemia of type 2 diabetes has been a matter of debate. In one of the initial studies, it was hypothesized that the increased secretory demand imposed on the ß-cell in type 2 diabetes resulted in the release of immature secretory granules containing disproportionate amounts of proinsulin, thereby resulting in elevated proinsulin concentrations (44). However, based on additional data obtained in healthy and diabetic humans as well as in animals under conditions of increased ß-cell secretory demand, an alternative explanation for these findings has been developed. It is our belief that the disproportionate proinsulinemia results from a primary ß-cell abnormality rather than increased secretory demand. In humans, the presence of natural or experimental insulin resistance is associated with increased ß-cell secretory demand, which results in hyperinsulinemia and hyperproinsulinemia (25, 45, 46, 59, 60). However, in all these studies the change in ß-cell peptide levels was proportionate, so that the quantity of immunoreactive insulin comprised of proinsulin-like molecules (the PI/IRI ratio) was not altered. In patients with type 2 diabetes the PI/IRI ratio is related to the ß-cell secretory defect and does not increase as body mass index increases, and, with it, ß-cell secretory demand (61). Moreover, in individuals with type 2 diabetes that have undergone marked weight loss, a 43% reduction in the fasting glucose concentration did not significantly reduce the proportion of proinsulin components in the fasting plasma (62). We believe, therefore, that the abnormality is proportional to the ß-cell defect and that small alterations in proinsulin release develop prior to the development of fasting hyperglycemia (63). Whether this alteration in peptide processing may affect not only proinsulin processing but also that of IAPP and might be the related to islet amyloid deposition is currently unknown (53).

Collectively, experimental observations based on several different approaches suggest that the early abnormalities in ß-cell function in type 2 diabetes are most likely due to some defect(s) in the glucose sensing and peptide processing system. Reduction in ß-cell mass would be a later event that is likely to contribute significantly to a further reduction in ß-cell function over time.

DEFECTIVE ß-CELL FUNCTION AS A PRECLINICAL FEATURE OF TYPE 2 DIABETES MELLITUS

Although abnormalities in ß-cell function and insulin sensitivity are well developed by the time hyperglycemia is evident, their relative roles in the pathogenesis of type 2 diabetes remain controversial (64, 65). Because defects in insulin sensitivity and insulin secretion may result in part from hyperglycemia (66), measurements in fully developed type 2 diabetes may not reflect the primary event. Studies in individuals at risk for type 2 diabetes offer one means to understand the early pathophysiology of the disease and help focus the search for genes and therapeutic targets.

Over the past 30 years, many studies have attempted to assess the relative roles of insulin secretion and insulin resistance in normal glucose-tolerant individuals with a first-degree relative with type 2 diabetes (64). The failure of these studies to resolve the relative roles of these two factors may result from at least three factors. First, many studies assessing insulin secretion have examined the response to oral glucose. While oral glucose was the first stimulus to be used, it is the least satisfactory as glucose levels cannot be adequately controlled during the oral glucose tolerance test, so that the glucose challenge to the ß-cell varies among individuals. Moreover, oral glucose administration is associated with activation of meal-related gut factors and neural transmitters that may impact the islet response. Therefore, it is not surprising that the correlation between simple measurements of insulin secretion assessed by an oral glucose tolerance test and those derived after the more reproducible intravenous glucose stimulus are weak (67-69). A second explanation for the discordant findings is genetic heterogeneity. As might be expected for an inherited disorder, not all individuals with a family history of diabetes show defects in either insulin sensitivity or insulin secretion. As an example, when African-American women with a parental history of type 2 diabetes were compared, those who had a history of gestational diabetes presented defects in insulin secretion and action compared to those who did not have a history of gestational diabetes (70). Therefore, studies comprising a small number of unrelated family members may be under-powered to find significant differences. Genetic heterogeneity among populations (71) and within different study populations (72, 73) may also help to explain the conflicting results. Finally, few studies have considered insulin secretion in the context of insulin sensitivity. Of note, in some of the reported studies suggesting the presence of insulin resistance as the key pathogenic finding, there was clear evidence of either poor matching of subjects or lack of demographic data to determine the appropriateness of matching (64, 65). The recognition that insulin sensitivity is determined by a number of different factors means that even matching individuals for some but not all of these factors may be potentially problematic.

The previously-described hyperbolic relationship between insulin sensitivity and secretion provides a means to compare ß-cell function in individuals with different degrees of insulin sensitivity. The disposition index, which is determined as the product of insulin sensitivity and insulin secretion and defines an individual's ß-cell response, can be used to estimate the adequacy of ß-cell function based on the prevailing insulin sensitivity (21). Using this approach we examined a relatively homogenous Caucasian population of first-degree relatives of type 2 sibling pairs (74). We found a broad range of both insulin sensitivity and ß-cell function that encompassed normal values. However, compared with normal controls in which the mean and median percentile score for the disposition index was 50, our sample of first degree relatives showed a mean percentile of 28.9. In this study, 45% of the relatives ranked in the lowest decile of the disposition index, rather than the expected 10% as occurs in a population of subjects with no family history of diabetes. These findings confirm those previously reported in non-obese offspring of Japanese type 2 diabetic patients (75). The findings were even more striking when we studied the role of obesity in a similar population (76). Based on the hyperbolic relationship between insulin sensitivity and insulin secretion, ß-cell function should increase with obesity to compensate for the reduced insulin sensitivity. Consistent with that relationship, both control and first degree relatives of patients with type 2 diabetes had a reduced insulin sensitivity and an increased ß-cell response in absolute terms. However, when the disposition index was determined it was observed that this measure was clearly decreased with obesity among family members but not among control individuals. Taken as a whole, our studies suggest that the relatives of individuals with type 2 diabetes appear to have inadequate ß-cell compensation for the prevailing insulin resistance, even when their glucose tolerance is still normal, and that this situation is aggravated when insulin sensitivity is further decreased by obesity. These findings are supported by those made by Pimenta *et al.*(77), who in a cross-sectional study demonstrated a 20-25% reduction in first and second phase insulin release in first-degree relatives of type 2 diabetic patients compared with controls who did not differ for insulin sensitivity by virtue of careful matching for age, sex and degree of obesity.

Similar cross-sectional analyses of insulin sensitivity and insulin secretion have been performed in individuals with impaired glucose tolerance (78), monozygotic twins of patients with type 2 diabetes (79), the elderly (26), women with polycystic ovary syndrome and a family history of type 2 diabetes (80), and women with a history of gestational diabetes (81), groups who are all at high risk of developing type 2 diabetes mellitus. Although insulin resistance is a common finding in those groups of individuals, when the magnitude of the insulin response to glucose is assessed relative to insulin sensitivity in each of these groups, ß-cell function can be demonstrated to be reduced (Figure 3).

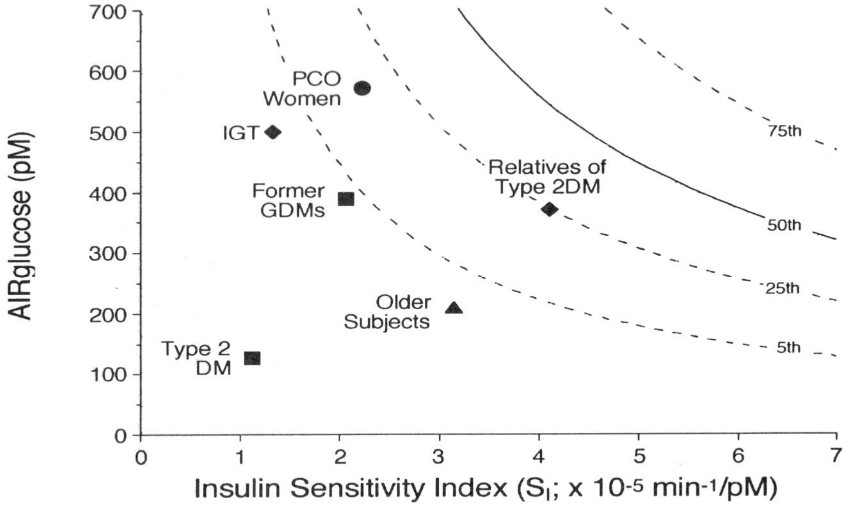

Figure 3: Percentile lines for the relationship between insulin sensitivity (S_I) and the first-phase insulin response (AIRglucose) based on data from 93 apparently healthy subjects (21). Mean data from six other studies are plotted. The ten subjects with type 2 diabetes are insulin resistant and have markedly impaired insulin secretion (87). Thirteen healthy older subjects demonstrate that aging is associated with insulin resistance and a reduction in ß-cell function (26). Reduced ß-cell function is also manifest in 8 women with a history of gestational diabetes (GDM) (81), 11 women with polycystic ovarian disease (PCO) and a family history of type 2 diabetes (80), 21 subjects with impaired glucose tolerance (IGT) (78), and in 14 subjects with a first-degree relative with type 2 diabetes mellitus (88). The reduction in ß-cell function in these latter five groups is compatible with their high risk of subsequently developing type 2 diabetes.

Data from prospective and longitudinal studies has recently confirmed the importance of impaired ß-cell function in the pathogenesis of type 2 diabetes and underscored that this is an early phenomenon in the process leading to hyperglycemia. Prospective studies indicate that both insulin sensitivity and insulin secretion may predict future diabetes (82-85). However, recent studies have demonstrated the value of the measurement of ß-cell compensation for the prevailing insulin resistance as a predictor of the future occurrence of the disease. In Latino women with a history of gestational diabetes, a ß-cell compensation index (derived from insulin sensitivity assessed by the hyperinsulinemic euglycemic clamp and the 30 minute insulin secretory response during the oral glucose tolerance test) measured antepartum, was a stronger predictor of future type 2 diabetes than measurements of insulin sensitivity and ß-cell function separately (85). In Caucasian non-diabetic post-menopausal women, a ß-cell compensation index calculated as the product of insulin sensitivity measured with the euglycemic clamp and the insulin response to intravenous arginine predicted future diabetes at three years of follow-up (86). Finally, in an epidemiological study in Pima Indians, simple indices of insulin secretion derived from oral glucose tolerance test were predictors of future conversion to diabetes when insulin sensitivity was taken into account (69).

The early occurrence of ß-cell secretory defects in the pathogenesis of type 2 diabetes has been recently demonstrated in a longitudinal study conducted in Pima Indians (89). In this study, forty-eight Pima Indians with normal glucose tolerance (NGT) were observed for approximately 5 years. On enrollment, these subjects were insulin resistant but maintained normal glucose tolerance as a result of increased insulin secretion. Over time, however, glucose tolerance deteriorated in 17 patients such that they

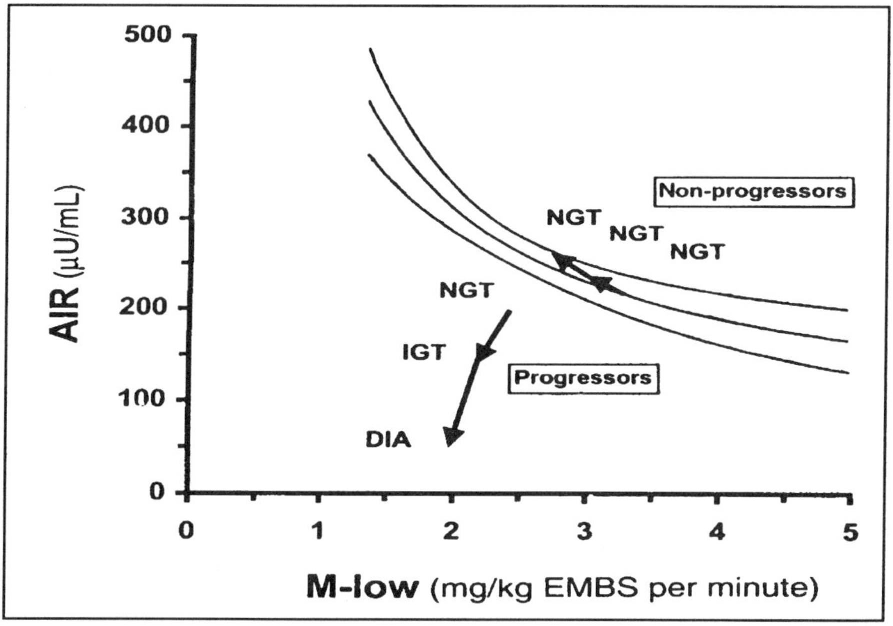

Figure 4: Changes in ß-cell function measured as the acute insulin response to glucose (AIR) relative to changes in insulin sensitivity measured by the clamp technique at a low insulin concentration (M-low). These measurements were made in 11 Pima Indians in whom glucose tolerance deteriorated from normal glucose tolerance (NGT) to impaired glucose tolerance (IGT) to diabetes (DIA) (progressors), and in 23 subjects who maintained normal glucose tolerance (NGT) throughout (non-progressors). The lines represent the prediction line and the lower and upper limits of the 95% confidence interval of the regression between the AIR and M-low as determined from a population of 277 Pima Indians with normal glucose tolerance. Reprinted from (89).

progressed from NGT to impaired glucose tolerance (IGT) to frank type 2 diabetes. The progression from NGT to IGT and from IGT to diabetes was associated with a 14% increase in body weight, a 14% decline in insulin-stimulated glucose disposal, and a 78% decrease in the insulin-secretory response. ß-cell function decreased by 31% during the transition from NGT to

IGT and by an additional 47% in the transition from IGT to diabetes in those individuals in which glucose homeostasis deteriorated, whereas it did not change over time in those who did not progress (Figure 4). This longitudinal study underscores the fact that defects in insulin secretion occur early in the development of the disease and that the inability of insulin secretion to compensate for a decrease in insulin sensitivity distinguishes individuals who develop diabetes from those who remain NGT. The data in Pima Indians contrasts with Warram *et al.*'s study in Caucasians (90), which is often cited as providing evidence that insulin resistance is the first abnormality in type 2 diabetes. However, in that study the role of insulin sensitivity to modulate ß-cell function was not accounted for. Thus, while the absolute insulin responses were similar in the subjects who did and did not progress to develop type 2 diabetes, the fact that the subjects who progressed were more insulin resistant is compatible with insulin secretion also being diminished at this very early stage in these individuals. That ß-cell secretory defects may indeed be critical in the pathogenesis of type 2 diabetes is further supported by the finding that low insulin secretion has been associated with an increase in future weight gain (91, 92). Therefore, it is tempting to speculate that the ß-cell secretory defect would create a vicious cycle where obesity would exacerbate the deficient insulin secretion in individuals at risk for type 2 diabetes.

A few studies have examined the ratio between plasma proinsulin and immunoreactive insulin (PI/IRI) and type 2 diabetes risk in groups recognized as having a greater chance of progressing to hyperglycemia. Non-diabetic Mexican-American subjects with a parental history of diabetes have been demonstrated to have an elevated PI/IRI ratio, suggesting that an increased ratio may be an indicator of ß-cell dysfunction in high risk subjects prior to the development of hyperglycemia (47). Evidence that an altered PI/IRI ratio may be a forerunner to type 2 diabetes comes from prospective studies in Japanese Americans. Those individuals who subsequently progressed to diabetes over a five year follow up period were demonstrated to have an elevated PI/IRI ratio prior to the development of the disease, at a time when they had either normal or impaired glucose tolerance (63). A similar observation has been made in older Finnish subjects who subsequently developed hyperglycemia (93).

GENETIC BASIS FOR THE ß-CELL SECRETORY DEFECTS

While the role of ß-cell dysfunction in the pathophysiology of type 2 diabetes has become clear, understanding the etiology of the underlying defects at the molecular and genetic levels has been more difficult. This is in part because type 2 diabetes is a complex metabolic disorder with both primary (i.e. genetic) and secondary (i.e. environmental and hyperglycemia-induced) causes, the relative contribution of each to the pathogenesis of the ß-cell defect and insulin resistance being a matter of debate (64, 65). The most convincing evidence for a genetic factor in type 2 diabetes derives from twin studies (94-96). Although there is some variation in the reported risk when comparing monozygotic and dizygotic twins, concordance is always higher for monozygotic than dizygotic twins. Further evidence for a genetic factor is the familial aggregation of type 2 diabetes in a variety of ethnic groups and a variation in the prevalence among these groups. Type 2 diabetes in different populations ranges from as high as 80% in Pima Indians whose parents both had early onset diabetes to estimates of approximately 5% in Caucasian-Americans, 10% in African-Americans, 25% in Mexican-Americans, and 35% in Pima Indians overall (71). However, although these data strongly suggest a genetic component in type 2 diabetes they do not resolve the issue of whether ß-cell dysfunction and/or insulin sensitivity have a genetic origin.

Vauhkonen *et al.* suggested that both insulin secretion and sensitivity are inherited and may differ between families (72). Reflecting the heterogeneity of type 2 diabetes, offspring of probands with a deficient insulin

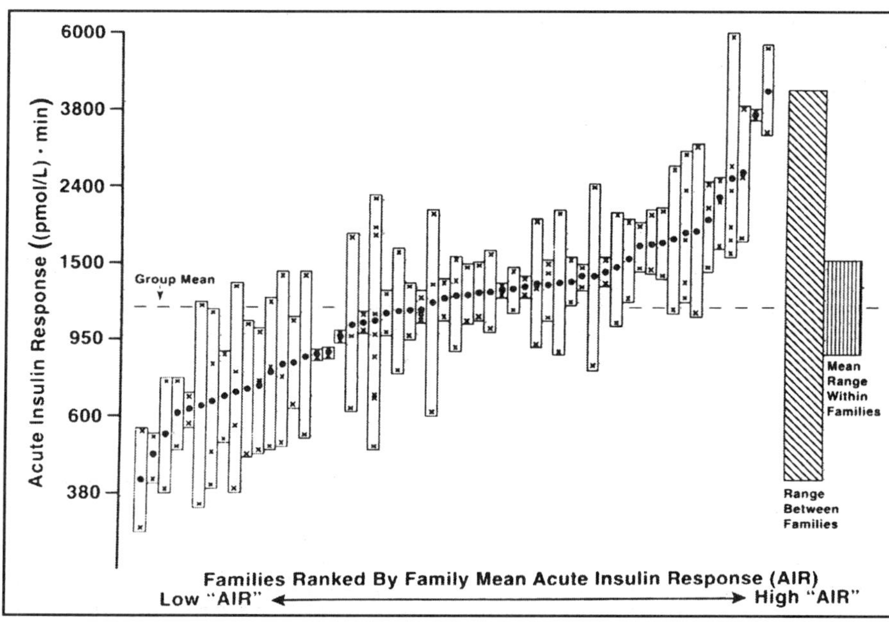

Figure 5: Acute insulin response (AIR) in non-diabetic Pima Indians grouped by family. Subjects (x) are grouped by family (vertical bars), and the 55 families are ranked by family mean AIR (black dots). The AIR was calculated as the mean plasma insulin concentration from 3, 4, and 5 minutes after an intravenous glucose tolerance test. The range of the mean family AIR and the mean range within families are indicated. Reprinted from (99).

secretion phenotype had an impaired insulin secretory capacity and normal insulin sensitivity, whereas offspring of probands with the insulin resistant phenotype had impaired insulin sensitivity but normal insulin secretory capacity. That a positive family history of type 2 diabetes is associated with altered ß-cell function also has been shown in many studies, suggesting the presence of a genetic determinant of ß-cell function (73, 97). Moreover, familial aggregation of insulin secretion has also been demonstrated (Figure 5) (98, 99). These studies in two different populations (Caucasians (98) and Pima Indians (99)) demonstrated familial aggregation of the acute insulin response as measured by an intravenous glucose tolerance test. Importantly, in these two reported studies the familial aggregation was not affected when measures of insulin sensitivity were taken into account.

Studies using heritability estimates also support a genetic basis for ß-cell function. Using the maximum likelihood method, Sakul *et al.* demonstrated the heritability of the acute insulin response in Pima Indians (100). The heritability of this early phase of insulin secretion was 80% and remained high (70%) after controlling for age, sex, body fat and insulin sensitivity. Although the heritability estimate of ß-cell function depended on which time point of this response was considered, it was larger than that of insulin sensitivity assessed by the hyperinsulinemic euglycemic clamp (49%). We reported similar findings in a cohort of first-degree relatives from families with two diabetic siblings using the same method for heritability estimation (74). In this cohort, diabetes showed 100% heritability, whereas ß-cell function and insulin sensitivity measured by minimal model analysis showed moderate heritability (33% and 29%, respectively). Interestingly, the disposition index (which accounts for the modulation of ß-cell function by insulin sensitivity) was the most heritable index, being 67% heritable in the whole population and 70% when only NGT individuals were included. A significant heritability of the glucose-induced insulin response has also been reported in offspring of diabetic sibling pairs (35%) (101) and monozygotic twins (55%) (102) of Finnish descent. In these two recent Finnish studies, the heritability estimate of insulin sensitivity was significantly lower than that of insulin secretion (20% and 37% respectively), which may explain at least in part the lower heritability estimates when insulin secretion was corrected for insulin sensitivity (21.5% and 41% respectively). The finding of moderate to high heritability of ß-cell function in different populations supports the concept that this is an important genetic determinant of glucose homeostasis and that unraveling the genetic bases for the ß-cell secretory defect(s) will be a key step in our understanding of the molecular basis for type 2 diabetes.

That a genetic defect in insulin secretion may be critical to type 2 diabetes is further supported by the description during the past decade of several monogenic forms of the disease. Both maturity onset diabetes of the young (MODY) (103) and maternally inherited diabetes and deafness (MIDD) (104) are associated with impaired ß-cell function (see Chapters 5 and 6). As reviewed above, glucokinase activity and mitochondrial metabolism are central to glucose metabolism in the ß-cell (Figure 1) (3, 105). MIDD is secondary to mutations in mitochondrial DNA (104), whereas MODY-2 has been demonstrated to be the result of mutations of the glucokinase gene. The genes responsible for other forms of MODY are transcription factors thought to play a role in both glucose metabolism and determination of ß-cell mass. Although mutations in the IPF-1 gene, which is related to MODY-4, have been suggested to predispose to the more common form of type 2 diabetes (106), these results have not been confirmed by others (107). Thus, there is presently little evidence for an association between MODY or MIDD genes and the more general form of type 2 diabetes. On the other hand, mutations in the SUR1 (108-111) and calpain 10 (112, 113) genes have recently been associated with type 2 diabetes in several populations. However, these genes, which are related to ß-cell function, still do not provide a genetic explanation for the ß-cell dysfunction observed in the vast majority of subjects with type 2 diabetes.

The heterogeneous nature of type 2 diabetes may help to explain the difficulty in identifying ß-cell genes as major predictors of the hyperglycemia (114). This difficulty is compounded by the fact that the ß-cell secretory defect may not be homogenous among different individuals (77). Thus, if we are to unravel the genetic bases for diabetes, appropriate phenotyping will be important to identify the genes responsible for ß-cell failure in type 2 diabetes.

CONCLUSION

Type 2 diabetes is a heterogeneous disease that results from the inability of the pancreatic ß-cell to secrete enough insulin to match the prevailing insulin sensitivity. The development of reliable techniques to quantify ß-cell function has identified the importance of this parameter for the development of the disease. Measurement of this parameter in selected populations may help to unravel the genetic basis of type 2 diabetes, a syndrome that for so long has had devastating consequences on those afflicted by it.

ACKNOWLEDGMENTS

This work was supported by NIH grants DK-02654, DK-17047, and RR-37 and by a Post-doctoral Fellowship from the Spanish Secretaria de Estado de Universidades, Investigación y Desarrollo.

REFERENCES

1. Kahn, S.E., and Porte, D., Jr. Pathophysiology of type II diabetes mellitus. In: Porte, D., Jr, Sherwin, R., editors. Diabetes Mellitus. New York: Elsevier; 1996. p 487-512.

2. Malaisse, W.J., Sener, A., Herchuelz, A., and Hutton, J.C. 1979. Insulin release: the fuel hypothesis. Metabolism. 28:373-86.
3. Matschinsky, F.M., Glaser, B., and Magnuson, M.A. 1998. Pancreatic beta-cell glucokinase: closing the gap between theoretical concepts and experimental realities. Diabetes. 47:307-15.
4. Malaisse, W.J., Rasschaert, J., Conget, I., and Sener, A. 1991. Hexose metabolism in pancreatic islets. Regulation of aerobic glycolysis and pyruvate decarboxylation. Int J Biochem. 23:955-9.
5. Aguilar-Bryan, L., and Bryan, J. 1999. Molecular biology of adenosine triphosphate-sensitive potassium channels. Endocr Rev. 20:101-35.
6. German, M.S., and Wang, J. 1994. The insulin gene contains multiple transcriptional elements that respond to glucose. Mol Cell Biol. 14:4067-75.
7. Davidson, H.W., Rhodes, C.J., and Hutton, J.C. 1988. Intraorganellar calcium and pH control proinsulin cleavage in the pancreatic beta cell via two distinct site-specific endopeptidases. Nature. 333:93-6.
8. Smeekens, S.P., Avruch, A.S., LaMendola, J., Chan, S.J., and Steiner, D.F. 1991. Identification of a cDNA encoding a second putative prohormone convertase related to PC2 in AtT20 cells and islets of Langerhans. Proc Natl Acad Sci U S A. 88:340-4.
9. Ward, W.K., Paquette, T.L., Frank, B.H., and Porte, D., Jr. 1986. A sensitive radioimmunoassay for human proinsulin with sequential use of antisera to C-peptide and insulin. Clin Chem. 32:728-733.
10. Kahn, S.E., and Halban, P.A. 1997. Release of incompletely processed proinsulin is the cause of the disproportionate proinsulinemia of NIDDM. Diabetes. 46:1725-32.
11. Nagamatsu, S., Nishi, M., and Steiner, D.F. 1991. Biosynthesis of islet amyloid polypeptide. Elevated expression in mouse beta TC3 cells. J Biol Chem. 266:13737-41.
12. Wolheim, C.B., Lang, J., and Regazzi, R. 1996. The exocytosis process of insulin secretion and its regulation by calcium and G-proteins. Diabetes Reviews. 4:298-319.
13. Skelly, R.H., Bollheimer, L.C., Wicksteed, B.L., Corkey, B.E., and Rhodes, C.J. 1998. A distinct difference in the metabolic stimulus-response coupling pathways for regulating proinsulin biosynthesis and insulin secretion that lies at the level of a requirement for fatty acyl moieties. Biochem J. 331:553-61.
14. Polonsky, K.S., Given, B.D., and Van Cauter, E. 1988. Twenty-four-hour profiles and pulsatile patterns of insulin secretion in normal and obese subjects. J Clin Invest. 81:442-8.
15. MacDonald, M.J., Al-Masri, H., Jumelle-Laclau, M., and Cruz, M.O. 1997. Oscillations in activities of enzymes in pancreatic islet subcellular fractions induced by physiological concentrations of effectors. Diabetes. 46:1996-2001.
16. Matthews, D.R., Lang, D.A., Burnett, M.A., and Turner, R.C. 1983. Control of pulsatile insulin secretion in man. Diabetologia. 24:231-7.
17. Yallow, R.S., and Benson, S.A. 1960. Immunoassay of endogenous plasma insulin in man. J Clin Invest. 39:1157-1175.
18. Karam, J.H., Grodsky, G.M., and Forsham, P.H. 1963. Excessive insulin response to glucose in obese subjects as measured by immunochemical assay. Diabetes. 12:197-204.
19. Porte, D., Jr., and Pupo, A.A. 1969. Insulin responses to glucose: evidence for a two pool system in man. J Clin Invest. 48:2309-2319.
20. Chen, M., and Porte, D., Jr. 1976. The effect of rate and dose of glucose infusion on the acute insulin response in man. J Clin Endocrinol Metab. 42:1168-75.
21. Kahn, S.E., *et al.* 1993. Quantification of the relationship between insulin sensitivity and beta- cell function in human subjects. Evidence for a hyperbolic function. Diabetes. 42:1663-72.
22. Ward, W.K., Beard, J.C., Halter, J.B., Pfeifer, M.A., and Porte, D., Jr. 1984. Pathophysiology of insulin secretion in non-insulin-dependent diabetes mellitus. Diabetes Care. 7:491-502.

23. Cerasi, E. 1975. Potentiation of insulin release by glucose in man. I. Quantitative analysis of the enhancement of glucose-induced insulin secretion by pretreatment with glucose in normal subjects. Acta Endocrinol (Copenh). 79:483-501.
24. Ward, W.K., Bolgiano, D.C., McKnight, B., Halter, J.B., and Porte, D., Jr. 1984. Diminished B cell secretory capacity in patients with noninsulin-dependent diabetes mellitus. J Clin Invest. 74:1318-28.
25. Kahn, S.E., *et al.* 1989. Increased beta-cell secretory capacity as mechanism for islet adaptation to nicotinic acid-induced insulin resistance. Diabetes. 38:562-8.
26. Kahn, S.E., *et al.* 1990. Effect of exercise on insulin action, glucose tolerance, and insulin secretion in aging. Am J Physiol. 258:E937-43.
27. Seaquist, E.R., and Robertson, R.P. 1992. Effects of hemipancreatectomy on pancreatic alpha and beta cell function in healthy human donors. J Clin Invest. 89:1761-6.
28. Kahn, S.E., *et al.* 1990. Treatment with a somatostatin analog decreases pancreatic B-cell and whole body sensitivity to glucose. J Clin Endocrinol Metab. 71:994-1002.
29. Ortiz-Alonso, F.J., Herman, W.H., Zobel, D.L., Perry, T.J., Smith, M.J., and Halter, J.B. 1991. Effect of epinephrine on pancreatic beta-cell and alpha-cell function in patients with NIDDM. Diabetes. 40:1194-202.
30. Byrne, M.M., *et al.* 1995. Altered insulin secretory responses to glucose in subjects with a mutation in the MODY1 gene on chromosome 20. Diabetes. 44:699-704.
31. Bagdade, J.D., Porte, D., Jr., Brunzell, J.D., and Bierman, E.L. 1974. Basal and stimulated hyperinsulinism: reversible metabolic sequelae of obesity. J Lab Clin Med. 83:563-9.
32. Beard, J.C., Ward, W.K., Halter, J.B., Wallum, B.J., and Porte, D., Jr. 1987. Relationship of islet function to insulin action in human obesity. J Clin Endocrinol Metab. 65:59-64.
33. Bergman, R.N., Phillips, L.S., and Cobelli, C. 1981. Physiologic evaluation of factors controlling glucose tolerance in man: measurement of insulin sensitivity and beta-cell glucose sensitivity from the response to intravenous glucose. J Clin Invest. 68:1456-67.
34. Kahn, B.B., and Rossetti, L. 1998. Type 2 diabetes--who is conducting the orchestra? Nat Genet. 20:223-5.
35. Kahn, S.E., *et al.* 1992. Exercise training delineates the importance of B-cell dysfunction to the glucose intolerance of human aging. J Clin Endocrinol Metab. 74:1336-42.
36. Kaiyala, K.J., Prigeon, R.L., Kahn, S.E., Woods, S.C., Porte, D., Jr., and Schwartz, M.W. 1999. Reduced beta-cell function contributes to impaired glucose tolerance in dogs made obese by high-fat feeding. Am J Physiol. 277:E659-67.
37. Lang, D.A., Matthews, D.R., Burnett, M., and Turner, R.C. 1981. Brief, irregular oscillations of basal plasma insulin and glucose concentrations in diabetic man. Diabetes. 30:435-9.
38. Polonsky, K.S., *et al.* 1988. Abnormal patterns of insulin secretion in non-insulin-dependent diabetes mellitus. N Engl J Med. 318:1231-9.
39. Matthews, D.R., Naylor, B.A., Jones, R.G., Ward, G.M., and Turner, R.C. 1983. Pulsatile insulin has greater hypoglycemic effect than continuous delivery. Diabetes. 32:617-21.
40. Perley, M.J., and Kipnis, D.M. 1967. Plasma insulin responses to oral and intravenous glucose: studies in normal and diabetic subjects. J Clin Invest. 46:1954-1962.
41. Brunzell, J.D., *et al.* 1976. Relationships between fasting plasma glucose levels and insulin secretion during intravenous glucose tolerance tests. J Clin Endocrinol Metab. 42:222-9.
42. Halter, J.B., Graf, R.J., and Porte, D., Jr. 1979. Potentiation of insulin secretory responses by plasma glucose levels in man: evidence that hyperglycemia in diabetes compensates for imparied glucose potentiation. J Clin Endocrinol Metab. 48:946-54.
43. Roder, M.E., Porte, D., Jr., Schwartz, R.S., and Kahn, S.E. 1998. Disproportionately elevated proinsulin levels reflect the degree of impaired B cell secretory capacity in patients with noninsulin-dependent diabetes mellitus. J Clin Endocrinol Metab. 83:604-8.
44. Ward, W.K., LaCava, E.C., Paquette, T.L., Beard, J.C., Wallum, B.J., and Porte, D., Jr. 1987. Disproportionate elevation of immunoreactive proinsulin in type 2 (non- insulin-

dependent) diabetes mellitus and in experimental insulin resistance. Diabetologia. 30:698-702.

45. Saad, M.F., *et al.* 1990. Disproportionately elevated proinsulin in Pima Indians with noninsulin- dependent diabetes mellitus. J Clin Endocrinol Metab. 70:1247-53.
46. Kahn, S.E., Leonetti, D.L., Prigeon, R.L., Boyko, E.J., Bergstrom, R.W., and Fujimoto, W.Y. 1995. Relationship of proinsulin and insulin with noninsulin-dependent diabetes mellitus and coronary heart disease in Japanese-American men: impact of obesity--clinical research center study. J Clin Endocrinol Metab. 80:1399-406.
47. Haffner, S.M., *et al.* 1994. Proinsulin and specific insulin concentration in high- and low-risk populations for NIDDM. Diabetes. 43:1490-3.
48. Galloway, J.A., *et al.* 1992. Biosynthetic human proinsulin. Review of chemistry, in vitro and in vivo receptor binding, animal and human pharmacology studies, and clinical trial experience. Diabetes Care. 15:666-92.
49. Halban, P.A. 1991. Structural domains and molecular lifestyles of insulin and its precursors in the pancreatic beta cell. Diabetologia. 34:767-78.
50. Saito, K., Yaginuma, N., and Takahashi, T. 1979. Differential volumetry of A, B and D cells in the pancreatic islets of diabetic and nondiabetic subjects. Tohoku J Exp Med. 129:273-83.
51. Kloppel, G., Lohr, M., Habich, K., Oberholzer, M., and Heitz, P.U. 1985. Islet pathology and the pathogenesis of type 1 and type 2 diabetes mellitus revisited. Surv Synth Pathol Res. 4:110-25.
52. Clark, A., *et al.* 1988. Islet amyloid, increased A-cells, reduced B-cells and exocrine fibrosis: quantitative changes in the pancreas in type 2 diabetes. Diabetes Res. 4:151-9.
53. Kahn, S.E., Andrikopoulos, S., and Verchere, C.B. 1999. Islet amyloid: a long-recognized but underappreciated pathological feature of type 2 diabetes. Diabetes. 48:241-53.
54. Opie, E. 1901. The relation of diabetes mellitus to lesions of the pancreas: hyaline degeneration of the islets of Langerhans. J Exp Med. 5:527-540.
55. Ward, W.K., Wallum, B.J., Beard, J.C., Taborsky, G.J., Jr., and Porte, D., Jr. 1988. Reduction of glycemic potentiation. Sensitive indicator of beta-cell loss in partially pancreatectomized dogs. Diabetes. 37:723-9.
56. Leahy, J.L., Bonner-Weir, S., and Weir, G.C. 1984. Abnormal glucose regulation of insulin secretion in models of reduced B- cell mass. Diabetes. 33:667-73.
57. Imamura, T., *et al.* 1988. Severe diabetes induced in subtotally depancreatized dogs by sustained hyperglycemia. Diabetes. 37:600-9.
58. Bonner-Weir, S., Trent, D.F., and Weir, G.C. 1983. Partial pancreatectomy in the rat and subsequent defect in glucose- induced insulin release. J Clin Invest. 71:1544-53.
59. Koivisto, V.A., Yki-Jarvinen, H., Hartling, S.G., and Pelkonen, R. 1986. The effect of exogenous hyperinsulinemia on proinsulin secretion in normal man, obese subjects, and patients with insulinoma. J Clin Endocrinol Metab. 63:1117-20.
60. Shiraishi, I., Iwamoto, Y., Kuzuya, T., Matsuda, A., and Kumakura, S. 1991. Hyperinsulinaemia in obesity is not accompanied by an increase in serum proinsulin/insulin ratio in groups of human subjects with and without glucose intolerance. Diabetologia. 34:737-41.
61. Roder, M.E., *et al.* 1999. Intact proinsulin and beta-cell function in lean and obese subjects with and without type 2 diabetes. Diabetes Care. 22:609-14.
62. Yoshioka, N., Kuzuya, T., Matsuda, A., and Iwamoto, Y. 1989. Effects of dietary treatment on serum insulin and proinsulin response in newly diagnosed NIDDM. Diabetes. 38:262-6.
63. Kahn, S.E., Leonetti, D.L., Prigeon, R.L., Boyko, E.J., Bergstrom, R.W., and Fujimoto, W.Y. 1995. Proinsulin as a marker for the development of NIDDM in Japanese- American men. Diabetes. 44:173-9.
64. Gerich, J.E. 1998. The genetic basis of type 2 diabetes mellitus: impaired insulin secretion versus impaired insulin sensitivity. Endocr Rev. 19:491-503.

65. Ferrannini, E. 1998. Insulin resistance versus insulin deficiency in non-insulin-dependent diabetes mellitus: problems and prospects. Endocr Rev. 19:477-90.
66. Yki-Jarvinen, H. 1992. Glucose toxicity. Endocr Rev. 13:415-31.
67. Howell, W.M., Prigeon, R.L., Fujimoto, W.Y., Kahn, S.E., and ADA GENNID Study Group. 1998. Comparison of estimates of insulin sensitivity and B-cell function derived from the oral glucose tolerance test versus intravenous glucose tolerance test and minimal model. Diabetes. 47:A197.
68. van Haeften, T.W., Dubbeldam, S., Zonderland, M.L., and Erkelens, D.W. 1998. Insulin secretion in normal glucose-tolerant relatives of type 2 diabetic subjects. Assessments using hyperglycemic glucose clamps and oral glucose tolerance tests. Diabetes Care. 21:278-82.
69. Hanson, R.L., *et al.* 2000. Evaluation of simple indices of insulin sensitivity and insulin secretion for use in epidemiologic studies. Am J Epidemiol. 151:190-8.
70. Osei, K., Gaillard, T.R., and Schuster, D.P. 1998. History of gestational diabetes leads to distinct metabolic alterations in nondiabetic African-American women with a parental history of type 2 diabetes. Diabetes Care. 21:1250-7.
71. Harris, M.I., Hadden, W.C., Knowler, W.C., and Bennett, P.H. 1987. Prevalence of diabetes and impaired glucose tolerance and plasma glucose levels in U.S. population aged 20-74 yr. Diabetes. 36:523-34.
72. Vauhkonen, I., Niskanen, L., Vanninen, E., Kainulainen, S., Uusitupa, M., and Laakso, M. 1998. Defects in insulin secretion and insulin action in non-insulin- dependent diabetes mellitus are inherited. Metabolic studies on offspring of diabetic probands. J Clin Invest. 101:86-96.
73. Alford, F.P., *et al.* 1998. Impact of family history of diabetes on the assessment of beta-cell function. Metabolism. 47:522-8.
74. Elbein, S.C., Hasstedt, S.J., Wegner, K., and Kahn, S.E. 1999. Heritability of pancreatic beta-cell function among nondiabetic members of Caucasian familial type 2 diabetic kindreds. J Clin Endocrinol Metab. 84:1398-403.
75. Doi, K., *et al.* 1997. Decreased glucose effectiveness but not insulin resistance in glucose-tolerant offspring of Japanese non-insulin-dependent diabetic patients: a minimal-model analysis. Metabolism. 46:880-3.
76. Elbein, S.C., Wegner, K., and Kahn, S.E. 2000. Reduced beta-cell compensation to the insulin resistance associated with obesity in members of Caucasian familial type 2 diabetic kindreds. Diabetes Care. 23:221-227.
77. Pimenta, W., *et al.* 1995. Pancreatic beta-cell dysfunction as the primary genetic lesion in NIDDM. Evidence from studies in normal glucose-tolerant individuals with a first-degree NIDDM relative. JAMA. 273:1855-61.
78. Cavaghan, M.K., Ehrmann, D.A., Byrne, M.M., and Polonsky, K.S. 1997. Treatment with the oral antidiabetic agent troglitazone improves beta cell responses to glucose in subjects with impaired glucose tolerance. J Clin Invest. 100:530-7.
79. Vaag, A., Henriksen, J.E., Madsbad, S., Holm, N., and Beck-Nielsen, H. 1995. Insulin secretion, insulin action, and hepatic glucose production in identical twins discordant for non-insulin-dependent diabetes mellitus. J Clin Invest. 95:690-8.
80. Ehrmann, D.A., Sturis, J., Byrne, M.M., Karrison, T., Rosenfield, R.L., and Polonsky, K.S. 1995. Insulin secretory defects in polycystic ovary syndrome. Relationship to insulin sensitivity and family history of non-insulin-dependent diabetes mellitus. J Clin Invest. 96:520-7.
81. Ward, W.K., Johnston, C.L., Beard, J.C., Benedetti, T.J., Halter, J.B., and Porte, D., Jr. 1985. Insulin resistance and impaired insulin secretion in subjects with histories of gestational diabetes mellitus. Diabetes. 34:861-9.
82. Lillioja, S., *et al.* 1993. Insulin resistance and insulin secretory dysfunction as precursors of non-insulin-dependent diabetes mellitus. Prospective studies of Pima Indians. N Engl J Med. 329:1988-92.

83. Chen, K.W., *et al.* 1995. Earlier appearance of impaired insulin secretion than of visceral adiposity in the pathogenesis of NIDDM. 5-Year follow-up of initially nondiabetic Japanese-American men. Diabetes Care. 18:747-53.
84. Haffner, S.M., Miettinen, H., Gaskill, S.P., and Stern, M.P. 1995. Decreased insulin secretion and increased insulin resistance are independently related to the 7-year risk of NIDDM in Mexican-Americans. Diabetes. 44:1386-91.
85. Buchanan, T.A., Xiang, A.H., Kjos, S.L., Trigo, E., Lee, W.P., and Peters, R.K. 1999. Antepartum predictors of the development of type 2 diabetes in Latino women 11-26 months after pregnancies complicated by gestational diabetes. Diabetes. 48:2430-6.
86. Larsson, H., and Ahren, B. 2000. Glucose intolerance is predicted by low insulin secretion and high glucagon secretion: outcome of a prospective study in postmenopausal Caucasian women. Diabetologia. 43:194-202.
87. Welch, S., Gebhart, S.S., Bergman, R.N., and Phillips, L.S. 1990. Minimal model analysis of intravenous glucose tolerance test-derived insulin sensitivity in diabetic subjects. J Clin Endocrinol Metab. 71:1508-18.
88. Kahn, S.E. 1996. Regulation of B-cell function in vivo. Diabetes Reviews. 4:372-389.
89. Weyer, C., Bogardus, C., Mott, D.M., and Pratley, R.E. 1999. The natural history of insulin secretory dysfunction and insulin resistance in the pathogenesis of type 2 diabetes mellitus. J Clin Invest. 104:787-94.
90. Warram, J.H., Sigal, R.J., Martin, B.C., Krolewski, A.S., and Soeldner, J.S. 1996. Natural history of impaired glucose tolerance: follow-up at Joslin Clinic. Diabet Med. 13:S40-5.
91. Gould, A.J., Williams, D.E., Byrne, C.D., Hales, C.N., and Wareham, N.J. 1999. Prospective cohort study of the relationship of markers of insulin resistance and secretion with weight gain and changes in regional adiposity. Int J Obes Relat Metab Disord. 23:1256-61.
92. Stone, L.M., Kahn, S.E., Deeb, S.S., Fujimoto, W.Y., and Porte, D., Jr. 1994. Glucokinase gene variations in Japanese-Americans with a family history of NIDDM. Diabetes Care. 17:1480-3.
93. Mykkanen, L., Haffner, S.M., Kuusisto, J., Pyorala, K., Hales, C.N., and Laakso, M. 1995. Serum proinsulin levels are disproportionately increased in elderly prediabetic subjects. Diabetologia. 38:1176-82.
94. Newman, B., Selby, J.V., King, M.C., Slemenda, C., Fabsitz, R., and Friedman, G.D. 1987. Concordance for type 2 (non-insulin-dependent) diabetes mellitus in male twins. Diabetologia. 30:763-8.
95. Kaprio, J., *et al.* 1992. Concordance for type 1 (insulin-dependent) and type 2 (non-insulin- dependent) diabetes mellitus in a population-based cohort of twins in Finland. Diabetologia. 35:1060-7.
96. Medici, F., Hawa, M., Ianari, A., Pyke, D.A., and Leslie, R.D. 1999. Concordance rate for type II diabetes mellitus in monozygotic twins: actuarial analysis. Diabetologia. 42:146-50.
97. Matsuda, A., and Kuzuya, T. 1996. The prevalence of low insulin responders to oral glucose load among groups with various patterns of family history of diabetes. Diabet Med. 13:S59-62.
98. Martin, B.C., and Soeldner, J.S. 1993. Familial clustering of first phase insulin secretion following intravenous glucose in nondiabetic offspring of NIDDM patients. Diabetes. 42:69A.
99. Janssen, R.C., Bogardus, C., Takeda, J., Knowler, W.C., and Thompson, D.B. 1994. Linkage analysis of acute insulin secretion with GLUT2 and glucokinase in Pima Indians and the identification of a missense mutation in GLUT2. Diabetes. 43:558-63.
100. Sakul, H., Pratley, R., Cardon, L., Ravussin, E., Mott, D., and Bogardus, C. 1997. Familiality of physical and metabolic characteristics that predict the development of non-insulin-dependent diabetes mellitus in Pima Indians. Am J Hum Genet. 60:651-6.

101. Watanabe, R.M., *et al.* 1999. Familiality of quantitative metabolic traits in Finnish families with non-insulin-dependent diabetes mellitus. Finland-United States Investigation of NIDDM Genetics (FUSION) Study investigators. Hum Hered. 49:159-68.
102. Lehtovirta, M., Kaprio, J., Forsblom, C., Eriksson, J., Tuomilehto, J., and Groop, L. 2000. Insulin sensitivity and insulin secretion in monozygotic and dizygotic twins. Diabetologia. 43:285-93.
103. Froguel, P., and Velho, G. 1999. Molecular genetics of maturity-onset diabetes of the young. Trends Endocrinol Metab. 10:142-146.
104. Ballinger, S.W., *et al.* 1992. Maternally transmitted diabetes and deafness associated with a 10.4 kb mitochondrial DNA deletion. Nat Genet. 1:11-5.
105. Wollheim, C.B. 2000. Beta-cell mitochondria in the regulation of insulin secretion: a new culprit in type II diabetes. Diabetologia. 43:265-77.
106. Macfarlane, W.M., *et al.* 1999. Missense mutations in the insulin promoter factor-1 gene predispose to type 2 diabetes. J Clin Invest. 104:R33-9.
107. Hansen, L., *et al.* 2000. Missense mutations in the human insulin promoter factor-1 gene and their relation to maturity-onset diabetes of the young and late-onset type 2 diabetes mellitus in caucasians. J Clin Endocrinol Metab. 85:1323-6.
108. Inoue, H., *et al.* 1996. Sequence variants in the sulfonylurea receptor (SUR) gene are associated with NIDDM in Caucasians. Diabetes. 45:825-31.
109. Hani, E.H., *et al.* 1997. Genetic studies of the sulfonylurea receptor gene locus in NIDDM and in morbid obesity among French Caucasians. Diabetes. 46:688-94.
110. Hansen, T., *et al.* 1998. Decreased tolbutamide-stimulated insulin secretion in healthy subjects with sequence variants in the high-affinity sulfonylurea receptor gene. Diabetes. 47:598-605.
111. t Hart, L.M., *et al.* 1999. Variants in the sulphonylurea receptor gene: association of the exon 16- 3t variant with Type II diabetes mellitus in Dutch Caucasians. Diabetologia. 42:617-20.
112. Sreenan, S.K., *et al.* 2000. Calpain-sensitive pathways in insulin secretion and action-a pathophysiologycal basis for type 2 diabetes? Diabetes. 49 (Suppl 1):A62.
113. Cox, N.J., Horikawa, Y., Oda, N., and Hanis, C.L. 2000. Genetic variation in the calpain 10 gene affects the susceptibility to type 2 diabetes in Mexican Americans. Diabetes. 49 (Suppl 1):A7.
114. McCarthy, M.I., Froguel, P., and Hitman, G.A. 1994. The genetics of non-insulin-dependent diabetes mellitus: tools and aims. Diabetologia. 37:959-68.

8
THE MOLECULAR BASIS OF INSULIN ACTION AND INSULIN RESISTANCE

Joseph Avruch, M.D.
Massachusetts General Hospital, Harvard Medical School, Boston MA 02114

INTRODUCTION

Type 2 diabetes (previously called non-insulin dependent diabetes, NIDDM) is a common, phenotypically heterogeneous syndrome that has a strong genetic basis, most clearly indicated by the roughly 70% concordance in identical sibs, a concordance at least twice as high as in nonidentical sibs, and also considerably higher than the 30-40% concordance observed in identical twins sets, wherein one sib has autoimmune Type 1 diabetes (1). Despite this convincing evidence for heritability, it is clear that environmental factors greatly affect the penetrance of the Type 2 diabetic phenotype. In particular, dietary composition, overall calorie excess leading to weight gain in adult life, and low physical activity each strongly promote the expression of Type 2 diabetes (2). Moreover, epidemiologic evidence points to strong correlations between several aspects of the intrauterine environment and prenatal nutritional experience and the occurrence of Type 2 diabetes as an adult. This has been well described in the Native American population known as the Pima Indians of Arizona; in comparing the offspring of Type 2 diabetic mothers, the presence of hyperglycemia in utero is associated with a much higher prevalence of diabetes in adult life than occurs if the mother became hyperglycemic only after the pregnancy. Infants of hyperglycemic diabetic mothers are hyperinsulinemic in utero and large at birth, reflecting the strong positive influence of insulin on fetal growth. Conversely, evidence both in the Pima and several other populations (UK, Hispanic-American) indicates that low birth weight (<2500gms) and low weight at one year also correlate positively with the emergence in adult life of a syndrome of insulin resistance, hypertension and excess atherosclerotic vascular disease (2-7).

A plausible hypothesis suggests that genetically endowed insulin resistance is manifest during fetal life as deficient body growth. Although growth impairment is eliminated during childhood, the insulin resistance remains, and, when compounded by obesity and physical inactivity in late adult life, becomes expressed as NIDDM (8). Conversely, most authorities currently favor a more Lamarckian view, based on the idea that metabolic systems, like neural development, are plastic during fetal and early postnatal life, and can be influenced by the ambient nutritional milieu. Low birth weight is thus proposed to reflect fetal malnutrition, which produces a permanent reprogramming of metabolism toward insulin resistance and limited beta cell reserve. Considerable support for this latter view is provided by studies in rodents which show that nutritional manipulations of the pregnant mother can promote the development of diabetes in the offspring and in turn the prevalence of diabetes in the second generation (9). Thus, a hyperglycemic intrauterine milieu, a small-for-date birth size, excessive weight gain as an adult, especially in an abdominal distribution, a diet high in refined carbohydrate and saturated fat and physical inactivity all independently contribute to the penetrance of the diabetic phenotype in adult life. Clearly, the majority of individuals who exhibit these predisposing features do not develop Type 2 diabetes; these environmental or acquired inputs must interact with the underlying genetic endowment in an additive or synergistic fashion, so as to bias nutrient metabolism toward a diabetic phenotype (10). In turn, several of these "environmental" conditions are themselves conditioned by genes, especially obesity (11), but also birth size (12) and possibly some aspects of energy expenditure, e.g., the level of "involuntary" physical activity (13). In view of the ongoing revolution in genomics, identification of the genes contributory to Type 2 diabetes is likely to be accomplished within the next decade. Nevertheless, once the identity and association of specific genes with susceptibility to Type 2 diabetes has been clearly ascertained, defining their relative contribution to the diabetic phenotype and the biochemical basis for their action will continue to present formidable challenges.

A crucial precondition to the identification of Type 2 diabetes genes and their mode of action will be the careful delineation of phenotype. Type 2 diabetes is defined at present entirely by the presence of fasting glycemia above a specific level, and by the delayed clearance of postprandial hyperglycemia in the absence of beta cell autoimmunity, pancreatic disease, or other known causes of nonketotic hyperglycemia. Approximately 80% of Type 2 diabetic subjects in the United States are obese (i.e., $\geq$ 30% above ideal body weight), whereas the minority of Type 2 diabetic subjects in Japan are obese. Physiologically, the syndrome in both populations is characterized by the concomitant occurrence of impaired insulin secretion and defective responsiveness to insulin at the target tissues relevant to nutrient metabolism i.e., skeletal muscle, liver and adipose tissue.

Considerable evidence indicates that hyperglycemia per se contributes to both of these defects and correction of hyperglycemia, whether accomplished by dietary manipulation, oral hypoglycemic agents or insulin injection, if sustained for days to weeks, will ameliorate, but not eliminate, both defects (14). Considerable debate has focussed on which of the residual, presumably preexisting defects in insulin action and beta cell function is the "primary" precursor, i.e., the genetically endowed component that predisposes to Type 2 diabetes in later life (15,16). Nearly all studies of individuals with normal glucose tolerance who are thought to be "genetic" prediabetics because both parents exhibit clinical Type 2 diabetes, show evidence for the presence of resistance to the hypoglycemic action of insulin. Nevertheless, subtle abnormalities in insulin secretion have also been observed in such prediabetic individuals. Nearly all examples of rare, monogenic forms of Type 2 diabetes, i.e., the MODY syndromes, are attributable to defective beta cell function (see Chapter 5). Moreover, it is well known that individuals with severe insulin resistance due to genetic defects in the insulin receptor or spontaneous anti-insulin receptor antibodies may exhibit only moderately impaired glucose tolerance, because compensatory insulin secretion is of sufficient vigor to maintain near-normoglycemia. An obvious inference is that although defective insulin action may be "primary" in the genesis of a large fraction of instances of Type 2 diabetes, the penetrance of fasting hyperglycemia is highly dependent on a coexisting defect in the beta cell, whether genetic or acquired. The possibility that the defects responsible for insulin resistance also underlie defective beta cell function has been highlighted by the finding that insulin itself acting through the beta cell insulin receptor, is a positive regulator of insulin gene transcription (17). Moreover, selective ablation of insulin receptor gene expression in the beta cell, using the cre-lox methodology, results in defective glucose-stimulated insulin secretion (18) (see Chapter 9). The purpose of this chapter is to review the concept of insulin "resistance" and current information regarding the biochemical pathways through which insulin regulates nutrient metabolism, especially glucose uptake. It is plausible to infer that the genetic loci ultimately shown to be linked to the insulin resistance that underlies Type 2 diabetes will encode elements that are directly involved in these pathways, or that act indirectly, through a series of steps, to interfere with the function of this pathway. Chapter 7 discusses the biology of the beta cell.

INSULIN REGULATION OF METABOLISM

A useful classification of insulin's actions on nutrient metabolism divides these into two major categories – anabolic and anticatabolic (19). The anabolic actions are those involving uptake of nutrients from the circulation into cells and their conversion to macromolecules and/or storage forms. Such actions include the stimulation of glucose transport into muscle and adipose tissue and its conversion to glycogen and potentially to triacylglycerol fatty acid through de novo fatty acid synthesis in liver and adipose tissue; the stimulation of amino acid transport into liver, muscle and adipose tissue, concomitant with the stimulation of protein synthesis initiation; stimulation of lipoprotein lipase expression, fatty acid uptake into adipose tissue, and triacylglycerol synthesis. In each instance, the stimulation of nutrient uptake and its channeling within the cell occur as parallel responses that share common upstream regulators, e.g., the insulin receptor itself, phosphatidylinositol 3-kinase (PI 3-kinase), etc. (see below), whose input diversifies into distinct biochemical pathways composed of elements that are subject to multiple other inputs, so that each of insulin's ultimate downstream targets can be independently regulated. Thus, GLUT4 mediated glucose entry and glycogen synthase are activated in parallel by insulin and neither event is dependent on the occurrence of the other; these processes are however functionally coupled because glucose-6-P generated from increased transport is both a precursor of UDP glucose, and an allosteric activator of glycogen synthase. Moreover, the activation of glucose transport itself reflects the operation of several individual component biochemical reactions that are each simultaneously but independently regulated; an increase in the rate of GLUT4 exocytosis to the cell surface, a somewhat smaller decrease in the rate of GLUT4 endocytosis back into the cell interior, and perhaps a change in the intrinsic activity of the GLUT4 transporter polypeptide (20). Similarly, the stimulation of protein synthesis is a complex, multistep process that involves several dozen polypeptides. Insulin activation is achieved through changes in the activity of amino acid transporters, several initiation factors as well as ribosome phosphorylation (21).

The anticatabolic actions of insulin are those that oppose the mobilization of energy stores, their hydrolysis, release into the circulation, and interconversion for the purpose of oxidative utilization. Examples include insulin inhibition of glycogenolysis in liver and muscle, inhibition of adipocyte triglyceride hydrolysis (lipolysis), inhibition of proteolysis in liver and skeletal muscle, inhibition of ketogenesis and gluconeogenesis by the liver. Each of these processes is strongly promoted by cAMP generated intracellularly in response to glucagon (in liver) or beta-adrenergic catecholamines (in adipose tissue and muscle). When insulin target tissues are incubated *in vitro*, the rate of these catabolic processes is very low in the absence of added catabolic hormone (i.e., a stimulus to cAMP production) and the inhibitory action of insulin is quantitatively small and may become indiscernible. However, these catabolic processes exhibit substantial "tonic" activity *in vivo* (presumably driven in part by basal secretion of various catabolic hormones and the activity of the autonomic nervous system) that is inhibitable by insulin. At a biochemical level, the anticatabolic actions of insulin, at least on carbohydrate and fat metabolism, are largely accounted for by the ability of insulin to inhibit the accumulation of cyclic AMP and to activate reactions that oppose the cAMP-directed protein phosphorylation mediated by the cyclic AMP dependent protein (Ser/Thr) kinase (e.g., by insulin activation of protein (Ser/Thr) phosphatases) (22).

An aspect of physiologic importance is the relative sensitivity of the various metabolic pathways to insulin. It has been appreciated for many years that the concentration of insulin required for half maximal inhibition of catabolic responses, e.g., lipolysis, is ten-fold or more lower than for the stimulation of anabolic responses, e.g. activation of glucose transport (19). This is true whether examined using a single cell type *in vitro* under conditions wherein it is certain that insulin-induced responses reflect the activation of a single homogenous set of insulin receptors (23), or *in vivo,* in the whole organism (24). Physiologically, such differential responsiveness is entirely consistent with insulin's role as the primary regulator of nutrient utilization in both the fasted and fed states. Thus, when food is taken in, plasma glucose rises stimulating insulin secretion by the beta cell; the resulting high levels of insulin are sufficient to promote anabolism, i.e., the rapid uptake and storage of nutrients. During the interprandial interval, blood glucose falls, insulin secretion recedes and insulin levels fall below those necessary to promote glucose transport into skeletal muscle and adipose tissue. This is an appropriate adaptation to absent food intake, as a continued vigorous uptake of glucose out of the circulation during fasting for the purpose of storage in insulin-sensitive tissues such as skeletal muscle would only serve to divert blood glucose from the insulin-nonresponsive tissues, especially the CNS. The resulting fall in blood glucose would endanger the metabolism of the brain, which is entirely dependent on circulating glucose for its oxidative energy needs. Nevertheless, a continued restraint on catabolism remains necessary during fasting, so that energy stores are released at the slowest rate compatible with the maintenance of cerebral metabolism, thereby preserving an adequate energy supply for the longest possible interval until food again becomes available. This restraint of catabolism is provided by insulin, at concentrations far below those capable of promoting anabolism. The lack of such restraint is reflected by the syndrome of diabetic ketoacidosis, i.e., the uncontrolled lipolysis, ketogenesis, gluconeogenesis and proteolysis that occurs as a consequence of the nearly complete deficiency of insulin action resulting from the profound loss of beta cell function in Type 1 diabetes.

The implication of this differential sensitivity to insulin of anabolism vs. anticatabolism for the phenotype of insulin "resistant" states is simply that partial deficiencies of insulin action (due either to diminished insulin secretion or altered tissue responsiveness) will be manifest primarily as impaired anabolism, i.e., inadequate glucose uptake and storage at postprandial insulin concentrations, whereas the restraint of catabolism (e.g., lipolysis, ketogenesis) remains essentially undisturbed. This provides much of the explanation for the evolving metabolic profile of Type 2 diabetes, where impaired postprandial glucose clearance occurs initially with little or no evidence of accelerated catabolism, e.g., gluconeogenesis or ketosis. Thus, the nondiabetic offspring of Type 2 diabetic parents, or the nondiabetic with a Type 2 diabetic identical sib, exhibit a modest impairment in insulin-stimulated glucose uptake into skeletal muscle, but no detectable defect in the insulin suppression of hepatic glucose output. As the insulin resistance worsens, and especially when the insulin resistance becomes compounded by defective insulin-secretion, a lessening of the anticatabolic restraint becomes evident, chiefly by an increased rate of hepatic gluconeogenesis, a major determinant of fasting blood glucose (25). Ketogenesis usually remains suppressed throughout, although rarely, sufficient stress-induced secretion of catabolic hormones can overwhelm the residual insulin effect to produce ketoacidosis in a Type 2 diabetic subject.

Although classically considered a hormone concerned with metabolic regulation, insulin is closely related in structure and functional capability to the growth factors and developmental regulators, insulin-like growth factor-1 (IGF-1) and IGF-2. Similarly, the insulin receptor is highly homologous to the receptor for IGF-1 (IGF-1R) and each receptor, although it binds its cognate ligand with 30-100 fold higher affinity than the other ligand, can be fully activated by either ligand. The IGF1R binds IGF-1 and IGF-2 with comparably high affinity. The insulin receptor is expressed as two isoforms, A and B, which differ only by the presence of 12 amino acids, encoded by exon 11, that are present at the carboxyterminus of the α subunit in the B isoform (26) . Whereas the two insulin receptor isoforms bind insulin in a fairly similar manner, the shorter insulin receptor-A isoform, which is the form predominantly expressed in embryonic tissues, has a ten-fold higher affinity for IGF-2 than does insulin receptor-B; insulin receptor-A binds IGF-2 nearly as well as it binds insulin (27). IGF-2 is the dominant growth factor in fetal life, and probably signals through both the IGF-1R and the insulin receptor-A, i.e., insulin receptor-A probably contributes to fetal growth. The downstream responses to insulin receptor (A or B) activation are qualitatively the same whether insulin or IGF-2 is the ligand employed. Moreover, the kinase domains of the insulin receptor and IGF-1R exhibit nearly 85% identity in amino acid sequence, and the downstream responses to activation of the two different receptors, examined on the same cell background, are also very similar, differing somewhat in quantitative potency; the IGF1R is more active than the insulin receptor in promoting mitogenesis and inhibiting apoptosis, but there is little evidence to indicate major qualitative differences (28,29). The insulin receptor and the IGF-1R both initiate a broad array of responses that are typical of all ligands acting through receptor tyrosine kinases in cell culture settings. Not only are nutrient uptake and protein synthesis activated, but cell cycle dynamics are altered, usually with an acceleration of cell cycle progression, leading to cell division, or occasionally by cell cycle arrest followed by cellular differentiation. Although such responses to insulin are often viewed as "artifacts" resulting from overexpression of the insulin receptor tyrosine kinase in an "inappropriate" cell background, they more likely reflect an aspect of insulin action that occurs *in vivo*, only during embryonic or fetal development. Despite the current interest in the role of insulin signalling during fetal life as a determinant of insulin resistance in adulthood, the discussion that follows will focus primarily on those signalling pathways that underlie the regulation of nutrient metabolism in the adult organism, as this is the physiologic program whose derangement typifies Type 2 diabetes.

INSULIN SIGNAL TRANSDUCTION PATHWAY

All of insulin's actions are initiated by the binding of insulin to a single receptor, a member of the transmembrane receptor tyrosine kinase family (Fig. 1) (30). The insulin receptor is encoded by a single gene on

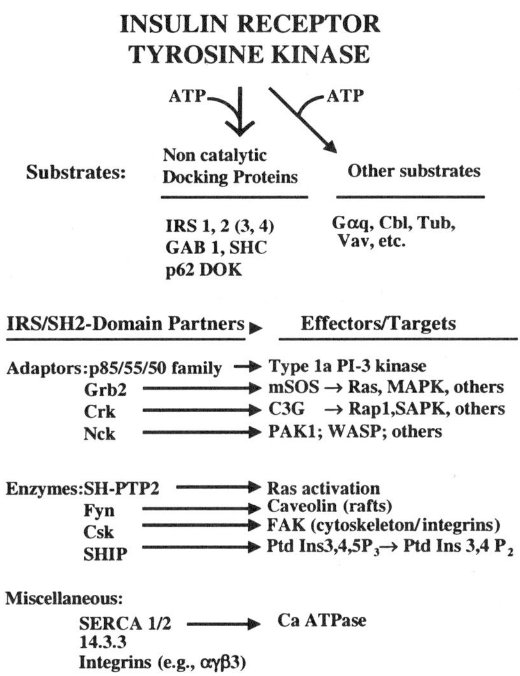

Figure 1. Signaling molecules in the insulin-stimulated signal transduction pathway.

chromosome 9, whose 22 exons encode two proreceptor polypeptides of 1343 or 1355 amino acids, reflecting alternative expression of exon 11. The proreceptor polypeptide is processed posttranslationally into a heavily glycosylated extracellular "alpha" subunit (719 or 731 amino acids), which bears the insulin binding site, and a transmembrane "beta" subunit (620 amino acids), whose extracellular, glycosylated extension is covalently linked to the alpha subunit through disulfide bonds, and whose intracellular extension, approximately 400 amino acids in length, encompasses three domains, a juxtamembrane segment (about 50 amino acids), a tyrosine kinase domain (about 250 amino acids) and a noncatalytic carboxyterminal tail (about 100 amino acids). The mature receptor is assembled at the cell surface in the form of two ($\alpha\beta$) structures covalently linked through disulfide bonds between the two α subunits. Each $\alpha\beta$ structure subunit can bind insulin with a K_D of somewhat over 10^{-8}M, however physiologic action occurs through the binding of insulin to a single, high affinity site (K_D approximately 10^{-9}M) generated by the two $\alpha\beta$ assemblies. Binding of insulin to this site causes the disinhibition of the tyrosine kinase domain, followed instantly by an extensive transmolecular phosphorylation of one beta subunit by its partner, that involves at least 6 of the 13 tyrosine residues on the beta subunit intracellular extension, distributed in all three domains. Transphosphorylation of a cluster of three tyrosine's situated on a segment in catalytic subdomain VIII, known as the "activation" loop, is crucial for activation of the receptor kinase itself; in fact, once this loop undergoes multiple tyrosine phosphorylation, insulin may be removed from the α subunit binding site with no loss in receptor kinase activity. Insulin receptor kinase inactivation requires the action of protein tyrosine phosphatase. Such a situation may occur physiologically when the activated receptor enters an endocytic compartment; acidification of the vesicle interior will result in dissociation of insulin, however the receptor kinase, which is directed into the cytosol, remains active until tyrosine dephosphorylation of the "activation" loop occurs. The phosphorylation of receptor tyrosine residues outside the catalytic domain, although not crucial to activation of the kinase, is nevertheless important to receptor signalling. This is best understood for tyrosine 960, the beta subunit tyrosine located in the juxtamembrane domain in the motif, NPXY. Phosphorylation of this tyrosine creates a binding site for the PTB (phosphotyrosine binding) domains found in several insulin receptor substrate proteins, such as the IRS proteins and Shc; elimination of Tyr 960 does not impair insulin activation of receptor kinase activity, however the mutation of 960 prevents phosphorylation of these protein substrates in vivo, and essentially all downstream signalling (31). The function of the two phosphotyrosines in the beta subunit noncatalytic carboxyterminal tail is less well understood; in cell culture systems, mutation of these residues to nonphosphorylatable amino acids, or truncation of the tail itself, appears to unbalance the relative intensity of signal outflow into metabolic versus mitogenic pathways.

The insulin receptor subfamily, including IGF-1R and the insulin-related receptor (IRR), differs in several ways from other members of the receptor tyrosine kinase (RTK) family that are important to its function as a signal transducer. In the absence of ligand, most other RTKs exist as monomers, which dimerize upon ligand binding, thus permitting transphosphorylation of the intracellular extensions. Although the insulin receptor is an obligatory covalent $(\alpha\beta)_2$ dimer in the absence of insulin, it is likely that insulin binding promotes a further apposition of the two $\alpha\beta$ segments within the dimer. Because the insulin receptor is an obligatory covalent $(\alpha\beta)_2$ dimer the tendency toward transphorylation and autoactivation in the absence of ligand is likely to be high. As initially suggested from enzymological and mutational analyses (reviewed in 32), structural studies have established that the insulin receptor possesses an exceptionally efficient autoinhibitory mechanism, wherein the unphosphorylated activation loop actually obstructs the ATP-binding site, greatly suppressing ligand-independent autophosphorylation. The binding of insulin to the extracellular domain somehow dislodges the activation loop from the ATP-site, permitting autophosphorylation and kinase activation to proceed. The multiple tyrosine phosphorylation of the activation loop not only prevents the return to an inactive configuration on removal of insulin, but also probably contributes to the configuration of the polypeptide substrate-binding site (33). The advantages conferred by the preassembly of the insulin receptor as an obligatory dimer may be in the speedier activation that occurs after ligand addition, and in the creation of an additional layer of regulation – i.e., through the need for phosphatase action in addition to ligand removal to achieve receptor kinase inactivation.

The new receptor phosphotyrosines generated upon insulin binding act to create a binding site for polypeptides that contain domains capable of specific binding to short amino acid sequences that contain a phosphotyrosine (34). The first such domains to be defined were called Src homology-2 (SH2) domains, so-called because they are found in each member of the Src subfamily of nonreceptor tyrosine kinases. SH2 domains bind to motifs containing phosphotyrosine and the 4-6 amino acids immediately carboxyterminal (35). PTB domains bind to phosphotyrosine in the motif NPXY (36,37). SH2 domains have been identified in numerous catalytic proteins that act as effectors of RTK signalling and in noncatalytic proteins that act as adaptors by bridging phosphotyrosine motifs to catalytic effector proteins. Examples of such SH2 domain-containing adaptors include the p85/55/50 family of SH2 domain-containing adaptors for Type 1a PI 3-kinases; Grb2, an adaptor for the guanylnucleotide exchanger mSOS (an activator of Ras and possibly Rac) and perhaps other partners; Crk and Nck, which each bind multiple candidate effectors. Once recruited to the receptor through their SH2 domains, some effectors undergo activation by tyrosine phosphorylation, e.g., phospholipase Cγ (PLCγ), whereas others are activated in an allosteric manner (e.g., PI-3K). Moreover, these effectors are brought in apposition with their substrates, e.g., Ptd Ins 4,5P_2 or Ras-GDP. The recruitment and activation of these effectors as mediated by the phosphotyrosine-SH2 domain interaction serves to generate a diverse set of secondary signals. In effect, the initial signal of tyrosine phosphorylation is translated into an array of chemically and functionally distinct signals going downstream, primarily in the form of lipid-derived messengers such as diacylglycerol (DAG), inositol trisphosphate (IP_3), PI-3,4,5P_3 etc. and activated forms of small GTPases, such as Ras-GTP, Rac-GTP etc.

Insulin-stimulated insulin receptor tyrosine autophosphorylation does not cause recruitment of known effectors to the insulin receptor that are sufficient to initiate signalling downstream (31). Rather, the insulin receptor mobilizes these effectors through the tyrosine phosphorylation of its substrate proteins, primarily the family of four insulin receptor substrate (IRS) polypeptides (discussed below), Shc, GAB1 and perhaps others yet to be identified (38). These insulin receptor substrates, once tyrosine phosphorylated by the activated insulin receptor tyrosine kinase, serve as the indispensable docking sites for recruitment and activation of the secondary signal generators. The reliance of insulin receptor signaling on its ability to phosphorylate substrates, especially those of the IRS family, has been demonstrated most clearly in cell lines of hematopoietic origin (32D cells) engineered to express abundant levels of (recombinant) insulin receptor but which lack expression of endogenous IRS polypeptides. These cells exhibit very weak insulin activation of a few downstream targets (e.g. Ras-MAPK activated through the insulin receptor-catalyzed tyrosine phosphorylation of the substrate Shc) and no activation at all of most pathways (PI 3-kinase, protein kinase B (PKB), p70 S6 kinase, glycogen synthase, protein synthesis initiation, mitogenesis, etc.). Responses to insulin can be restored by introduction of one of the IRS polypeptides (40). The coupling to glucose transport has not been evaluated.

When insulin receptors bearing mutations that delete or inactivate the kinase domain coexist with normal insulin receptors, the obligatory dependence of insulin receptor signaling on substrate tyrosine phosphorylation results in an interruption of signal transmission downstream; the inactive insulin receptor acts as a dominant inhibitor of the active insulin receptor gene product (41). Assuming equal abundance of active and inactive $\alpha\beta$ assemblies, half of the receptor $(\alpha\beta)_2$ dimers will contain one wildtype and one mutant receptor. Insulin receptor dimers consisting of one active and one mutant inactive kinase are almost completely deficient for signalling. The inactive $\alpha\beta$ halfdimer cannot transphosphorylate and activate the normal $\alpha\beta$, as is required to enable the normal $\alpha\beta$ to phosphorylate exogenous substrates. Moreover, although the mutant inactive $\alpha\beta$ can be transphosphorylated by the active $\alpha\beta$, insulin receptor autophosphorylation per se does not confer on the mutant inactive $\alpha\beta$ any ability to signal downstream. The clinical expression of this scenario is encountered in individuals who carry one allele encoding an inactive insulin receptor kinase, who exhibit insulin receptor kinase activity approximately 25-30% that of individuals with two normal alleles. Although clearly insulin resistant, these heterozygotes are usually not diabetic because compensatory hyperinsulinemia generates sufficient insulin receptor kinase activity to maintain near normal signalling downstream.

Insulin Receptor Substrates

Given the indispensable nature of insulin receptor-catalyzed substrate phosphorylation for insulin signalling, the identification of substrates and the demonstration of their specific participation in metabolic regulation is a critical task. The first substrate to be identified was IRS-1, a 180kDa predominantly cytosolic polypeptide that undergoes rapid tyrosine phosphorylation in response to insulin and IGF1 but not other RTK ligands (31). Four members of this polypeptide family have now been characterized. IRS-1, IRS-2 and IRS-4 are similar in architecture and size, at 1243, 1322 and 1257 amino acids in length respectively. IRS-1 and 2 are widely expressed, whereas IRS-4 is expressed primarily in pituitary. Other members of this family of phosphotyrosine-based docking proteins include IRS-3 and the more distantly related GAB1 and p62 DOK, respectively 482, 482 and 694 amino acids in length. Common to these proteins is the presence of a Pleckstrin Homology (PH) domain near the aminoterminus. In the IRS polypeptides, the PH domain is followed by a phosphotyrosine-binding (PTB) domain; the greatest conservation in amino acid sequence (40-45%) within this protein family occurs in this aminoterminal region. Each of the IRS polypeptides as well as GAB1 require an intact PH domain in order to undergo insulin-stimulated tyrosine phosphorylation in vivo, although direct binding of the PH domain to the insulin receptor has not been observed. The IRS polypeptides interact directly, through their PTB domain, with the juxtamembrane NPXY(P) motif on the autophosphorylated insulin receptor. IRS-2 also contains a novel domain (amino acids 591-786) that binds to the tyrosine phosphorylated activation loop of the insulin receptor. The amino acid sequence of the IRS polypeptides carboxyterminal to the PTB domain exhibits rather little (30-35%) conservation in overall sequence, however IRS 1,2 and 4 each contains 16-21 tyrosines, 8-9 of which are situated in the context YMXM or YXXM; the shorter IRS-3 contains roughly half this number. The YXXM/YMXM motifs are optimal both for the substrate specificity of the insulin receptor kinase, as well as for the binding of the SH2 domains of the p85/p55/50 adaptor family of the class 1a PI 3-kinases (42). In addition, the IRS polypeptides are multiply phosphorylated by the insulin receptor in a processive manner, including at tyrosines situated in motifs quite divergent from those most rapidly phosphorylated by the insulin receptor kinase. The diversity of phosphotyrosine-containing sequence motifs on the IRS polypeptides thereby enables the recruitment of proteins containing a wide array of SH2 domain-containing polypeptides, in addition to the p85/p110 PI 3-kinase heterodimer. Known IRS partners include the tyrosine phosphatase SH-PTP2, the nonreceptor tyrosine kinase Fyn, the adaptors Grb2, Crk and Nck, All three adaptors bind numerous candidate effectors; the identity of the physiologically relevant partners of Crk and Nck, first identified as oncogenes, are not known. By contrast considerable biochemical and genetic evidence indicates that mSOS, a Ras-specific guanyl nucleotide exchange enzyme, is a physiologic partner of Grb2. Recruitment of the Grb2/mSOS complex is the mechanism by which the insulin receptor promotes activation (i.e., GTP-charging) of the small GTPase, Ras. The activated insulin receptor also phosphorylates the adaptor Shc at a single tyrosine, creating a binding site for Grb2. In fact, Shc mediated recruitment of Grb2/mSOS may be the dominant pathway for insulin activation of Ras in some cell backgrounds, as it is for many RTKs. One effector commonly activated by other RTK but very poorly recruited by the IRS proteins is PLCγ (43); thus, an increase in diacylglycerol or cytosolic Ca^{++} (from intracellular stores) are not features of insulin signalling.

What Actions of Insulin are Mediated by the IRS Polypeptides?

Current information based on the phenotype of murine IRS gene knockout models (reviewed in detail in Chapter 9) indicates that IRS-1 and IRS-2 are each required for normal growth and glucose homeostasis. Both IRS-1 and IRS-2 knockout mice exhibit clear cut insulin resistance; IRS-1 deficient mice develop robust compensatory hyperinsulemia whereas IRS-2 deficient mice progress to diabetes because of an impaired beta cell compensation (44). The phenotype of IRS-3 knockout mice is essentially normal, including insulin regulation of glucose transport in isolated primary adipocytes, where IRS-3 is normally abundant (45). IRS-4 knockout mice show only subtle defects in growth, reproduction and glucose homeostasis (46). Thus, although each IRS polypeptide, if overexpressed in primary adipocytes, has the ability to promote GLUT4 translocation in the absence of insulin, only IRS-1 and IRS-2 appear to play a substantial role in intact mice. In the case of IRS-3, selective mutation of the four YXXM motifs to FXXM abolishes its ability to promote GLUT4 translocation (47). Consequently, it is plausible to conclude that the IRS polypeptides acting through their ability to recruit effectors through Y(P)XXM motifs (presumably the p85/p110 PI 3-kinase but perhaps others also) are physiologic mediators of insulin's program of metabolic regulation.

Interestingly, some responses to insulin may also be signaled through phosphotyrosine-independent actions of the IRS polypeptides (48). Thus, in the 32D hematopoietic cell line, activation of recombinant insulin receptors promotes mitogenesis only if an IRS polypeptide is also present. A mutant IRS-1 polypeptide, lacking all 18 tyrosines (IRS 18F) does not undergo insulin-stimulated tyrosine phosphorylation, fails to recruit PI 3-kinase or activate the p70 S6 kinase, but nevertheless, supports insulin-stimulated ^3H-thymidine incorporation at 20-60% of the maximal extent seen in 32D cells expressing wildtype IRS-1, although only at very high concentrations of insulin. Conversely, reintroduction of three YMXM motifs into IRS-1 18F restores the insulin-activation of PI 3-kinase and mitogenesis in a manner indistinguishable from wildtype IRS-1. A carboxyterminally truncated IRS-1 polypeptide containing the PH and PTB domains but no tyrosine phosphorylation sites, although unable to support insulin activation of PI 3-kinase, can nevertheless mediate insulin-stimulated phosphorylation of protein kinase B (PKB) Ser473 (see below), stimulation of mitogenesis (at 30-40% of maximal), and protection from apoptosis (49). Although there is no measurable insulin-induced increase in PI 3-kinase activity in a p85 immunoprecipitate, the in vivo responses to insulin in cells expressing these mutants are completely inhibited by the PI 3-kinase inhibitor, LY294002. Thus the IRS polypeptide appears to enable the insulin receptor to signal some responses and perhaps couple some isoform of PI 3-kinase, independently of IRS tyrosine phosphorylation.

Are There Insulin Receptor Substrates Other than IRS Polypeptides Important for Metabolic Regulation?

The evidence presently available does not permit a dogmatic conclusion as to whether insulin receptor substrates critical for metabolic regulation exist, apart from the IRS polypeptides. Nevertheless, some data support the view that such "alternative" substrates may be involved in the pathway through which insulin activates glucose transport. L6 myocytes engineered to respond to IL-4 show IL-4-stimulated IRS tyrosine phosphorylation comparable to that elicited by insulin, yet IL-4 fails to elicit GLUT4 translocation (50). Microinjection of anti IRS-1 antibody or peptides capable of inhibiting interaction of IRS-1 with the insulin receptor each inhibited by about 50% insulin-stimulated membrane ruffling (a PI 3-kinase-dependent response) in 3T3 L1 adipocytes and fibroblasts and insulin-stimulated mitogenesis in fibroblasts, without inhibiting insulin-stimulated GLUT4 translocation (51). Similarly, a more robust, adenoviral-mediated, overexpression of a peptide which inhibited interaction of IRS-1 with the insulin receptor almost completely inhibited insulin-induced IRS tyrosine phosphorylation and PI 3-kinase, p70 S6 kinase and MAP kinase activation without affecting insulin-induced PKB activation and GLUT4 translocation. The responses to insulin occurring in the presence of the dominant inhibitor of IRS-1 are nevertheless inhibited by wortmannin, indicating the existence of an IRS-independent mechanism for activation of PI 3-kinase (52,53). A number of studies have shown that the nonhydrolyzable GTPγS (54), as well as several G protein-coupled receptors acting through Gαq, (e.g., endothelin), promote GLUT4 translocation in 3T3 L1 adipocytes through a mechanism that is sensitive to inhibition by tyrosine kinase inhibitors and microinjection of anti-P-Tyr antibodies (55,56). Microinjection of an anti-Gαq antibody, or the Gαq-GTPase-activating protein (GAP), RGS2, into 3T3 L1 cells each inhibits insulin-stimulated GLUT4 translocation by 60-75%, whereas adenoviral-mediated overexpression of a constitutively active Gαq (Q209L) activates endogenous PI 3-kinase, and also increases glucose uptake in a wortmannin-inhibitable manner to 70% of the maximal level induced by insulin. Insulin stimulates Gαq tyrosine phosphorylation, and tyrosine phosphorylation has been reported to promote Gαq activation. Based on these data, it is proposed that Gαq, perhaps acting through a nonreceptor tyrosine kinase such as Src rather than an IRS polypeptide, is the critical intermediate recruited by insulin for the activation of that component of PI 3-kinase activity relevant to the insulin-induced translocation of GLUT4 to the surface membrane (57). The plausibility of this proposal is enhanced by recent work demonstrating the existence of a multiplicity of mechanisms through which G protein coupled receptors can recruit effectors previously associated exclusively with RTK signalling such as Src kinases, Ras, PI 3-kinase and others (58). Whether Gαq functions upstream or parallel to PI 3-kinase is currently unclear, inasmuch as stable expression of active Gαq (Q209L) in 3T3-L adipocytes promotes a wortmannin-resistant GLUT4 translocation without a concomitant activation of PI 3-kinase (59). A comparison of insulin-stimulated glucose transport in mice with selective skeletal muscle deficiency of Gαq versus IRS-1 or IRS-2 should be helpful in defining the relative contributions of these intermediates to insulin-stimulated glucose transport.

PI 3-kinase Activity is Indispensable for Insulin's Program of Metabolic Regulation

The demonstration that PI 3-kinase is indispensable to insulin's program of metabolic regulation has enabled the development of relatively specific pharmacologic and recombinant inhibitors and recombinant, constitutively active forms of the catalytic subunit of the PI 3-kinase. Similar tools have also been applied to the examination of the role of the Ras GTPase, and its major downstream effector pathway, the Raf/MAP kinase cascade, in metabolic regulation. This latter work (reviewed in 60) established in a convincing way that despite the central place of Ras and MAP kinase in the control of mitogenesis and cell differentiation, this pathway contributes insignificantly to the classical actions of insulin in the minute-to-minute control of carbohydrate and fat metabolism. In contrast, inhibition of PI 3-kinase using the chemical inhibitors wortmannin (61) or Ly294002 (62) interrupts essentially all of insulin's rapid effects on the control of nutrient metabolism including both the anabolic actions, e.g., activation of glucose transport, glycogen synthase, protein synthesis initiation, etc., and the anticatabolic actions, e.g., activation of the cAMP phosphodiesterase, inhibition of adipocyte lipolysis and hepatic gluconeogenesis, etc. Similarly, dominant inhibitory mutants of the p85 adaptor of PI 3-kinase (63), and microinjection of specific antibodies to the p110α PI 3-kinase catalytic subunit also block glucose transport and the other responses examined thusfar, except the activation of glycogen synthase (64).

The biochemical evidence compiled in mammalian systems pointing to the central role of PI 3-kinase in insulin action has been strongly supported by genetic work in invertebrates. The most comprehensive genetic evidence bearing on the identity of the components of the insulin-signal transduction system comes from work in the nematode *C. elegans*. Loss of function mutations in the insulin receptor/IGF1R homolog, Daf2 (65), leads to two phenotypes – one is the constitutive occurrence of an alternative developmental program known as the dauer larvae, an inert, spore-like state that occurs physiologically when early developing larvae are overcrowded or deprived of food. A second phenotype is uncovered if temperature-sensitive Daf2 loss-of-function mutants are allowed to develop at the permissive temperature and shifted to the nonpermissive temperature in adult life; the adult Daf2 mutant worms exhibit a substantial lengthening of lifespan. Thus, a wildtype Ins/IGF-1R limits and shortens longevity in *C. elegans*. A variety of strategies have uncovered the components of the signal transduction system downstream of the *C. elegans* insulin/IGF-1 receptor Daf2; in order of their site of action, these include – Age1, the PI 3-kinase (p110) catalytic subunit (66); PTEN, a D3 Ptd Ins phosphatase (67); the protein (Ser/Thr) kinases Ptd Ins 3,4,5P3-dependent kinase 1 (PDK1) (68) and PKB (69); and the forkhead (FKH) transcription factor, Daf16. Interestingly, an IRS homolog has not yet emerged from this classical genetic analysis in *C. elegans*, although mutations in the *Drosophila* IRS homolog, Chico, produce defects in cell size and growth similar to those resulting from mutations in the *Drosophila* insulin receptor (70). The *C. elegans* pathway identified downstream of Daf2 (insulin receptor/IGF1R) appears to be devoted entirely to the negative regulation of the Daf 16 transcription factor, inasmuch as loss-of-function mutations in Daf 16 reverse completely the phenotypes resulting from loss-of-function mutations in the upstream elements in the pathway (71). Biochemical studies have established that Daf16 and its mammalian homologs are direct substrates for PKB in vitro (72-75); thus, it appears that in *C. elegans*, Daf 16 is the dominant, if not the sole physiologic target of PI 3-kinase and PKB. It should be emphasized that the significance of FKH related proteins to insulin regulation of metabolism is not known at present (76-77), and metabolic regulation of energy storage and utilization in the nematode is quite different than in mammals. In fact, the phenotypes associated with insulin receptor/IGF1R loss-of-function in *C. elegans*, i.e., developmental arrest in diapause and increased longevity in the adult, are not those seen with insulin, insulin receptor, IRS-1 or combined IGF1R/IGF2R gene deletion in mice, man or *Drosophila* (reviewed in 44 and Chapter 9), suggesting that a broader set of PKB substrates, or additional, parallel pathways downstream of the insulin receptor exist in these organisms. Nevertheless, the conserved architecture of the insulin/IGF1R signaling pathway in *C. elegans*, in comparison to that constructed from biochemical studies in mammalian cells, provides very strong support for the conclusion that PI 3-kinase (as well as PDK1, PKB and PTEN) serve a central physiologic role downstream of the insulin receptor.

Persuasive although indirect evidence indicates that one or more signalling outflows in addition to PI 3-kinase is in fact required to fully recapitulate insulin's program of metabolic regulation. In *C. elegans*, activating mutations in PKB are much more potent suppressors of Age 1 (PI 3-kinase) loss-of-function mutants, than of Daf2 (insulin receptor) loss-of-function mutants (69). In mammalian cells, the PI 3-kinase inhibitors, wortmannin and LY 294002, e.g., do not suppress insulin activation of mitochondrial Pyruvate Dehydrogenase (PDH), an important component of the lipogenic response (78). Overexpression of an inhibitory mutant of the p85 adaptor subunit of PI 3-kinase in CHO-IR cells, blocks insulin activation of glucose transport, but not glycogen synthase, whereas wortmannin blocks both processes (63). Moreover, although overexpression of various constitutively active recombinant forms of class 1a PI 3-kinase is sufficient to activate many (but not all, e.g., glycogen synthase) pathways activated by insulin, the downstream effects elicited in response to continuous, high grade PI 3-kinase activity do not show the same extent of activation relative to one another as occurs with insulin and may, in part, be recruited indirectly through mechanisms not ordinarily engaged by the more modest increases in PI 3-kinase activity incurred by insulin (64, 79-83). Activation of PI 3-kinase in 3T3 L1 cells by a variety of ligands other than insulin, e.g., PDGF or EGF, fails to promote GLUT4 translocation in cells responsive to insulin (84,85). Interestingly, despite comparable activation of PI 3-kinase activity, insulin generates much higher steady state levels of Ptd Ins 3,4,5P_3 product in 3T3 L1 cells than does EGF or PDGF (86).

The most compelling evidence (87) for the existence of a second insulin-stimulated signal that is necessary, in addition to PI 3-kinase, for the activation of glucose transport is the finding that a cell permeant Ptd Ins 3,4,5P_3 analog is unable to activate glucose transport by itself, but can overcome the wortmannin-induced inhibition of insulin-stimulated glucose transport. Conceivably, the failure of PDGF, EGF and IL-4 to promote GLUT4 translocation may reflect their inability to recruit this PI 3-kinase-independent pathway, as compared to insulin. No information is available currently as to the identity of this "second" signal, apart from the certainty that it is unrelated to the Ras MAPK pathway.

PI 3-kinases

The primary signaling molecule synthesized by PI 3-kinase appears to be Ptd Ins 3,4,5P_3, which increases rapidly after insulin addition (64,88,89). Ptd Ins 3,4,P_2 accumulates more slowly, and may arise from the action of a 5' OH phosphatase on Ptd Ins 3,4,5P_3, such as the SH_2 domain-containing protein SHIP, or de novo from Ptd Ins or Ptd Ins 4P by the action of a class 1 or class 2 PI 3-kinase. Ptd Ins 3,4,5P_3 functions as a membrane-bound signalling molecule, like DAG or Ras GTP, and termination of the Ptd Ins 3,4,5P_3 signal requires the action of a 3'OH phosphatase.

Several subfamilies of Ptd Ins 3 kinases have been identified (64,88,90). The subfamily called class 1 is homologous to the *C. elegans* PI 3-kinase, Age1, and, thus, includes the primary isoforms recruited directly downstream of the insulin receptor. Four class 1 isoforms are currently known, each approximately 110kDa, each containing a lipid kinase catalytic domain near the carboxyterminus and a binding domain for Ras-GTP in the aminoterminal third of the polypeptide. Three of the four class 1 subfamily members (α,β,δ) are regulated by RTKs through the family of p85/55/50 SH_2 domain-containing adaptors, and are designated class 1a. Each of the p85/55/50 adaptor polypeptides contains two SH_2 domains and the class 1a p110 catalytic subunits bind tightly, to a segment of the adaptor situated between the two SH_2 domains. The p85 isoforms (α and β) differ from the shorter p55/50 variants by the presence of a unique aminoterminal extension, which contains a BCR-like domain, and a binding site for the Rho subfamily of small GTPases. The single class 1b PI 3-kinase catalytic polypeptide (p110γ) is not regulated by RTKs, but by the $\beta\gamma$ complex of heterotrimeric G proteins; p110γ does not bind a p85/55/50 adaptor, but rather a p101 polypeptide.

Class 1 PI 3-kinases are believed to phosphorylate only Ptd Ins 4,5,P_2 in vivo, to give the membrane bound lipid signal, Ptd Ins 3,4,5P_3. (88). The recruitment of class 1a PI 3-kinase occurs through the binding of p85/55/50 SH_2 domains to IRS phosphotyrosines in YMXM or YXXM motifs. Optimal activation of Type 1a p110 catalytic activity occurs through an allosteric mechanism that depends on the simultaneous engagement of both p85 SH_2 domains by a properly spaced set of Y(P)XXM or Y(P)MXM motifs on the same polypeptide. The simultaneous ligation of both p85/55/50 SH_2 domains results in synergistic activation, and properly spaced tandem YXXM sites exist on the IRS polypeptides (91). Once recruited to the vicinity of the membrane, it appears that occupancy of the Ras binding domain on p110 by Ras-GTP augments PI 3-kinase activity an additional 3-5 fold (92). It should be noted that class 1a PI 3-kinases also possess an intrinsic serine kinase activity, capable of phosphorylating the p85 adaptor subunit and of p110 autophosphorylation; the latter is autoinhibitory to the Ptd Ins kinase activity (64,88,90). The significance of the intrinsic p110 serine kinase to downstream signalling is uncertain, although it has been reported that a p110γ mutant devoid of lipid kinase activity and unable to activate PKB in vivo can nevertheless promote MAPK activation (93).

The class 2 PI 3-kinase polypeptide is approximately 170 kDa, lacks a Ras-binding domain but contains a modified C2 domain carboxyterminal to the catalytic domain, that is capable of Ca^{++} independent binding of phosphatidyl (Ptd) serine. Type 2 PI 3-kinase does not bind to either the p85/55/50 or p101 adaptor polypeptides, however class 2 PI 3-kinase is activated by insulin (94), through an as-yet-unidentified mechanism. Class 2 PI 3-kinase can phosphorylate Ptd Ins and Ptd Ins 4P, but not Ptd Ins 4,5,P_2. Class 3 PI 3-kinases phosphorylate only Ptd Ins to give Ptd Ins 3P. Although not initially considered a signalling molecule because it shows little change in overall abundance after ligand stimulation (88), it is now clear that Ptd Ins 3P may serve as a precursor to the "signalling" polyphosphoinositides, Ptd 3,4,P_2, Ptd Ins 3,4,5P_3 and the newly described Ptd 3,5P_2 (95). Moreover, Ptd Ins 3P is bound specifically by proteins containing so-called FYVE domains, many of which participate in endosome targetting; Ptd Ins 3P is in fact critical to Rab-mediated endosome docking, and thus to GLUT4 translocation (88,96).

1. PDK1
   a. Activation loop kinase for AGC subclass kinases:
      PKB (α,β,γ)/cAkt
      P70 S6 kinase (a,b)
      PKCs: conventional (α,β,γ)
      novel (δ,ε,θ)
      atypical (ζ,λ)
      PRKs, SGKs, Rsks
   b. Non kinase substrates
      Cardiac: F2,6Pase/PFK-2
      ? Others

2. PKBs/cAKT
   a. Glycogen synthase kinase 3
      (inhibited, ∴ increased glycogen)
   b. cAMP phosphodiesterase 3b
      (activated, ∴ decreased cAMP)
   c. Endothelial nitric oxide synthase
      (activated, ∴ increased blood flow)
   d. ? Increased glucose transport (GLUT4)
   e. Forkhead transcription factors (Daf16, FKHR, AFX)
      (inactivate, ∴ increased longevity, ? mechanism)
   f. Antiaptosis (BAD, caspases, FKHR, others)

3. Atypical PKCs (λ, ζ)
   a. ? Increased glucose transport
   b. ? Others

4. Dbl family guanyl nucleotide exchangers
   a. activate Rac, cdc42, ?Rho
      rearrange actin cytoskeleton
      activate protein kinase cascades

Figure 2. Direct effectors of Ptd Ins 3,4,5P_3.

Downstream Effectors of the Ptd Ins 3,4,5P$_3$ Signal

Considerable effort has focused on identification of Ptd Ins 3,4,5P$_3$ effectors (Fig. 2). An important early insight was the realization that PH domains are capable of specific binding to polyphosphoinositides and inositol polyphosphates (97-100). Ptd Ins 4,5P$_2$, which represents only about 5% of all Ptd Ins moieties, is nevertheless, twenty-fold more abundant than all 3' OH phosphorylated forms of Ptd Ins (88). Thus, *bona fide* Ptd Ins 3,4,5P$_3$ binding partners must posses a substantially higher affinity for Ptd Ins 3,4,5P$_3$ (or Ptd Ins 3,4,P$_2$) over Ptd Ins 4,5P$_2$. In fact, a subset of PH domain-containing proteins do show selective binding of Ptd Ins 3,4,5P$_3$ or Ptd Ins 3,4P$_2$, consistent with the view that each of these is a likely candidate to be a physiologic PI 3-kinase effector (99). Among the candidate direct Ptd 3,4,5P$_3$ effectors, those that are best supported as physiologic effectors of insulin signal transduction are the protein kinases PKB/cAkt and PDK1 followed by the atypical isoforms of protein kinase C (PKC), λ and ζ. Other protein (Ser/Thr) kinases, such as glycogen synthase kinase-3 (GSK-3) and the p70 S6 kinase, are regulated in response to insulin in a wortmannin-sensitive manner, but do not interact directly *in vitro* with Ptd Ins 3,4,5P$_3$, These kinases have been shown to be situated downstream of a direct Ptd Ins 3,4,5P$_3$ effector. Thus, GSK-3, an inhibitor of glycogen synthase, is negatively regulated by insulin *in vivo* through a wortmannin-sensitive pathway, and is phosphorylated and inhibited *in vitro* by PKB, a direct Ptd Ins 3,4,5P$_3$ effector (101). p70 S6 kinase, a positive regulator of protein synthesis initiation, is activated by insulin in a wortmannin-sensitive manner *in vivo*, and phosphorylated and activated *in vitro* by PDK1, a direct Ptd Ins 3,4,5P$_3$ effector (102-103).

PKB and PDK1

Although genetic evidence in *C. elegans* identified PKB (69) and PDK1 (68) as gene products functioning downstream of the PI 3-kinase Age1, earlier biochemical experiments in mammalian systems had identified these protein kinases as likely Ptd Ins 3,4,5P$_3$ effectors. cAkt/PKB was described in 1991 as the cellular homolog of the vAkt oncogene, a protein kinase in the AGC subclass whose catalytic domain is about 40% identical to those of the PKCs, PKAs, p70 S6 kinase and the N-terminal catalytic domain of RSK (104-106). Three PKB gene products exist in mammals; each is 50-55 kDa, with a catalytic domain situated close to the carboxyterminus and a noncatalytic aminoterminal segment containing a PH domain. A series of reports in 1995 (107-109) established that PKB is activated rapidly by insulin, PDGF and other growth factors in a wortmannin-sensitive manner, independent of Ras/GTP. In addition PKB exhibits a specific, high affinity interaction with liposomes containing 3'OH phosphorylated Ptd Ins, that is mediated through the PKB-PH domain, with somewhat higher affinity for Ptd

Ins 3,4,P_2 over Ptd Ins 3,4,5P_3 (110). The binding of Ptd Ins 3,4,5P_3 to PKB *in vitro* does not per se cause activation, but is necessary to allow the activating phosphorylations (111,112,113). Two phosphorylation sites are crucial to PKBα activation, Thr308, in the activation loop of the catalytic domain, and Ser473, situated in a hydrophobic motif (FXXF<u>S</u>Y) carboxyterminal to the catalytic domain (114). A 55kDa protein kinase capable of phosphorylating Thr308 *in vitro*, in a reaction completely dependent on the presence of Ptd Ins 3,4,5P_3, was purified and named Ptd Ins 3,4,5P_3-dependent kinase 1 (PDK1) (115). The molecular structure of PDK1 revealed a catalytic domain of the AGC subclass located in the aminoterminal half of the polypeptide, and a noncatalytic carboxyterminal segment encompassing a PH domain that binds 3,4,5P_3 with high affinity (113). PDK1 itself appears to be constitutively active, *in vivo* and *in vitro* (116). The binding of Ptd Ins 3,4,5P_3 to PDK1 does not alter the catalytic activity of PDK1, but does promote its colocalization with PKB; of equal importance, the binding of Ptd Ins 3,4,5P_3 to the PKB-PH domain induces a conformational change in PKB that makes Thr 308 available for phosphorylation by PDK1. PDK1 is able to phosphorylate the activation loop of nearly all of the AGC subfamily of kinases *in vitro* including those of the p70 S6 kinase, Rsk N-terminal catalytic domain, all subclasses of PKC, the serum-glucocorticoid induced kinase (SGK), and PKA (116). The physiologic relevance for several of these candidate PDK1 targets has been established by demonstration that embryonic stem cells deficient in PDK1 fail to exhibit activation of PKB, p70 S6 kinase and RSK, whereas the activity of PKA remains intact; PKCs have not yet been evaluated (117). Thus, PDK1 is a *bona fide* effector of PI 3-kinase, that is recruited to sites of Ptd Ins 3,4,5P_3 synthesis, where it phosphorylates substrates based on Ptd Ins 3,4,5P_3 co-localization and the availability of the phosphorylation site. Of note, PDK1 not only binds the lipid signal, but also binds directly to its targets through a motif FXXF(S/T(P)/D/E)F, that corresponds to the Ser473 site on PKB. Homologous motifs are found on PKCs, PRKs, p70 S6 kinase and RSK but not PKA. When this motif contains a Ser or Thr, as in the case of PKB, p70 S6 kinase and the novel PKCs, the creation of a high affinity PDK1 binding site requires (Ser/Thr) phosphorylation, a reaction that is catalyzed by one or more as-yet-unidentified protein kinases; the insulin-activated kinase directed at this site (Ser473) in PKB has been tentatively named PDK2. It should be noted that PDK1 can also phosphorylate and activate at least one probable physiologic substrate that is not a protein kinase – cardiac 6-phosphofructose-2 kinase (PFK2); a comparable modification of PFK2 occurs *in vivo* in response to insulin and underlies the insulin stimulation of cardiac glycolysis (118). Thus, PDK1 may have substrates other than protein kinases, including some that directly mediate metabolic responses.

PKB is a classical multifunctional effector protein kinase of broad specificity, in the mold of PKA and MAP kinase (117,119,121). Over 40 agonists capable of PKB activation have been described, including several that employ PI 3-kinase-independent pathways, such as cAMP and Ca^{++} regulated mechanisms. The discovery that activating mutations in *C. elegans*' PKBs could suppress the phenotypes resulting from loss of function mutations in PI 3-kinase (Age1) provided independent evidence that PKB is in fact a physiologically significant component of the insulin/IGF1 signal transduction pathway, at least upstream of the *C. elegans* forkhead domain transcription factor Daf16. In fact, PKB can directly phosphorylate Daf16, as well as its mammalian homologs, FKHR and FKHRL1, and thereby negatively regulate the DNA binding activity as well as the nuclear localization of these forkhead transcription factors. Nevertheless, the role of this PKB-regulated subfamily of FKH transcription factors in insulin's program of metabolic regulation in mammalian cells is not known.

A number of PKB substrates clearly relevant to insulin regulation of metabolism have been identified. One such target is glycogen synthase kinase 3 (GSK-3), a 50 kDa protein kinase first identified as a potent negative regulator of glycogen synthase activity. Many GSK-3 substrates in addition to glycogen synthase are now known. Insulin causes wortmannin-sensitive inhibition of GSK-3 by promoting phosphorylation of a single serine near the GSK-3 aminoterminus; PKB can catalyze this phosphorylation both *in vitro* and *in vivo*. Thus PKB-mediated inhibition of GSK-3 may underlie, in part, insulin activation of glycogen synthase (GS). Considerable evidence exists for other mechanisms operative in the insulin activation of GS, especially an insulin-induced increase in GS phosphatase activity. By example, insulin activates GS in 3T3-L1 adipocytes in a wortmannin-sensitive fashion, however constitutively active PKB does not promote activation of GS, perhaps because of the low expression of GSK3 (122). Such phenomena do not undercut the likelihood that the pathway from insulin receptor to PKB to GSK-3 is a mode of physiologic regulation, but rather illustrates the multiple pathways that the insulin receptor can recruit to reach physiologic targets.

PKB can also phosphorylate and activate the cAMP phosphodiesterase isoform PDE3B that is activated by insulin in liver and adipose tissue. Mutation of a single PDE3B serine abrogates the response to insulin *in vivo* and to PKB, both *in vivo* and *in vitro*. Moreover, dominant inhibitory forms of recombinant PKB block insulin activation of PDE3B. Through its ability to suppress cAMP levels, PDE3B is an especially important element in the apparatus responsible for insulin's anticatabolic actions on glucose and fatty acid metabolism, specifically, the inhibition of lipolysis and gluconeogenesis (123).

As to the role of PKB more broadly in the responses attributed to PI 3-kinase in mammalian cells, the ability of constitutively active forms of both PKB and PI 3-kinase to act as dominant oncogenes establishes their pro-mitogenic action. Moreover, both PKB and PI 3-kinase are potent anti-apoptotic agents (120). Evidence has been presented in support of a variety of apoptotic effectors/regulators as direct PKB substrates and probable mediators of PKB's anti-apoptotic actions e.g., the Bcl2 homolog BAD, caspase 9 (and perhaps other caspases), the IκB kinase (necessary for generation of the anti-apoptotic transcription factor NFκB) and the FKHR transcription factors (reviewed in 117,120).

The Regulation of Glucose Transport Downstream of PI 3-kinase

In response to the very strong biochemical and genetic evidence for PKB as a physiologic effector downstream of the insulin receptor and PI 3-kinase, a large number of reports have examined the role of PKB in insulin activation of glucose transport. Essentially all reports agree that overexpression or conditional activation of PKB in 3T3-L1 adipocytes or the L6 myoblast cell line promotes strong activation of glucose transport and translocation of GLUT4 to the surface membrane (124,127). There is, however, considerable disagreement as to whether recombinant dominant inhibitors of PKB are capable of suppressing insulin-stimulated GLUT4 translocation in a specific manner. The main concern with the use of recombinant inactive PKB constructs as inhibitors is that they may interact with Ptd Ins 3,4,5P_3 itself, and block all PI 3-kinase effectors (not just PKB). In fact, the amount of Ptd Ins 3,4,5P_3 needed to engage other effectors relative to that required for PKB activation is not known, nor is the degree of PKB activation necessary to elicit each of its downstream effects known. By example, a recombinant, inactive PKB was reported to inhibit insulin activation of endogenous PKB, and to strongly suppress insulin-stimulated GLUT4 translocation without inhibiting another PI 3-kinase mediated, response, i.e., membrane ruffling (a Rac-GTP mediated response) (126). Conversely, another study showed that a somewhat different inactive recombinant PKB produced inhibition of endogenous PKB sufficient to suppress the insulin activation of protein synthesis completely and the activation of p70 S6 kinase partially, but gave no inhibition of insulin-stimulated amino acid or glucose transport (128). These discrepancies may arise from purely technical considerations; thus if different downstream responses have differential requirements for the vigor of PKB activation, as is known to be true for PKA, and the different dominant inhibitors generate differing degrees of PKB inhibition, then these apparently discordant results may all be compatible with a crucial role for PKB in GLUT4 translocation. Although the weight of evidence favors a role for PKB, it is nevertheless possible that the stimulatory effect elicited by PKB on glucose transport reflects a very indirect, nonphysiologic response to a potent oncogene, and the inhibition produced by overexpression of inactive PKB polypeptides may reflect a general sequestration of Ptd Ins 3,4,5P_3. If so, then the component of GLUT4 translocation that is mediated by Ptd Ins 3,4,5P_3 could be due, entirely or in part, to a Ptd Ins 3,4,5P_3 effector other than PKB.

The idea that insulin promotes GLUT4 translocation through several pathways, only one of which is regulated by PKB, is a plausible and attractive explanation for the many conflicting reports. In 3T3-L1 cells, insulin promotes externalization of GLUT4, GLUT1 and the transferrin receptor (TfnR), whereas a constitutively active PKB promotes externalization of GLUT4 only; moreover, Botulinum toxin (B or E)-catalyzed cleavage of vesicle SNAP protein reduces insulin-stimulated GLUT4 externalization by 65%, but abolishes the response of GLUT4 to PKB completely; Botulinum toxin E had no effect on TfnR mobilization (129). Thus, different outflows from Ptd Ins 3,4,5P_3 may control separate components of the GLUT4 recycling mechanism in response to insulin.

PKCs and PRKs

Atypical PKCs (aPKCs) and possibly novel PKCs (nPKCs) are currently the major alternative candidate effectors of Ptd Ins3,4,5P_3 action on GLUT4 translocation (130,131). A number of reports describe the ability of nPKCs (δ) and/or aPKCs (both ζ and λ) (132,133) to promote GLUT4 translocation in a variety of cell backgrounds, including primary adipocytes, L6 myocytes and NIH 3T3 cells (134-138). The ability of chemical and recombinant inhibitors of the PKCs to suppress GLUT4 translocation in response to insulin, but not hyperosmolality or growth hormone provides additional evidence for the role of these kinases in the insulin response. The mechanism by which insulin regulates these kinases however is poorly understood.

The PKCs are the largest of the protein kinase families within the AGC class of (Ser/Thr) protein kinases, and can be subclassified into three main subfamilies, whether using amino acid sequence alignment or the known mode of regulation (130,131). The architecture of the entire PKC family is characterized by a carboxyterminal catalytic domain that shares 40-50% identity across the entire family, and a more variable non-catalytic aminoterminal regulatory segment that contains two more highly conserved domains, a C1 domain, which contains two tandem zinc-finger motifs and a C2 domain. The "classical" PKCs (α,β,γ) are regulated by diacylglycerol (DAG), Ca^{++} and Ptd Ser. The more carboxyterminal of the two tandem zinc finger motifs in the C1 domain of the classical PKCs (cPKCs) binds DAG; the C2 domain binds Ptd Ser in a Ca^{++} dependent fashion. The nPKCs (δ,ε,η, Φ) are regulated by DAG in a Ca^{++} independent fashion, whereas the aPKCs (ζ and λ) do not bind either DAG or Ca^{++}. The protein kinase C-related kinases (PRKs) have 50% identity to the PKCs in their catalytic domain, but have a more divergent structure in their aminoterminal regulatory domain, which contains a C2 but no C1 segment; the PRKs contain a set of aminoterminal motifs not found in the PKCs that enable binding to activated forms of the Rho GTPases, RhoA and/or Rac1.

All PKCs require phosphorylation for activity (139-144). The complex sequence of phosphorylations required by the cPKCs is necessary to achieve proper folding and subcellular localization of the PKC polypeptides, but does not appear to provide a mode of regulation in response to extracellular stimuli. In contrast, phosphorylation does represent a mode of regulation for the nPKCs and aPKCs (139-141). The cPKCs and nPKCs undergo a sequence of phosphorylations initiated by phosphorylation of the activation loop, probably catalyzed by PDK1, followed by phosphorylation at two sites carboxyterminal to the catalytic domain, one of which is in a Ser Pro motif, and the other is situated within a hydrophobic motif homologous to that surrounding PKBα Ser473. In the cPKCs, these two C-terminal phosphorylations occur constitutively through an autophosphorylation that is triggered by the PDK1-catalyzed phosphorylation of the activation loop; thereafter cPKC activation occurs entirely through DAG binding (142,143). By contrast, the phosphorylation of the homologous hydrophobic site in the nPKCs appears to be catalyzed by one or more as yet unidentified protein kinases (144). The phosphorylation of the nPKCs by PDK1 is stimulated by both Ptd Ins 3,4,5P_3 and DAG, in an additive manner; in addition, recent evidence indicates that the phosphorylation of the C terminal FXXFSY site in the nPKCs is independently regulated by extracellular stimuli. Thus, the nPKCs are activated by DAG together with PDK1 and one or more (FXXFS/TY) kinases. The regulation of the aPKCs is uncertain; phosphorylation of the activation loop, which is probably catalyzed by PDK1, is necessary for activity, with the major regulatory step in aPKC activation, based on present information, appearing to be colocalization with PDK1 and PDK1-catalyzed aPKC phosphorylation (144). The PRKs are also substrates for PDK1. Regulation of the PRKs is mediated by binding to active Rho GTPases, phospholipids and PDK1-catalyzed phosphorylation, although the relative contribution of each input to receptor-induced PRK activation is not yet clear (145).

Several lines of evidence point to the nPKCs, aPKCs and possibly PRKs as effectors of PI 3-kinase. Thus, each of these kinases have been shown to interact with or undergo activation in response to Ptd Ins3,4,5P_3 or Ptd Ins 3,4,P_2 *in vitro* in preference to Ptd Ins4,5P_2 (146,147). As to regulation *in vivo*, a number of reports have demonstrated insulin and mitogen activation of the nPKCs and aPKCs; e.g., insulin activates PKCε and promotes its translocation to the membrane in fetal chick neurons, and activates and translocates PKCδ in primary cultures of neonatal rat skeletal myocytes (132). Insulin, EGF and PDGF have each been reported to activate the atypical PKCλ and ζ through wortmannin-sensitive, PI 3-kinase dependent pathways (148-150). Earlier reports established that insulin does not engender significant DAG accumulation nor support activation of the cPKCs. Such results support the conclusion that Ptd Ins 3,4,5P_3 is the likely mediator of insulin activation of the nPKCs and aPKCs. Whether insulin activation of the nPKCs and aPKCs occurs through a Ptd Ins 3,4,5P_3-induced allosteric effect, colocalization with and phosphorylation by PDK1 at the membrane, and/or colocalization with another membrane-based activator (e.g., a tyrosine kinase) (151) is unknown.

In summary, a considerable body of evidence supports the participation of PKB, PKCζ and/or λ, and perhaps PKCδ as mediators of insulin-stimulated GLUT4 translocation. The case for PKB as a physiologic mediator is strongest for several reasons: (1) the genetic evidence in invertebrates pointing to PKB as a physiologic effector of insulin receptor/IGF-1R signaling; (2) the almost complete understanding of the mechanism by which PKB is recruited and activated by the Ptd Ins 3,4,5P_3 signal (with the identity of the Ser473 kinase "PDK2" as the major unanswered question); and (3) the substantial number of probable physiologic PKB substrates already identified (e.g., GSK3, PDE-3B, FKHR, etc.). It should be mentioned, moreover, that PKB has been shown to phosphorylate and activate endothelial nitric oxide synthase (NOS) and is, thus, a candidate to mediate the insulin-induced increase in skeletal muscle blood flow that contributes significantly to the overall magnitude of glucose uptake *in vivo*. Conversely, the assignment of PKCs as effectors of insulin action cannot yet be made confidently, because: (1) insight into the regulation of the PKCs by Ptd Ins 3,4,5P_3 is much less advanced than for PKB; e.g., a specific binding site on PKCs for Ptd Ins 3,4,5P_3 has not been identified, and the rather modest activation *in vitro* by Ptd Ins 3,4,5P_3 alone as well as by PDK1-catalyzed phosphorylation leaves the physiologic importance of these phenomena open to question; (2) a lack of independent genetic evidence in support of a role for PKCs acting downstream of the insulin receptor and/or PI 3-kinase; and (3) the paucity of known direct nPKC or aPKC substrates clearly related to insulin action (although there is a report assigning to PKCζ a key role in the insulin stimulation of protein synthesis initiation) (152). Nevertheless, focusing only on glucose transport, the force of evidence in support of a role for PKBs and PKCs is similar, and, as a more detailed understanding of the molecular basis for GLUT4 recycling develops, it would not be surprising to find that both kinase subfamilies participate in the regulation of this process, either in a sequential or additive way, through different targets and/or different pathways that regulate the overall GLUT4 vesicle sorting phenomenon.

Other Insulin Receptor Targets Relevant to Glucose Transport

The activation of glucose transport is the most characteristic, and one of the most physiologically important actions of insulin. Consequently, a detailed understanding of the pathways employed by the insulin receptor to achieve this response is likely to reveal most or all of insulin's crucial signalling pathways. Unfortunately the molecular machinery controlling the trafficking of GLUT4 to and from the plasma membrane is incompletely understood (153-155) and thus the site(s) at which this process is regulated by insulin remain largely obscure. The majority of GLUT4 is located intracellularly in unstimulated adipose and muscle cells, mostly in a vesicular compartment whose composition appears to be distinct from that of the recycling endosomes that bear the TfnR and GLUT1. The mechanism for the intracellular sequestration of GLUT4 into this unique compartment is unclear, however at least one other protein, the insulin-responsive aminopeptidase (IRAP) is also resident in this vesicle. Insulin stimulation causes an approximately 10-20 fold increase in the rate of GLUT4/IRAP exocytosis, and a much smaller (2-4 fold) decrease in the rate of GLUT4 endocytosis. It is unclear whether the effect of insulin on GLUT4 exocytosis involves primarily a release of GLUT4 vesicles from a site of sequestration, a facilitation of the tethering/docking and fusion of the GLUT4 vesicle to the plasma membrane, or both. The intracellular GLUT4 is probably mobilized into a vesicle by the action of coat proteins, which may be recruited by GTP-occupied forms of the Arf GTPase and by the Arf-GTP-induced activation of phospholipase D, which enables vesicle budding (156,157). The targeting/docking and fusion of GLUT4 vesicles to the plasma membrane probably involves a set of vesicle-specific receptors (v-snares) and cognate plasma membrane binding partners (t-snares), aided by soluble factors, (e.g., NSF and SNAPS and Rab-GTPases) (158-162). The Rab GTP complexes recruit effectors necessary for the accurate tethering of vesicles to their target membrane and participates in the restructuring of the cytoskeleton that is required to enable docking (158,159). The ultimate fusion step appears to be mediated by the binding of v- and t-snares (160-163), however a variety of proteins appear to regulate accessibility of the v-and t-snares, e.g., Munc 18 and the recently described Synip (164); the association of these proteins with the t-snare is regulated by insulin. Which of these steps provide critical targets for the activation of GLUT4 exocytosis in response to insulin is not known. The discovery of Arf-specific guanyl nucleotide exchangers (e.g., GRP-1, cytohesin) that contain PH domains which bind Ptd Ins 3,4,5P_3 with high affinity provides one attractive candidate (165) and points to a site of regulation at the mobilization of GLUT4 vesicles. Consistent with this, insulin activates phospholipase D in cells overexpressing insulin receptor, but not in 3T3-L1 cells (166). Regulation of the docking process is also likely. An insight into the role of Ptd Ins 3P in vesicle transport has been provided by the discovery that the Rab 5 GTP effector, Early Endosomal Antigen-1 (EEA1), which is necessary for Rab 5-mediated vesicle transport, contains an FYVE finger domain, that binds specifically to Ptd Ins 3P; the ability of EEA-1 to bind Ptd Ins3P is necessary to enable snare-mediated vesicle fusion (96).

GLUT4 endocytosis, although stimulated by insulin to a much smaller extent than exocytosis, is not abrogated by inhibitors of PI 3-kinase. The regulated steps in endocytosis are not known. The GTPase Dynamin functions to pinch off the recycling endocytic vesicles, and is necessary for GLUT4 endocytosis; a GTPase deficient Dynamin mutant blocks GLUT4 internalization (167). Dynamin undergoes insulin-stimulated tyrosine phosphorylation, however the effect of phosphorylation on Dynamin function is not known.

Although the translocation of GLUT4 appears to be the dominant mechanism by which insulin activates transport, a body of indirect evidence indicates that once arrived at the plasma membrane, GLUT4 must still undergo an "activation" step. Thus, wortmannin inhibits glucose uptake in 3T3-L1 cells at tenfold lower concentration than that necessary for the inhibition of translocation (168). This suggests that the maintenance of GLUT4 transport activity requires higher concentrations of Ptd Ins 3,4,5P_3 than does GLUT4 translocation. Alternatively, a novel effector that has a higher affinity for wortmannin than PI 3-kinase may be necessary for GLUT4 activation.

The Rho family GTPases (RhoA-D, Rac1,2, cdc42, etc.) are important to cell division and growth, and particularly to the control of the actin cytoskeleton (169). The PI 3-kinases may provide a critical input to the control of the Rho family GTPases in response to specific stimuli. Consistent with this, insulin-induced membrane ruffling in cultured cells, a Rac-regulated function, is abrogated by the PI 3-kinase inhibitor wortmannin. Similarly, insulin activation of the cdc42/Rac-activated PAK1 protein kinase in L6 myotubes is blocked by wortmannin. The Rho family of small GTPases acts through the direct recruitment of Type 2 PI kinase and a variety of protein kinases. Most of the protein kinases controlled directly by the Rho subfamily, in addition to acting on substrates that regulate the assembly/disassembly of the actin cytoskeleton, also control cascades of MAP kinase-related protein kinases, i.e., the SAPKs/JNK and p38 kinase cascades, that like the Ras/Raf activated MAPKs, signal to transcriptional regulatory proteins and thereby control gene expression and ultimately determine cell phenotype. Although insulin has been observed to control the activity of many of the protein kinase pathways downstream of the Rho GTPases in a variety of cell backgrounds, there is little evidence at present as to the role of those kinases as positive effectors in insulin's programs of metabolic regulation in muscle liver and adipose tissue. An exception is the observation that inhibition of the insulin activation of the p38 kinase in 3T3-L1 and L6 myocytes inhibits insulin activation of glucose transport, without affecting insulin-stimulated GLUT4 translocation (170). Interestingly, insulin activation of p38 kinase is not sensitive to wortmannin.

Negative Regulation of Insulin Signaling

Complementing the activation of signaling pathways by insulin are the various mechanisms available to attenuate insulin signaling (Fig. 3).

Insulin Receptor Abundance

The insulin receptor is widely expressed, with 3000-5000 receptors present on most cells, and approximately tenfold higher numbers on the three

NEGATIVE REGULATION OF INSULIN SIGNALING

1. Insulin Receptor Abundance-Downregulation
   - a) insulin induced IR degradation
   - b) transcriptional regulation

2. Tyrosine Dephosphorylation
   - a) Protein Tyrosine Phosphatase 1b
   - b) transmembrane receptor PTPases
     e.g. LAR, RPTP α, T cell PTP

3. Insulin Receptor Substrate (Ser/Thr) phosphorylation
   - I) Inhibition of IRS Tyr phosphorylation
   - II) Inhibition of PI3 kinase docking

   a) Insulin: via PKB → ?mTOR
   b) Mitogens: via PKB → ?mTOR
   → MAPK
   via PKC → MAPKs
   c) Stress: via TNFR → SAPKs (?p38, others)
   via TOllR
   via IL-1R
   d) Nutrients: Glucose, FFA → ?DAGs → ?PKCs
   → Hexosamines →?
   e) Miscellaneous kinases - GSK-3, ?others

4. PTEN/MMAC- cleaves 3'OH phosphates from PIPs:
   Ptd Ins 3,4,5P $_3$ → Ptd Ins 4,5,P2
   Ptd Ins 3,4,5P $_2$ → Ptd Ins 4P

Figure 3. Factors which contribute to negative regulation of insulin signaling.

target tissues. The steady state number of insulin receptors on the cell surface is an important determinant of insulin sensitivity (A0.5), and many studies characterizing insulin resistant states in man and animal models have consistently detected modest decrements in the number of insulin binding sites on target cells in these states. The two relevant questions are: what is the mechanism of these decrements and what is their contribution to the insulin-resistance? As to the mechanism, little evidence supports impaired insulin receptor gene expression as the basis of the diminished insulin receptor number in Type 2 diabetes, or its precursor states; rather it appears that insulin receptor degradation is the major mechanism for downregulation. Insulin receptors are recycling continuously between the cell surface and an endosomal compartment, within which receptor-bound insulin is released following vesicle acidification. The ligand is directed to degradative pathways, whereas the receptor is partitioned in this endosomal compartment, either recycling to the cell surface, or entering a degradative pathway. In cell culture, the addition of insulin results in a decrease in the steady state level of total and cell surface insulin receptors, due to an increased rate of insulin receptor endocytosis and the diversion of a greater fraction of the recycling receptors into a degradative pathway (171). The magnitude of insulin receptor downregulation in the presence of saturating concentrations of extracellular insulin does not exceed 50% of the initial value. The biochemical mechanisms underlying ligand-induced internalization and degradation are not fully defined. The insulin receptor motif responsible for endocytosis via clathrin coated pits is the NPXY motif in the juxtamembrane region on the intracellular extension of the beta subunit; deletion of this motif diminishes the rate of insulin receptor endocytosis but does not reduce the insulin-induced increment in insulin receptor fractional degradation (172,173). Inactivation of the insulin receptor kinase ATP-binding site significantly diminishes both the rate of insulin-induced insulin receptor endocytosis, and the fractional degradation of the insulin receptor in the presence of insulin (174). Thus, degradation is accelerated by receptor autophosphorylation/ activation. Although the mechanism is uncertain, the SH2 domain containing insulin receptor substrate Cbl may be involved (175,176). Accelerated IRS degradation is another potential site of negative regulation; prolonged exposure of cells in culture to both insulin and glucocorticoids has been reported to increase the rate of IRS degradation (177). In clinical situations, all states of hyperinsulinemia are associated with a diminished steady state level of cell surface insulin receptor, whether the hyperinsulinemia is primary (e.g., due to insulin overproduction as in insulinoma or transgenic overexpression of insulin) or secondary to some preexisting mechanism of insulin "resistance".

As to the importance of such modest decrements in insulin receptor number to the genesis of insulin "resistance," studies *in vitro* using insulin–responsive isolated cells, e.g., primary isolated rat adipocytes, indicate that when measuring a downstream metabolic response to insulin e.g., activation of glucose transport or glycogen synthase, maximal activation is observed at insulin concentrations sufficient to occupy less than 10%, and probably less than 5% of the available insulin binding sites. This finding led to the concept of "spare" receptors, an unfortunately misleading term. All cellular insulin receptors, including those present in apparent "excess" of the number required for maximal activation of glucose transport, appear functionally equivalent. Activation of the insulin receptor occurs through an insulin-stimulated receptor autophosphorylation; once insulin binds, autophosphorylation and kinase activation is a highly concerted, essentially all-or-none reaction. Thus occupancy of 10% of receptors can be inferred to reflect the complete activation of 10% of receptors, while 90% of receptors remain inactive. If the receptor number is progressively diminished, one observes a shift of the A0.5 for the activation of glucose transport to progressively higher values with no change in Vmax, until total receptor number falls below the level of occupied receptors needed to elicit a maximal response, i.e., 5% to 10% of the original number. Thus although receptor number is an important determinant of A0.5, and insulin-resistant states are associated with a diminished number of insulin binding sites on target cells (usually adipocytes), in no instance is this decrement greater that 40-50% of normal levels (178,179); reductions of insulin receptor abundance of this magnitude produces minor degrees of insulin resistance (e.g., a twofold increase in A0.5 with no change in Vmax) and based on the behavior of various insulin receptor transgenic and gene deletion models in mice, is unlikely to contribute significantly to *in vivo* insulin resistance.

Tyrosine Dephosphorylation

Deactivation of insulin receptor and IRS-1 is mediated primarily by tyrosine dephosphorylation. The PTPase inhibitors, vanadate or peroxyvanadate added to cells in culture greatly enhance the subsequent response to insulin and, if given *in vivo* to diabetic rodents, promote hypoglycemia (180). Thus, the activity of PTPases and their access to the insulin receptor and IRS-1 greatly affect the duration and intensity of insulin receptor signalling. The identity of the PTPase(s) primarily responsible for insulin receptor tyrosine dephosphorylation remains uncertain. Insulin receptor tyrosine dephosphorylation occurs predominantly after insulin receptor internalization into endosomes (181,182). A variety of transmembrane, so-called "receptor" tyrosine phosphatases (LAR, PTPα) (183,184) and nonreceptor tyrosine phosphates (SH-PTP1, SH-PTP2, PTP-1B) have been shown to dephosphorylate the insulin receptor *in vitro* or on overexpression (185,186), however studies wherein the activity or abundance of specific PTPases has been reduced, either in cell culture (PTPα, SHP1, SHP2) (187,188) or in intact mice (LAR) (189) have failed to provide support for a physiologic role of these PTPases in insulin receptor tyrosine dephosphorylation. By contrast a significant body of work in cultured cells is consistent with an important role for PTP-1B as a negative regulator of insulin signalling (190), and this evidence is strongly reinforced by the phenotype of PTP-1B null mice (191). PTP-1B is localized to the endoplasmic reticulum through a domain near it C-terminus, with the phosphatase catalytic domain directed into the cytoplasm; thus situated, PTP-1B is a plausible candidate to mediate tyrosine dephosphorylation of the insulin receptor as the latter cycles through the endosomal compartment. PTP-1B null mice exhibit significantly enhanced insulin signalling, in association with an increased and more sustained insulin-induced insulin receptor and IRS tyrosine phosphorylation in liver and muscle. This is accompanied by a decrease in the glycemic excursion after glucose administration and a prolongation of the hypoglycemia engendered after an insulin injection. Moreover, contrary to expectation, the PTP-1B deficient mice, despite their enhanced responsiveness to insulin, fail to develop the obesity and insulin resistance that occurs in wildtype mice when placed on a high fat diet, despite comparable calorie intake. Interestingly, the insulin resistance seen in mice deleted of the gene encoding Gαi2 is accompanied by a substantial upregulation in the expression of PTP-1B (192).

Although the phenotype of PTP-1B null mice establish an important role for this phosphatase in the termination of insulin signalling, the relatively modest effects of PTP-1B gene deletion indicate that other PTPases can contribute to the control of insulin signalling; whether the other PTPases participate in the physiologic setting in wildtype mice (or man), or only serve as a backup in the PTP-1B null mice, is unknown. Characterization of the phenotypes of other PTP null models, singly and crossed into the PTP-1B null background, should clarify this issue.

PTEN/MMAC

PTEN was discovered as a candidate human tumor suppressor gene on chromosome 10q23; germline mutations in PTEN are found in patients with the Cowden syndrome, a state predisposed to breast and thyroid tumors. PTEN is a 403 amino acid protein most related in amino acid sequence to the dual specificity protein (Tyr and Ser/Thr) phosphatases (193). PTEN is highly and specifically active against the D-3 phosphorylated site on phosphoinositols and phosphatidylinositides, both *in vitro* and *in vivo* (194). Nearly all PTEN mutations associated with tumors occur in the phosphatase homology domain and result in catalytic inactivation. The best evidence as to the *in vivo* specificity is the finding that some PTEN mutations in Cowdens syndrome abolish phosphoinositide but not phosphotyrosine phosphatase activity (193,194). Additional support for the crucial role of PTEN as a negative regulator acting downstream of PI-3K is the identification of a loss-of-function mutant of *C. elegans* PTEN (Daf18) as a suppressor of both the Daf2 (insulin receptor) and Age1 (PI-3K) loss-of-function phenotype (67). In *Drosophila*, PTEN has been shown to act in opposition to Chico, a *Drosophila* IRS homologue, and PI3 kinase, and to be especially important in regulating the organization of the actin cytoskeleton (195). Despite the certainty as to the importance of PTEN in PI 3-kinase signalling, the role of PTEN in insulin-resistant states is unexplored.

Insulin Receptor/IRS Ser/Thr Phosphorylation

In addition to undergoing insulin-stimulated tyrosine phosphorylation, the insulin receptor and IRS polypeptides are both phosphorylated on Ser/Thr residues in resting cells and undergo substantial further (Ser/Thr) phosphorylation in response to insulin and other ligands; the extent of IRS phosphorylation is particularly striking. Several reports suggest that insulin receptor Ser/Thr phosphorylation significantly impairs insulin receptor tyrosine kinase activity both in cell culture and in insulin resistant states, e.g., in association with PCOS (196). Although attractive, little direct evidence supports the assignment of a negative regulatory function to insulin receptor (Ser/Thr) phosphorylation. By example, overexpression of a number of PKC isoforms results in a substantial increase in insulin receptor Ser phosphorylation with little change in insulin receptor tyrosine kinase activity measured *in vitro* (197). At this time the function of insulin receptor (Ser/Thr) phosphorylation, the identity of the sites of phosphorylation, either basally or in response to insulin and various other hormones and growth factors, and the identity of the kinases responsible for these modifications *in vivo* are all unresolved.

In contrast, a large and persuasive body of work indicates that IRS Ser/Thr phosphorylation is a ubiquitously encountered and potent mechanism for the inhibition of the signalling function of the IRS polypeptide. This inhibition occurs through interference with insulin receptor-catalyzed IRS tyrosine phosphorylation, and/or (more commonly) IRS docking of PI 3-kinase. An early example was the finding that overexpression of recombinant PKCs or activation of endogenous PKCs by active phorbol esters (PMA), although having no effect on insulin receptor kinase activity assayed *in vitro*, significantly reduced the insulin-stimulated increment in PI 3-kinase that could be adsorbed to antiphosphotyrosine antibodies (reflecting primarily IRS-associated PI 3-kinase) (198). Conversion of a single IRS-1 serine residue (S612) to Ala abrogates the inhibitory action of PMA (199). This serine is situated immediately carboxyterminal to a potential IRS tyrosine phosphorylation site that serves as a docking site for SH_2 domain of the p85 adaptor of PI 3-kinase. Further experiments identified a MAPK (ERK2) as the likely immediate effector of this action of PMA (200). Hormonal activators of cPKCs, e.g., endothelin and angiotensin II, can also downregulate IRS-1 tyrosine phosphorylation through a MAPK-directed mechanism (201). In addition, hyperglycemia induces a state of insulin resistance that is reversed in part by inhibitors of PKC. Several additional IRS (Ser/Pro) motifs have been identified as likely sites of MAPK-catalyzed IRS-1 phosphorylation; conversion of IRS-1 Ser632, 662 and 731 to Ala enhances basal and insulin stimulated IRS-1-associated PI 3-kinase activity. Thus, MAPK catalyzed phosphorylation at serine residues adjacent to potential SH_2 docking sites is a well-defined mode for the negative regulation of IRS-1 signalling.

A number of stimuli induce IRS (Ser/Thr) phosphorylation leading to diminished IRS-1 tyrosine phosphorylation/PI 3-kinase association through pathways that do not involve MAP kinase. The protein Ser/Thr phosphatase inhibitor okadaic acid activates a large number of phosphorylation-dependent protein kinases and potently downregulates IRS-1; the okadaic acid-induced inhibition of IRS-1, however, is not abrogated by mutation of serines 612, 632, 662 and 731 or by the MAPK inhibitor PD98059 (202). A particularly intriguing effector of IRS Ser/Thr phosphorylation is TNFα which strongly inhibits IRS tyrosine phosphorylation and downregulates IRS function in cultured adipocytes and hepatocytes. TNFα is overexpressed by adipose tissue in various states of obesity, and has been proposed as an effector of obesity-induced insulin resistance (203,204). TNFα activates a variety of proline-directed Ser/Thr kinases in addition to, and more potently than MAPK, e.g., SAPK/JNK and p38 kinase, as well as the protein kinases in the IκB kinase pathway. The SAPKs are strong candidates for the immediate effector of TNFα-induced IRS-1 (Ser/Thr) phosphorylation; SAPKγ/JNK1 but not p38 kinase binds to IRS-1, and catalyzes a phosphorylation adjacent to the IRS PTB domain at Ser307 (205). Conversion of Ser307 to Ala abrogates the ability of TNFα to inhibit insulin-stimulated IRS-1 tyrosine phosphorylation. Several mechanisms have been proposed to account for TNFα-induced IRS downregulation in addition to phosphorylation in the PTB domain inhibiting the insulin receptor/IRS interaction (206), e.g., phosphorylation of Ser/Pro motifs adjacent to potential SH_2 docking sites, or TNFα-induced conversion of IRS into an inhibitor of the insulin receptor kinase. The contribution of TNFα to the insulin resistance of obesity, although attractive (207,208), is currently uncertain, because conflicting results have been observed concerning the development of insulin resistance in rodents given exogenous TNFα, and in various TNFR-null mice subjected to overfeeding (209,210). A limited body of data in man attempting to neutralize endogenous TNFα have not provided support for this very interesting hypothesis.

Sustained hyperinsulinemia is invariably accompanied by some degree of insulin resistance. Insulin itself is a potent inducer of IRS (Ser/Thr) phosphorylation, which is likely to represent one mechanism of physiologic downregulation. Insulin-induced IRS (Ser/Thr) phosphorylation occurs through a wortmannin-sensitive pathway. Although the PI 3-kinase p110 catalytic subunit can itself act as a serine kinase toward IRS-1, the primary pathway of insulin-induced IRS (Ser/Thr) phosphorylation appears to flow through PKB (201). The downregulation of IRS-1 tyrosine phosphorylation and PI 3-kinase docking by PKB overexpression is abrogated by mutation of the IRS-1 Ser at 632, 662 and 731; each is a Ser/Pro motif, entirely distinct from sites directly phosphorylated by PKB. A similar wortmannin-sensitive IRS inhibitory pathway is activated by PDGF, and the IRS-1 inhibition induced by PDGF and PKB are both largely abolished by rapamycin, a highly selective inhibitor of the mTOR kinase activity (201). A proline-directed kinase activity is associated with (or intrinsic to) mTOR and has been reported to be modestly stimulated by insulin and PKB. Thus, mTOR may represent the insulin-stimulated IRS-1 kinase, although other as yet unidentified IRS (Ser/Thr) kinase activities have been described. In addition, PKB itself can directly phosphorylate IRS-1 at four sites within the IRS PTB domain; conversion of these sites to Ala substantially accelerates the rate of IRS-1 tyrosine dephosphorylation, suggesting that PKB in addition to impairing IRS tyrosine phosphorylation can also prolong the duration of IRS activation (212). Which of these effects predominates in physiologic or pathologic states remains to be defined. Another (Ser/Thr) kinase capable of phosphorylating and negatively regulating IRS-1 is GSK3 (213). Under usual conditions, insulin signalling suppresses GSK3 activity by a PKB-catalyzed mechanism. Overexpression of a nonsuppressible form of GSK3 increases IRS-1 serine phosphorylation and strongly suppresses insulin-stimulated tyrosine phosphorylation of both the insulin receptor and IRS-1. GSK3 activity is both positively and negatively regulated by a variety of pathways in addition to insulin and other ligands, and its role in modulating insulin sensitivity in physiologic or pathologic states is unclear (214). Contributions by other, as yet unidentified IRS (Ser/Thr)kinases are quite likely (215,216). The role of phosphoserine-dependent binding of 14-3-3 proteins in the negative regulation of IRS function remains to be more fully elucidated (217-219).

In summary, IRS (Ser/Thr) phosphorylation is a ubiquitous mechanism for downregulation of insulin signalling. The major mechanisms involve phosphorylation within or adjacent to the PTB domain, which interferes with IRS/insulin receptor interaction, and phosphorylation adjacent to SH_2 domain docking sites.

Miscellaneous and indirect influences on insulin signaling

A number of gene products influence insulin responsiveness *in vivo* or in cell culture through biochemical mechanisms that are poorly understood (Table 1). The transcription factors of the PPARγ subfamily are targets of

Table 1. Miscellaneous modifiers of insulin signaling

Gene Product	*In vivo* evidence (Man, Mouse)
PPARγ	Extensive
Monogenic obesity – e.g., leptin	Complex and mostly indirect via obesity
AP2 – Adipocyte fatty acid binding protein	Yes (mouse)
GFAT – Glutamine-Fructose 6P amidotransferase	Yes (mouse)
PC1 – Plasma cell membrane glycoprotein-1	Some (man)
Grb7/10/14	No
PEA-15	No

the thiazolidinedione class of "insulin-sensitizing" drugs (220). Inasmuch as these drugs are agonists, it is presumed that PPARγ action promotes insulin sensitivity. Consistent with this view, dominant inhibitory PPARγ mutations in man produce severe insulin resistance and diabetes in the absence of obesity (221), and the severe obesity associated with a heterozygous PPARγ mutation that removes a negative regulatory site of MAPK phosphorylation is unaccompanied by diabetes (222). Surprisingly, however, mice heterozygous for PPARγ deficiency exhibit enhanced insulin sensitivity and are refractory to the induction of insulin resistance by a high fat diet (223, 224). A polymorphism in the PPARγ N terminal region (Pro12 Ala), found in 15% of several North American and European populations, appears to confer protection from diabetes (see Chapter 10) (222). The Ala12 variant appears to have diminished transcriptional activating activity (226). Thus, the role of PPARγ in determining insulin sensitivity, the targets of this transcriptional regulator, and the precise mode of action of the thiazolidinediones remains uncertain.

Leptin is a hormone secreted by adipose tissue in proportion to the filling of adipocyte triglyceride stores (227). Leptin promotes satiety, energy expenditure, hypothalamic gonadatrophin secretion and insulin responsiveness. Lack of leptin or inactivating mutations in the leptin receptor (as seen in the OB mouse and DB mouse, respectively) results in obesity, diabetes, low energy expenditure and abnormalities in the hypothalamic-pituitary gonadal axis; rare instances of leptin deficiency in man produce a similar syndrome. The mechanisms by which leptin deficiency promotes diabetes are unclear; however, it should be emphasized that human obesity is accompanied by constitutively high levels of circulating leptin, and, while evidence of impaired leptin signaling is harder to ascertain, leptin deficiency per se is a very rare cause of human diabetes, except perhaps in the setting of the rare lipodystrophy-associated diabetic syndromes. The insulin-resistant diabetes associated with a murine model of partial lipodystrophy is cured by injection of leptin (228, 229). In contrast, a murine model with a more severe insulin-resistant diabetes in association with virtually complete lipoatrophy, although also severely leptin deficient, is not cured of their diabetes by leptin, given either at physiological or pharmacologic doses (230, 231). This syndrome can be reversed, however, by transplantation of near physiologic amounts of adipose tissue (232). In these lipoatrophic mice, the ability of insulin to promote IRS tyrosine phosphorylation and activation of PI 3-kinase in skeletal muscle is severely reduced (233). Thus, in the setting of severe lipodystrophy, leptin deficiency does not appear to be the primary determinant of the diabetic state.

AP2 is a 12 kDa adipocyte-specific, intracellular fatty acid binding protein. Homozygous deletion of AP2 in the mouse does not produce a phenotype; however, induction of obesity through overfeeding the AP2-null mice fails to cause increased expression of TNFα in adipose tissue and fails to result in insulin-resistance, as occurs in the comparably overfed wild-type mice (234). Thus, the adipocyte fatty acid binding protein AP2 is necessary for the development of insulin resistance in the setting of obesity.

Glutamine Fructose-6-Phosphate Amidotransferase (GFAT) is an enzyme that catalyzes the first and rate-limiting step in the production of hexosamines. Considerable evidence supports the hypothesis that hyperglycemia induces insulin resistance, at least in part, by increasing flux through the hexosamine pathway (235). FFA also increase flux through this pathway in skeletal muscle (236), and overexpression of GFAT in skeletal muscle per se induces insulin resistance (237). Thus, the activity of the glucosamine pathway, perhaps serving to signal nutrient sufficiency (238), promotes adaptations that, while not fully defined, result in insulin resistance.

The Grb 7/10/14 insulin receptor class of SH2 domain containing adaptor proteins are polypeptides of roughly 400 amino acids that contain a central PH domain and carboxyterminal SH_2 domain. The latter enables binding to the activated insulin receptor through the activation loop. Overexpression of these polypeptides in cell culture systems appears to inhibit insulin signalling; however their physiologic function is unknown (239,240). PC1 is a nucleotide phosphodiesterase which is located in the plasma membrane and whose catalytic site is directed into the extracellular space. The abundance of PC1 on the cell surface is negatively correlated with insulin signalling in cell culture in some (241), but not all (242), studies. PEA-15, a 15 kDa phosphoprotein overexpressed in skeletal muscle of Type 2 diabetics (243), inhibits insulin-stimulated glucose transport and GLUT4 translocation in cultured muscle cells and also inhibits TNFα- and Fas-induced apoptosis in a PKC dependent manner. The role of these molecules in insulin resistance associated with Type 2 diabetes remains to be determined.

1. Acquired as an initial endowment
   a. genes – the "Thrifty Genotype"
   b. fetal/neonatal nutritional milieu – the "Thrifty Phenotype"

2. Acquired by living in the "First World"
   a. obesity (FFA and adipocyte polypeptides)
   b. physical inactivity/deconditioning (loss of oxidative capacity)

3. Acquired by misfortune
   a. endocrine diseases (Cushing's Syndrome, Acromegaly, etc.)
   b. acute and chronic inflammatory diseases – inflammatory cytokines
   c. trauma and burns – inflammatory cytokines

4. Pregnancy – primarily placental lactogen

5. Hyperglycemia - ? hexosamine-mediated

Figure 4. Etiologic categories of insulin resistance

Insulin Resistance in Type 2 Diabetes

Insulin resistance accompanies many different physiologic and pathophysiologic states with different etiologic factors accounting for the insulin resistance (Fig. 4). Unlike Type 2 diabetes mellitus, however, insulin resistance does not have a formal quantitative definition. At a clinical level, the term is usually used to indicate a subnormal ability of insulin to decrease serum glucose. Epidemiologic studies of nondiabetic individuals often use the presence of an elevated fasting insulin concentration to indicate the presence of insulin resistance, in effect employing a single point measurement at the normal fasting glucose level. Although high values of fasting insulin are inferred to reflect an impedance to insulin-regulated glucose uptake, in reality the levels of fasting insulin are near the bottom of the *in vivo* dose-response curve for glucose transport and better reflect the combined impact of several anti-catabolic actions of insulin, especially inhibition of proteolytic production of gluconeogenic precursors, inhibition of hepatic gluconeogenesis and glycogenolysis and inhibition of lipolysis (which indirectly affects fasting glucose through the stimulatory effect of FFA on hepatic gluconeogenesis). A measure more reflective of the efficiency of insulin-activated glucose transport is the ratio of the glucose excursion during an oral or intravenous glucose tolerance test, to the concomitant excursion in insulin level. The reliability of this ratio as an index of insulin "resistance" is, however, essentially lost in the presence of coexistent defects in insulin secretion. Even when insulin secretion is intact, the inability to control either the glucose or insulin concentration limits the utility of this parameter. A more specific test of the efficacy of insulin action *in vivo* is the classic "insulin tolerance" test, wherein a fixed dose of insulin, e.g., 0.1 U/kg, is administered intravenously as a bolus followed by measurements of blood glucose at frequent intervals over sixty minutes. In nondiabetic subjects, the nadir in blood glucose is reached at about thirty minutes, and its level is determined by the alacrity of glucose uptake by skeletal muscle and the vigor of the "counterregulatory" secretion of pancreatic glucagon and adrenal medullary epinephrine, triggered by the falling plasma glucose, which act to promote hepatic glycogenolysis (glucagon) and limit muscle glucose uptake (epinephrine). Although not influenced by endogenous insulin secretion, this test suffers from many deficiencies, including its essentially qualitative nature, the inability to specify the level of plasma insulin stimulus, and the contribution of the counterregulatory response in addition to insulin-stimulated glucose uptake.

The gold standard for the measurement of insulin "action" *in vivo* is the glucose clamp (244-247). This test employs the simultaneous intravenous infusion of insulin (at any dose desired) and glucose, the latter in amounts that maintain the blood glucose at the initial fasting concentration, as guided by frequent blood glucose measurements. As insulin levels increase and muscle glucose transport is activated, the distribution of glucose utilization shifts so that even with elevations of insulin only several-fold over basal, over 80% of the infused glucose is taken up by skeletal muscle, the majority of which is converted to glycogen. A pseudo-steady state level of glucose infusion is attained by 60-120 minutes after a plateau insulin concentration is achieved, and this rate of glucose infusion or "M" value is taken as a direct measure of whole-body insulin-stimulated glucose uptake at that plasma insulin concentration (determined by radioimmunoassay). Refinements of this protocol involve infusion of labelled glucose to enable quantification of the rate of endogenous glucose production by isotope dilution (248), or the rate of oxidative glucose metabolism by collection of expired CO_2 (249); direct assessment of the concentration of specific muscle metabolites e.g. glucose-6-phosphate or the rate of muscle glycogen deposition, using ^{31}P or ^{13}C NMR over leg muscles (250,251); and muscle biopsy for assessment of metabolite levels, and specific enzyme activities (e.g., insulin receptor kinase or glycogen synthase). Somatostatin may be infused to suppress endogenous insulin secretion. This methodology allows the construction of formal dose-response curves; however, given the duration and technical complexity of each study, construction of such curves is rarely feasible in a single subject; rather pooled data in carefully selected groups enables valid conclusions (248,252). The relevant parameters of such a comparison are the concentration of insulin that gives half-maximal activation in the rate of glucose uptake (A0.5) and the maximal rate of glucose uptake achievable (Vmax). Insulin "resistance" is an increase in A0.5 beyond the normal range; Vmax is often also found to be diminished, however in clinical situations, a decrease in Vmax without an increase in A0.5 is rarely, if ever, encountered. In young, lean nondiabetic Caucasian subjects, maximal M values are observed at 5-10 nM concentrations of insulin, starting from levels of 0.05-0.1 nM (248,252). Obese nondiabetic individuals show a greater dispersion in A0.5 than do lean subjects, so that mean A0.5 is increased; alternatively, obese individuals may be viewed as two groups, with one exhibiting essentially normal A0.5 and a second group with clearly increased A0.5, i.e., insulin resistance. Vmax is generally preserved in nondiabetic obese individuals (253). In the presence of impaired glucose tolerance, A0.5 is increased, and Vmax is depressed uniformly. These abnormalities are more marked in frank Type 2 diabetes, with A0.5 increased as much as 10-fold and Vmax depressed by 40-50% (254). Restoration of near-normoglycemia for several weeks improves, but does not restore, "M" to nondiabetic levels (252).

The glucose clamp measures the integrated effect of a series of insulin responses including the ability of insulin to promote delivery of glucose to skeletal muscle by increasing muscle blood flow, the insulin activation of the transport step per se, and the activation of muscle glycogen synthase. The increase in blood flow reflects a vasodilatory response that is dependent on insulin activation of endothelial nitric oxide synthase. Inhibition of NO synthesis in lean nondiabetic subjects diminishes "M" by 20-30% (255). The vasodilatory response to insulin is markedly impaired in insulin resistant obese (256) and Type 2 diabetic subjects (257,258). Studies employing ^{13}C and ^{31}P NMR indicate that intracellular glucose-6-phosphate (G6P) levels are increased by hyperinsulinemia (259,260), with little or no change in the very low level of intracellular free glucose (<0.1mM) (261,262). This finding indicates that although glucose transport and glycogen synthase are activated coordinately (263), the accelerated deposition of glycogen is being "pushed" by the activation of transport, rather than being "pulled" by the activation of glycogen synthase, as the latter would cause a drop in G6P. Thus, transport activation is the dominant permissive step in insulin action, as first proposed in the classic studies of Levine and colleagues (264). Baseline muscle G6P levels and the increment caused by insulin are both low in Type 2 diabetic subjects, indicating that, as in the nondiabetic subjects, the glucose transport step is the primary rate-determining step in glucose uptake (259,260,262) and that impairment in transport is the major cause of the diminished glucose uptake. Nevertheless, direct measurements of muscle blood flow and muscle glycogen synthase activity obtained during euglycemic, hyperinsulinemic glucose clamp studies in insulin-resistant obese or Type 2 diabetic individuals show increases in A0.5 and decreases in Vmax, and the changes in these parameters for blood flow and glycogen synthase parallel the changes seen in overall glucose uptake ("M") (255,257). The concordance between the changes in blood flow, glucose transport and glycogen synthase activity in the diabetic subjects is consistent with the view that all three parameters are regulated by the insulin receptor through a common signalling pathway, and their reduction in insulin resistant states reflects a shared mechanism and/or site of inhibition. As discussed previously, all three responses require insulin activation of PI 3-kinase. Nevertheless, the specific biochemical steps operating downstream of PI 3-kinase for the activation of glucose transport and skeletal muscle glycogen synthase are, as yet, incompletely understood.

What are the dominant determinants of insulin sensitivity, and what can be concluded from present information as to the biochemical steps that are predominantly impaired in the common states of insulin-resistance seen in prediabetes, obesity and frank Type 2 diabetes? The sensitivity of the three insulin target tissues to insulin is certainly attributable in part to the relatively high number of IR expressed on target cells, e.g., 10,000-40,000/cell on the highly responsive rat adipocyte, as compared to 3000-5000 IR in a typical poorly responsive cell, such as a cultured fibroblast. Nevertheless, the relationship of biologic response to receptor number is not necessarily linear. Introduction of 10,000-40,000 recombinant insulin receptor into a fibroblast does not per se reduce the A0.5 for insulin activation of glycogen synthase to the level observed in the adipocyte. As discussed previously, reduction in the number of insulin receptors on target cells will steadily increase A0.5 but must exceed 50% in skeletal muscle and 90% in adipose tissue to reduce

Vmax; this reflects the substantial amplification that occurs concomitant with intracellular signal transmission. Thus the abundance, availability and functional state of the intracellular elements are probably of greater importance in determining A0.5 and, especially, Vmax than is receptor number.

The abundance and functional state of the intermediate signalling elements will affect primarily the sensitivity of the response to insulin (A0.5) whereas the size of the metabolic response that can be elicited by insulin (Vmax) will be influenced more strongly and selectively by the abundance and functional state of the final target, e.g., the number of GLUT4 transporters or glycogen synthase polypeptides. In fact, considerable evidence indicates that both the abundance of GLUT4, and the ability of a variety of stimuli other than insulin (e.g., exercise hypoxia, Ser/Thr phosphatase- and Tyr phosphatase-inhibitors) to activate glucose transport in skeletal muscle from Type 2 diabetic subjects, *in vitro* and *in vivo*, is relatively unimpaired (265,266). Thus the impedance to insulin action appears to reside upstream of GLUT4 and the translocation apparatus per se. Moreover, although the insulin resistant states accompanying pre-Type 2 diabetes, impaired glucose tolerance or frank Type 2 diabetes are defined by the presence of defective glucose uptake, evidence of a parallel impairment in the anticatabolic actions of insulin, specifically in the ability of insulin to inhibit hepatic gluconeogenesis and adipocyte lipolysis, emerges as the insulin resistance becomes more severe (267,268). This indicates strongly that the genesis of insulin resistance in these states is attributable primarily to interruption at one or more of the proximal steps in insulin signal transduction pathways common to both the anabolic and anticatabolic actions, rather than at more distal steps in these pathways (e.g., in the genes encoding GLUT4, glycogen synthase or gluconeogenic enzymes). The anabolic and anticatabolic actions of insulin both require activation of PI 3-kinase. The differential sensitivity of these responses to insulin must be attributable to the abundance or properties of signalling elements positioned distal to the PI 3-kinase/Ptd Ins 3,4,5P_3 signal, or in a parallel pathway; the specific molecular determinants of the differential sensitivity are not known.

The components of the signalling apparatus downstream of the insulin receptor likely to be critical to insulin sensitivity include e.g., the specific activity of the insulin receptor kinase, the concentration of insulin receptor substrates and their availability for insulin receptor-catalyzed tyrosine phosphorylation; the lifetime of insulin receptor and IRS phosphotyrosines as influenced by the activity of phosphotyrosine phosphates; the concentration of secondary signal generators, such as PI 3-kinase, and the ability of such SH2 domain-containing effectors to be recruited onto phosphotyrosine motifs; the efficiency of coupling PI 3-kinase activation into the generation of Ptd Ins 3,4,5P_3; and Ptd Ins 3,4,5P_3 recruitment and activation of its targets, such as PKB.

The majority of studies in insulin-resistant obese and Type 2 diabetic individuals demonstrate the presence of impaired activation of IRS-associated, or antiphosphotyrosine-precipitable PI 3-kinase in response to insulin in the skeletal muscle (e.g. 269, 270). Interestingly, PKB activation is not consistently impaired despite diminished activation of PI 3-kinase (269), although decreased PKB activity at maximal insulin may be evident (270). Despite the decrease in PI 3-kinase activity, activation of MAP kinase, which is very modest in insulin-stimulated skeletal muscle (and is much more strongly activated by exercise) appears unaltered (270). The mechanisms responsible for the decreased insulin activation of PI 3-kinase appear to be a modest decrease in overall insulin-induced IRS tyrosine phosphorylation together with a more marked decrease in PI 3-kinase docking to the IRS polypeptides. Such a defect can be induced in insulin-responsive nondiabetic subjects during a euglycemic, hyperinsulinemic glucose clamp by a sustained elevation of plasma FFA (271) produced by the administration of a triglyceride infusion plus heparin (to activate lipoprotein lipase). Such an infusion overcomes the marked fall in plasma FFA that otherwise occurs due to the insulin inhibition of lipolysis during a hyperinsulinemic clamp; after 1-2 hours of sustained plasma FFA elevation, a decrease in glucose clearance becomes evident with "M" values reduced by 30-40% compared to those seen in the absence of the TG/heparin infusion (271,272). The biochemical mechanism by which FFA cause this effect is of considerable interest. The mechanism proposed by Randle and colleagues in 1963, the so-called "glucose-fatty acid cycle", suggested that FFA oppose glucose utilization because FFA oxidation inhibits pyruvate dehydrogenase and promotes an increase in cytosolic citrate, which causes an inhibition of phosphofructokinase (PFK-1), the rate limiting step in glycolysis; this results in an increase in G-6-P, inhibition of hexokinase and glucose uptake (273). Although the ability of FFA to inhibit glucose utilization in skeletal muscle is now firmly established, the mechanism proposed by Randle and coworkers has not been borne out by more recent work, which reveals that FFA infusion results is a major decrease in skeletal muscle G6P levels; this indicates that the major site of FFA inhibition of glucose utilization is at the glucose transport step rather than in glycolysis (260,262). In addition, the TG/heparin infusion results in a marked decrease in the IRS-associated PI 3-kinase activity, measured in skeletal muscle biopsies taken before and during the infusion (271). It has been proposed that the accumulation of intracellular fatty acyl CoA, perhaps by diversion into DAG, promotes activation of the novel PKC (θ,d,ε) isoforms that are found in skeletal muscle, resulting in IRS phosphorylation on Ser/Thr, as described in cell culture (274). Additional evidence as to the mechanism is required, as is an explanation for the lag in the appearance of the FFA-induced inhibition of glucose transport. Nevertheless, these studies provide an attractive model for one mechanism of obesity-induced insulin resistance, inasmuch as the expanded adipose depot, especially the more lipolytically active abdominal fat depots, provide a continuous infusion of FFA into the circulation in proportion to their mass.

CONCLUSIONS

The insulin signal transduction pathway is a multistep process, beginning at a single insulin receptor, which projects information downstream through an arborizing, progressively enlarging network of positive and negative regulators. The initial signal of tyrosine phosphorylation recruits a diverse set of secondary signal generators, with Ptd Ins kinases and small GTPases as the best-characterized examples at present. These secondary signals recruit protein (Ser/Thr) kinases, which, in turn, control cascades of protein (Ser/Thr) kinases, protein (Ser/Thr) phosphatases and other small GTPases, whose ultimate targets are the enzymes and transporters that carry out the actual reactions of nutrient metabolism. Insulin controls the pathways regulating nutrient metabolism at multiple steps. In addition, each of the regulated steps is usually controlled by insulin through several independent mechanisms, discussed at length for glucose transport. A similar situation prevails for the activation of glycogen synthase, where insulin inhibits the activity of protein kinases that inactivate glycogen synthase, such as GSK3 and PKA, and also augments glycogen synthase phosphatase activity, by altering phosphatase colocalization with glycogen synthase, by deactivating glycogen synthase phosphatase inhibitory proteins, etc. The signalling pathway from the insulin receptor to the IRS polypeptides to the recruitment of PI 3-kinase (p85/55/50 p110 heterodimer) is established with certainty as a crucial part of the metabolic control pathway; PKB appears to be indispensable for at least a subset of the responses downstream of PI 3-kinase; the other critical effectors of PI 3-kinase are less well established, but probably include one or more subfamilies of PKCs, especially atypical PKCs ζ and λ. Some evidence supports the existence of a pathway from the insulin receptor to GLUT4 that parallels and bypasses the IRS proteins, which may involve Gαq. The number of insulin receptor-initiated outflows operating in parallel to PI 3-kinase is not known, either for the activation of glucose transport or for the regulation of other aspects of nutrient metabolism; the molecular nature of such parallel pathway(s) is mostly undefined, although current evidence indicates that Ras-GTP is not involved, whereas Gαq and the p38 MAPK bear special consideration as candidate effecter elements.

Despite the remaining uncertainties concerning the identity of the necessary positive effectors in the insulin signalling pathway, multiple mechanisms for termination, feedback inhibition and negative crossregulation of the insulin signal by other signal transduction pathways have been identified. It is plausible to anticipate that the insulin resistance underlying obesity and Type 2 diabetes will reflect the interactions between the genetically programmed abnormalities in the abundance and/or activity of the positive and negative regulators, and their responsiveness to environmentally-induced perturbations, especially adipocyte overfilling, excess circulating FFA and glucose, and reduced muscular work. It is likely that defective function at multiple sites will be found within a single individual, and these sites are likely to differ in different subsets of Type 2 diabetes. The common, quantitatively significant defects known at this time (in order of diminishing importance) involve deficiencies in the IRS-mediated activation of PI 3-kinase, impaired tyrosine phosphorylation of IRS polypeptides, decreased specific activity of the insulin receptor kinase, and a decreased number of surface insulin receptor. The likelihood is high that further significant abnormalities await description, pending more complete understanding of the insulin signalling pathway. Moreover, the interconnections between the brain, pancreatic islet, adipocyte, skeletal muscle and liver in nutrient homeostasis are so tight that perturbation at one site invariably elicits offsetting adjustments and adaptations at one or more of the other sites; thus the initiating abnormalities underlying insulin-resistance could well originate at any of these sites. This chapter has described the molecular elements currently known to be responsible for insulin signal transduction, as well as the negative regulatory inputs to this pathway currently appreciated.

REFERENCES

1. Reeves M and Hamman RF. "Risk factors for non-insulin dependent diabetes. In: "*Diabetes in America 2nd*" pp 179-220. National Institutes of Health NIDDK/Bethesda MD, National Diabetes Data Group, ed., 1995.
2. Pratley RE. Gene Environment interactions in the pathogenesis of Type 2 diabetes mellitus: Lesson learned from the PIMA Indians Proc Nutr Soc 1988; 57:175-178.
3. Barker DJ, Clark PM, Cox LJ, Fall C, Osmond C, Winter PD. Fetal and infant growth and impaired glucose tolerance at age 64. BMJ 1991;303:1019-1022.
4. Rich-Edward JW, Codlitz GA, Stampfer MJ, et. al. Birthweight and the risk for type 2 diabetes mellitus in adult women. Ann Intern Med 1999;130:278-284.
5. Carlsson S, Persson PG, Alvarsson M, Efendic S, Norman A, Svanstrom L, Ostenson CG, Grill V. Low birth weight, family history of diabetes, and glucose intolerance in Swedish middle-aged men. Diabetes Care 1999; 22:1043-1047.
6. Mi J, Law C, Zhang KL, Osmond C, Stein C, Barker D. Effects of infant birth weight and maternal body mass index in pregnancy on components of the insulin resistance syndrome in China. Ann Intern Med 2000; 32:253-260.
7. Lindsay RS, Dabelea D, Roumain J, et al. Type 2 diabetes and low birth weight: the role of paternal inheritance in the association of low birth weight and diabetes. Diabetes 2000; 49:445-449.
8. Hattersley AT and Tooke JE. The fetal insulin hypothesis: an alternative explanation of the association of low birth weight with diabetes and vascular disease. Lancet 1999; 353:1789-1792.
9. Barker DJP. The fetal origins of type 2 diabetes mellitus. Ann of Int Med 1999;130:322-324.

10. Neel JV, Weder AB, Julius S. Type II diabetes, essential hypertension and obesity as "syndromes of impaired genetic homeostasis". The "Thrifty Genotype: hypothesis enters the 21st century. Persp Biol Med 1998; 42:44-74.
11. North MA. Advances in the molecular genetics of obesity. Curr Opin Gen Develop 1999; 9:283-288.
12. Hattersley AT, Beards F, Ballentype E, Appleton M, Harvey R, Ellard S. Mutations in the glucokinase gene of the fetus result in reduced birth weight. Nat Genet 1998; 19:268-270.
13. Ravussin E, Gautier JF. Metabolic predictors of weight gain. Int J Obes Relat Metab Disord 1999; 1:37-41.
14. Rosetti L, Ciaccari A, DeFronzo RA. Glucotoxicity. Diabetes Care 1990;13:610-630.
15. Ferrannini E. Insulin resistance vs. insulin deficiency in NIDDM: Problems and prospects. Endo Rev 1998; 19:477-490.
16. Gerich JE. The genetic basis of type 2 diabetes mellitus: Impaired insulin secretion versus impaired insulin sensitivity. Endo Rev 1998; 19:491-503.
17. Leibiger IB, Leibiger B, Moede T, Berggren PO. Exocytosis of insulin promotes insulin gene transcription via the insulin receptor/PI 3-kinase/p70 S6 kinase and CaM kinase. Mol Cell 1998;1:933-938.
18. Kulkarni RN, Bruning JC, Ninnay JN, Posti C, Magnuson MA Kahn CR. Tissue-specific knockout of the insulin receptor in pancreatic beta cells creates an insulin secretory defect similar to that in type 2 diabetes. Cell 1999; 96:329-339.
19. Cahill GF. The physiology of insulin in man. Diabetes 1971; 20:785-799.
20. Pessin JE, Thurmon DC, Elmendorf JS, Coker KJ, Okada S. Molecular basis of insulin-stimulated GLUT4 vesicle trafficking. J Biol Chem 1999; 274:2593-2596.
21. Proud CG, Denton RM. Molecular mechanisms for the control of translation by insulin. Biochem J 1997; 328: 329-341.
22. Londos G, Honnor RC, Dhillon GS. CAMP-dependent protein kinase and lipolysis in rat adipocytes: III. Multiple modes of insulin regulation of lipolysis and regulation of insulin responses by adenylate cyclase regulators. J Biol Chem 1985;260:15139-15145.
23. Fain JN, Kovacev VP, Scow RO. Antilipolytic effect of insulin in isolated fat cells of the rat. Endocrinology 1966; 78:773-778..
24. Campbell PJ, Carlson MG, Hill JO, Nurjhan N. Regulation of free fatty acid metabolism by insulin in humans: role of lipolysis and reesterification. Am J Physiol 1992; 263;1063-1069.
25. Weyer C, Bogardus C, Mott DM, Pratley RE. The natural history of insulin secretory dysfunction and insulin resistance in the pathogenesis of Type 2 diabetes mellitus. J Clin Invest 1999;104:787-794.
26. Moller DE, Yokata A, Caro JF, Flier JS. Tissue specific expression of two alternatively spliced insulin receptor mRNAs in man. Mol Endo 1989; 3:1263-1269.
27. Frasca F, Pandini G, Scalia P, Sciacca L, Mineo R, Costantino A, Goldfine ID, Belfiore A, Vigneri R. Insulin receptor isoform A, a newly recognized, high-affinity insulin-like growth factor II receptor in fetal and cancer cells. Mol Cell Biol 1999;19:3278-3288.
28. Chen H, Yan GC, Gishizky ML. Identification of structural characteristics that contribute to a difference in antiapoptotic function between human insulin and insulin-like growth factor I receptors. Cell Growth Diff 1998; 9:939-947.
29. Blakesley VA, Scrimgeour A, Esposito D, LeRoith D. Signaling via the insulin-like growth factor-I receptor: Does it differ from insulin receptor signaling? Cytokine Growth Factor Rev 1996; 7:153-159.
30. Lee J, Pilch LJ. The insulin receptor: structure, function, and signaling. Am J Physiol 1994; 266:C319-334.
31. White MF, Kahn CR. The insulin signaling system. J Biol Chem 1994; 269: 1-4.

32. Avruch J. The insulin receptor kinase: Structure-function relationships. In: Molecular and Cellular Biology of Diabetes Mellitus, Vol II: Insulin Action, Draznin B, Melmed S, LeRoith D, eds, New York:Alan R. Liss, 1989, pp. 65-77.
33. Hubbard SR, Mohammadi M, Schlessinger J. Autoregulatory mechanisms in protein tyrosine kinases. J Biol Chem 1998; 11987-11990.
34. Fantl WJ, Johnson De, Williams LT. Signaling by receptor tyrosine kinases. Annu Rev Biochem 1993; 62:453-481.
35. Pawson T. Protein modules and signaling networks. Nature 1995; 373:573-580.
36. Kavanaugh WM, Williams LT. An alternative to SH2 domains for binding tyrosine-phosphorylated proteins. Science 1994; 266:1862-1865.
37. Blaikie P, Immanuel D, Wu J, Li N, Yajnik V, Margolis B. A region in Shc distinct from the SH_2 domain can bind tyrosine phosphorylated growth factor receptors. J Biol Chem 1994; 269:32031-32034.
38. Yenush L, White MF. The IRS-signalling system during insulin and cytokine action, Bioessays 1997; 19:491-500.
39. Tzahar E, Yarden Y. The ErbB-2/HER2 oncogenic receptor of adenocarcinomas: From orphanhood to multiple stromal ligands. Biochim Biophys Acta 1998; 1377: 25-37
40. Myers MG Jr, Grammer TC, Wang LM, Sun XJ, Pierce JH, Blenis J, White MF. Insulin receptor substrate-1 mediates phosphatidylinositol 3' – kinase and p70S6k signaling during insulin, insulin-like growth factor-1, and interleukin-4 stimulation. J. Biol Chem 1994; 269:28783-28789.
41. Taylor SI. Lilly lecture: molecular mechanisms of insulin resistance. Lessons from patients with mutations in the insulin-receptor gene. Diabetes 1992; 41:1473-1490.
42. Songyang Z, Cantley L. Recognition and specificity in protein tyrosine kinase-mediated signalling. TIBS 195; 20:470-475.
43. Kayali AG, Eichhorn J, Haruta T, Morris AJ, Nelson JG, Vollenweider P, Olefsky JM, Webster JG. Association of the insulin receptor with phospholipase C-γ (PLCγ) in 3T3 L1 adipocytes suggests a role for PLCγ in metabolic signaling by insulin. J Biol Chem 1998; 273:13808-13813.
44. Lamothe B, Baudry A, Desbois, Lamotte L, Bucchini D, DeMeyts P, Joshi RL. Genetic engineering in mice: impact on insulin signalling and action. Biochem J 1998; 335:193-204.
45. Liu SC, Wang Q, Lienhard GE, Keller SR. Insulin receptor substrate 3 is not essential for growth or glucose homeostasis. J Biol Chem 1999; 274:18093-18099.
46. Fantin VR, Wang Q, Lienhard GE, Keller SR. Mice lacking insulin receptor substrate 4 exhibit mild defects in growth, reproduction, and glucose homeostasis. Am J Physiol 2000; 278:E127-133.
47. Zhou L, Chen H, Xu P, Cong LN, Sciacchitano S, Li Y, Graham D, Jacobs AR, Taylor SI, Quon MJ: Action of insulin receptor substrate-3 (IRS-3) and IRS-4 to stimulate translocation of GLUT4 in rat adipose cells. 1999; Mol Endocrinol 13:505-514.
48. Myers MG Jr., Zhang Y, Aldaz GAI, Grammer T, Glasheen EM, Yenush L, Wang LM, Sun XJ, Blenis J, Pierce JH, White M. YMXM motifs and signaling by an insulin receptor substrate 1 molecule without tyrosine phosphorylation sites. Mol Cell Biol 1996;16:4147-4155.
49. Yenush L, Zanella C, Uchica T, Bernal D, White MF. The pleckstrin homology and phosphotyrosine binding domains of insulin receptor substrate 1 mediate inhibition of apoptosis by insulin. Mol Cell Biol 1998; 18:6784-6794.
50. Isakoff SJ, Taha C, Rose E, Marcusohn J, Klip A, Skolnik EY. The inability of phosphatidylinositol 3-kinase activation to stimulate GLUT4 translocation indicates additional signaling pathways are required for insulin-stimulated glucose uptake. Proc Natl Acad Sci 1995;92:10247-10251.

51. Morris RJ, Martin SS, Haruta T, Nelson JG, Vollenwieder P, Gustafson TA, Mueckler M, Rose DW Olefsky JM. Evidence for an insulin receptor substrate 1 independent insulin signaling pathway that mediates insulin-responsive glucose transporter (GLUT4) translocation. Proc Natl Acad Sci 1996; 93: 8401-8406.
52. Sharma PM, Egawa K, Gustafson TA, Martin JL, Olefsky JM. Adenovirus-mediated overexpression of IRS-1 interacting domains abolishes insulin-stimulated mitogenesis without affecting glucose transport in 3T3 L1 adipocytes. Mol Cell Biol 1997; 17:7386-7389.
53. Sharma PM, Eqawa K, Huang Y, Martin JL, Huvar I, Boss GR, Olefsky JM.. Inhibition of phosphatidylinositol 3-kinase activity by adenovirus-mediated gene transfer and its effect on insulin action. J. Biol Chem 1998; 17:18528-18537.
54. Elmendorf JS, Chen D, Pessin JE. Guanosine 5'-O (3-thiotriphosphate) GTPγS stimulation of GLUT4 translocation is tyrosine kinase-dependent. J Biol Chem 1998; 273: 13289-13296.
55. Kishi K, Hayashi H, Wang L, Kamohara S, Tamaoka K, Shimizu T, Ushikubi F, Narumiya S, Ebina Y. G-q-coupled receptors transmit the signal for GLUT4 translocation via an insulin-independent pathway. J Biol Chem 1996; 271: 26561-26568.
56. Imamura T, Ishibashi K-I, Dalle S, Ugi S, Olefsky JM. Endothelin-1-induced GLUT4 translocation is mediated via Gq/11 protein and phosphatidylinositol 3-kinase in 3T3-L1 adipocytes. J Biol Chem 1999; 274:33691-33695.
57. Imamura T, Vollenweider P, Egawa K, Clodi M, Ishibashi K, Nakashima N, Ugi S, Adams JW, Brown JH, Olefsky JM. G alpha-q/11 protein plays a key role in insulin-induced glucose transport in 3T3-L1 adipocytes. Mol Cell Biol 1999; 19:6765-6774.
58. Luttrell LM, Daaka Y, Lefkowitz RJ. Regulation of tyrosine kinase cascades by G-protein-coupled receptors. Curr Opin Cell Biol 1999; 11:177-183.
59. Kanzaki M, Watson RT, Artemyev NO, Pessin JE. The trimeric GTP-binding protein (G(q)/G(11)) alpha subunit is required for insulin-stimulated GLUT4 translocation in 3T3L1 adipocytes. J Biol Chem 2000; 275:7167-7175.
60. Denton RM, Tavare JM. Does mitogen-activated-protein kinase have a role in insulin action? The cases for and against. Eur J. Biochem. 1995;227:597-611.
61. Yano H, Nakanishi S, Kimura K, et al. Inhibition of histamine secretion by wortmannin through the blockade of phosphatidylinositol 3–kinase in RBL–2H3 cells. J. Biol. Chem. 1993;268:25846-25856.
62. Cheatham B, Vlahos CJ, Cheatham L, Wang L, Blenis J, Kahn CR. Phosphatidylinositol 3-kinase activation is required for insulin stimulation of pp70 S6 kinase, DNA synthesis, and glucose transporter translocation. Mol Cell Biol 1994;14:4902-4911.
63. Sakaue H, Hara K, Noguchi T, Matozaki T, Kotani K, Ogawa W, Yonezawa K, Waterfield MD, Kasuga M. Ras-independent and wortmannin sensitive activation of glycogen synthase by insulin in Chinese hamster ovary cells. J Biol Chem 1995; 270:11304-11309.
64. Shepherd PR, Withers DJ, Siddle K. Phosphoinositide 3-kinase: the key switch mechanism in insulin signaling. Biochem. J. 1998 ;333:471-490.
65. Kimura K, Tissenbaum HA, Liu Y, Ruvkun. Daf-2, an insulin-receptor like gene that regulates longevity and diapause in caenorhabditis elegans. Science 1997;277:942-946.
66. Morris JZ, Tissenbaum HA, Ruvkun G. A phosphatidylinositol-3-OH kinase family member regulating longevity and diapause in Caenorhabditis elegans. Nature 1996;382:536-538.
67. Ogg S, Ruvkun S. The C. elegans PTEN homolog, DAF-8, acts in the insulin receptor-like metabolic signaling pathway. Mol. Cell 1998;2:887-893.

68. Paradis S, Ailion M, Toker A, Thomas JH, Ruvkun G. A PDK1 homolog is necessary and sufficient to transduce AGE-1PI3 kinase signals that regulate diapause in Caenorhabditis elegans. Genes & Devel. 1999;13:1438-1452.
69. Paradis S, Ruvkun G. Caenorhabditis elegans Akt/PKB transduces insulin receptor-like signals from AGE-1 PI3 kinase to the DAF-16 transcription factor. Genes Dev. 1998;12:2488-2498.
70. Bohni R, Riesgo-Escovar J, Oldham S, Brogiolo W, Stocker H, Andruss BF, Beckingham K, Hafen E. Autonomous control of cell and organ size by CHICO, a *Drosophila* homolog of vertebrate IRS-4. Cell 1999; 97:865-875.
71. Ogg S, Paradis S, Gottlieb S, Patterson GI, Lee L, Tissenbaum HA, Ruvkun G. The fork head transcription factor DAF-16 transduces insulin-like metabolic and longevity signals in C. elegans. Nature 1997;389:994-999.
72. Brunet A, Bonni A, Zigmond MJ, Lin MZ, Juo P, Hu LS, Anderson MJ, Arden KC, Blenis J. Greenberg ME. Akt promotes cell survival by phosphorylating and inhibiting a Forkhead transcription factor. Cell 1999;96:857-868.
73. Kops GJ, de Ruiter ND, De Vries-Smits AM, Powell DR, Bos JL. Burgering BM. Direct control of the Forkhead transcription factor AFX by protein kinase B. Nature. 1999;398:630-634.
74. Rena G, Guo S, Cichy SC, Unterman TG, Cohen P. Phosphorylation of the transcription factor forkhead family member FKHR by protein kinase B. J. Biol. Chem. 1999;274:17179-17183.
75. Biggs WH 3rd, Meisenhelder J, Hunter T, Cavenee WK, Arden KC. Protein kinase B/Akt-mediated phosphorylation promotes nuclear exclusion of the winged helix transcription factor FKHR1. Proc. Natl Acad. Sci. 1999;96:7421-7426.
76. Gu S, Rena G, Cichy S, He X, Cohen P, Unterman T. Phosphorylation of serine 256 by protein kinase B disrupts transactivation by FKHR and mediates effects of insulin on insulin-like growth factor-binding protein-1 promoter activity through a conserved insulin response sequence. J. Biol. Chem. 1999;274:17184-17192.
77. Tang ED, Nunez G, Barr FG, Guan K-L. Negative regulation of the forkhead transcription factor FKHR by Akt. J. Biol. Chem. 1999; 274:16741-16746.
78. Moule SK, Edgell NJ, Welsh GI, Diggle TA, Foulstone EJ, Heesom KJ, Proud CG, Denton RM. Multiple signaling pathways involved in the stimulation of fatty acid and glycogen synthesis by insulin in rat epididymal fat cells. Biochem. J. 1995;311:595-601.
79. Katagiri H, Asano T, Ishihara H, Inukai K, Shibasaki Y, Shibasaki Y, Kikuchi M, Yazaki Y, Oka Y. Overexpression of catalytic subunit p110αof phosphatidylinositol 3-kinase increases glucose transport activity with translocation of glucose transporters in 3T3-L1 adipocytes. J Biol Chem 1996; 271: 16987-16990.
80. Martin SS, Haruta T, Morris AJ, Klippel A, Williams LT, Olefsky JM. Activated phosphatidylinositol 3-kinse is sufficient to mediate actin rearrangement and GLUT4 translocation in 3T3-L1 adipocytes. J Biol Chem 1996; 271:17605-17608.
81. Klippel A, Reinhard C, Kavanaugh WM, Apell G, Escobedo M-A, Williams LT. Membrane localization of phosphatidylinositol 3-kinase is sufficient to activate multiple signal-transducing kinase pathways. Mol Cell Biol 1996; 16:4117-4127.
82. Tanti J-F, Gremeaux T, Grillo S, Calleja V, Klippel A, Williams LT, Van Obberghen E, Le Marchand-Brustel Y. Overexpression of a constitutively active form of phosphatidylinositol 3-kinase is sufficient to promote GLUT4 translocation in adipocytes. J Biol Chem 1996; 271:25227-25232.
83. Frevert EU, Kahn BB. Differential effects of constitutively active phosphatidylinositol 3-kinase on glucose transport, glycogen synthase activity, and DNA synthesis in 3T3 –L1 adipocytes. Mol Cell Biol 1997; 17:190-198.
84. Robinson LJ, Razzack ZF, Lawrence JC Jr., James DE. Mitogen-activated protein kinase activation is not sufficient for stimulation of glucose transport or glycogen synthase in 3T3-L1 adipocytes. J. Biol. Chem. 1994;268:26422-26427.

85. Staubs PA, Nelson JG, Reichart DR,Olefsky JM. Platelet-derived growth factor inhibits insulin stimulation of insulin receptor substrate-1-associated phosphatidylinositol 3-kinase in 3T3-L1 adipocytes without affecting glucose transport. J. Biol. Chem. 1998;273:2513925147.
86. Nave BT, Haigh RJ, Hayward AC, Siddle K, Shepherd PR. Compartment-specific regulation of phosphoinositide 3-kinase by platelet-derived growth factor and insulin in 3T3-L1 adipocytes. Biochem. J. 1996;318 :55-60.
87. Jiang T, Sweeney G, Rudolf MT, Klip A, Traynor-Kaplan A, Tsien RY. Membrane-permeant esters of phosphatidylinositol 3,4,5-trisphosphate. J. Biol. Chem. 1998;273:11017-11024.
88. Rameh LE, Cantley LC. The role of phosphoinositide 3-kinase lipid products in cell function. J. Biol. Chem. 1999;274:8347-8350.
89. Van der Kaay J, Batty IH, Cross DAE, Downes CP. A novel, rapid, and highly sensitive mass assay for phosphatidylinositol 3,4,5-Trisphosphate (Ptd Ins (3,4,5)P^{-}_{3} production in rat skeletal muscle *in Vivo.* J Biol Chem 1997; 272:5477-5481.
90. Vanhaesebroeck B, Leevers SJ, Panayotou G, Waterfield MD. Phosphoinositide 3-kinases: a conserved family of signal transducers. Trends in Biochem. Sci. 1997;22:267272.
91. Rordorf-Nikolic T, Van Horn DJ, Cehn D, White MF, Backer JM. Regulation of phosphatidylinositol 3'-kinase by tyrosyl phosphoproteins. Full activation requires occupancy of both SH2 domains in the 85-kDA regulatory subunit. J Biol Chem 1995; 24:270:3662-3662.
92. Rodriquez-Vicianna P, Warne PH, Vanhaesenbroeck B, Waterfield MD, Downward J. Activation of phosphoinositide 3-kinase by interaction with Ras and by point mutation. EMBO J 1996;15:2442-2451.
93. Bondeva T, Priola L, Bulgarelli-Leva G, Rubio I, Wetzker R, Wymann MP. Bifurcation of lipid and protein kinase signals of PI-3K gamma to the protein kinases PKB and MAPK. Science 1998; 282:293-296.
94. Brown RA, Domin J, Arcaro A, Waterfield MD, Shepherd PR. Insulin activates the alpha isoform of class II phosphoinositide 3-kinase. Journal of Biological Chemistry. 1999;274:14529-14532.
95. Zhang X, Loijens JC, Boronenkov IV, Parker GJ, Norris FA, Chen J. Thum O.Prestwich GD, Majerus PW, Anderson RA. Phosphatidylinositol-4-phosphate 5-kinase isozymes catalyze the synthesis of 3-phosphate-containing phosphatidylinositol signaling molecules. J. Biol. Chem. 1997;272:17756-17761.
96. Wurmser AE., Gary JD, Emr SD. Phosphoinositide 3-kinases and their FYVE domain-containing effectors as regulators of vacuolar/lysosomal membrane trafficking pathways. J. Biol. Chem. 1999;274:9129-9132.
97. Mayer BJ, Ren R. Clark KL Baltimore D. A putative modular domain present in diverse signaling proteins. Cell. 1993;73:629-630.
98. Haslam RJ, Koide HB, Hemmings BA. Pleckstrin domain homology Nature. 1993;363:309-310.
99. Rameh LE, Arvidsson AK, Carraway KL 3rd, Couvillon AD, Rathbun G, Crompton A, VanRenterghem B, Czech MP, Ravichandran KS, Burakoff SJ, Wang DS, Chen CS, Cantley LC. A comparative analysis of the phosphoinositide binding specificity of pleckstrin homology domains. J. Biol. Chem. 1997;272:22059-22066.
100. Fruman DA, Rameh LE, Cantley LC. Phosphoinositide binding domains: embracing 3-phosphate. Cell. 1999;97:817-820.
101. Cross DA, Watt PW, Shaw M., van der Kaay J, Downes CP, Holder JC, Cohen P. Insulin activates protein kinase B, inhibits glycogen synthase kinase-3 and activates glycogen synthase by rapamycin-insensitive pathways in skeletal muscle and adipose tissue. FEBS Letters. 1997;406:211-215.

102. Alessi DR, Kozlowski MT, Weng Q-P, Morrice N, Avruch J. 3-Phosphoinositide-dependent protein kinase 1 (PDK1) phosphorylates and activates the p70 S6 kinase *in vivo* and *in vitro*. Curr. Biol. 1997;8:69-81.
103. Pullen N. Dennis PB. Andjelkovic M. Dufner A. Kozma SC. Hemmings BA. Thomas G. Phosphorylation and activation of p70s6k by PDK1 Science. 1998;279:707-710.
104. Jones PF, Jakubowicz T, Pitossi FJ, Maurer F, Hemmings BA: Molecular cloning and identification of a serine/threonine protein kinase of the second-messenger subfamily. Proc Natl Acad Sci 88: 1991;4171-4175.
105. Coffer PJ, Woodgett JR: Molecular cloning and characterisation of a novel putative protein-serine kinase related to the cAMP-dependent and protein kinase C families. Euro J Bioch 1991;201:475-481.
106. Bellacosa A, Testa JR, Staal SP, Tsichlis PN: A retroviral oncogene, Akt, encoding a serine-threonine kinase containing an SH2-like region. Science. 1991;254: 274-277.
107. Franke TF, Yang SI, Chan TO, Datta K: Kazlauskas A. Morrison DK.
108. Kaplan DR, Tsichlis PN. The protein kinase encoded by the Akt proto-oncogene is a target of the PDGF-activated phosphatidylinositol 3-kinase. Cell. 1995;81: 727-736.
109. Burgering BM, Coffer PJ: Protein kinase B (c-Akt) in phosphatidylinositol-3-OH kinase signal transduction. Nature 1995;376: 599-602.
110. Kohn AD, Kovacina KS, Roth RA: Insulin stimulates the kinase activity of RAC-PK, a pleckstrin homology domain containing ser/thr kinase. EMBO Journal. 1995;14:4288-4295.
111. Franke TF, Kaplan DR, Cantley LC, Toker A. Direct regulation of the Akt proto-oncogene product by phosphatidylinositol-3,4-bisphosphate Science. 1997;275:665-668.
112. Kohn AD, Takeuchi F, Roth RA: Akt, a pleckstrin homology domain containing kinase, is activated primarily by phosphorylation. J Biol Chem 1996;271: 21920-21926.
113. James Sr, Downs CP, Gigg R, Grove SJ, Holmes AB, Alessi DR. Specific binding of the Akt-1 protein kinase to phosphatidylinositol 3,4,5-trisphosphate without subsequent activation. Biochem J 1996; 315:709-713.
114. Alessi DR, Deak M. Casamayor A, Caudwell FB, Morrice N, Norman DG, Gaffney P, Reese CB, MacDougall CN, Harbison D, Ashworth A. Bownes M. 3-Phosphoinositide-dependent protein kinase-1 (PDK1): structural and functional homology with the Drosophila DSTPK61 kinase. Curr. Biol. 1997;7:776-789.
115. Alessi DR, Andjelkovic M, Caudwell B, Cron P, Morrice N, Cohen P. Hemmings BA: Mechanism of activation of protein kinase B by insulin and IGF-1. EMBO 1996;15: 6541-6551.
116. Alessi DR, James SR, Downes CP, Holmes AB, Gafrey PRJ, Reese CB, Cohen P: Characterization of a 3-phosphoinositide-dependent protein kinase which phosphorylates and activates protein kinase Bα. Curr Biol 1997;7: 261-269.
117. Vanhaesenbroeck B, Alessi DR. The PI3K-PDK1 connection: more than just a road to PKB. Biochem J 2000; 346:561-576.
118. Williams MR, C Arthur JS, Balendran A, van der Kaay J, Poli V, Cohen P, Alessi DR. the role of 3-phosphoinositide –dependent protein kinase 1 in activating AGC kinases defined in embryonic stem cells. Curr Biol 2000; 10:439-448.
119. Bertrand L, Alessi DR, Deprez J, Deak M, Viaene E, Rider MH, Hue L. Heart 6-phosphofructo-2-kinase activation by insulin results from Ser-466 and Ser-483 phosphorylation and requires 3-phosphoinositide-dependent kinase-, but not protein kinase B. J Biol Chem 1999; 274:30927-30933.
120. Coffer PJ, Jin J, Woodgett JR. Protein kinase B (c-Akt): a multifunctional mediator of phosphatidylinositol 3-kinase activation. Biochem J 1998; 335 1-13.
121. Datta SR, Brunet A, Greenberg ME. Cellular survival: a play in three Akts. Genes & Dev 1999; 13:290-2927.

122. Kandel ES, Hay N. The regulation and activities of the multifunctional serine/threonine kinase Akt/PKB. Exp Cell Res 1999; 253:210-229.
123. Brady MJ, Bourbonais FJ, Saltiel AR. The activation of glycogen synthase by insulin switches from kinase inhibition to phosphatase activation during adipogenesis in 3T3-L1 cells. J. Biol. Chem. 1998;273:14063-14066.
124. Kitamura T, Kitamura Y, Kuroda S, Hino Y, Ando M, Kotani K, Honishi H, Matsuzaki H, Kikkawa U, Ogawa W, Kasuga. Insulin-induced phosphorylation and activation of cyclic nucleotide phosphodiesterase 3B by the serine-threonine kinase Akt. Mol Cell Biol 1999;19:6286-6296.
125. Cong L-N, Li Y, Zhou L, McGibbon MA, Taylor SI, Quon MJ. Physiological role of Akt in insulin-stimulated translocation of GLUT4 in transfected rat adipose cells. Mol Endo 1997; 11:1881-1890.
126. Kohn AD, Summers SA, Birnbaum MJ, Roth RA. Expression of a constitutively active Akt Ser/Thr kinase in 3T3-L1 adipocytes stimulates glucose uptake and glucose transporter 4 translocation. J Biol Chem 1996; 271:31372-31378.
127. Wang Q, Somwar R, Bilan J, Liu Z, Jin J, Woodgett JR, Klip A. Protein kinase B/Akt participates in GLUT4 translocation by insulin in L6 myoblasts. Mol Cell Biol 1999; 4008-4018.
128. Hill MM, Clark SF, Tucker DF, Birnbaum MJ, James DE, Macaulay SL. A role for protein kinase B□/Akt2 in insulin-stimulated GLUT4 translocation in adipocytes. Mol Cell Biol 1999; 19:7771-7781.
129. Kitamura T, Ogawa W, Sakaue H, Hino Y, Kuroda S, Takata M, Matsumoto M, Maeda T, Honishi H, Kikkawa U, Kasuga M. Requirement for activation of the serine-threonine kinase Akt (protein kinase B) in insulin stimulation of protein synthesis but not of glucose transport. Mol Cell Biol 1998; 18:3708-3717.
130. Foran PGP, Fletcher LM, Oatey PB, Mohammed N, Dolly JO, Tavare JM. Protein kinase B stimulates the translocation of GLUT4 but not GLUT1 or transferrin receptors in 3T3-L1 adipocytes by a pathway involving SNAP-23, synaptobrevin-2 and/or cellubrevin. J Biol Chem 1999; 274:28087-28095.
131. Mellor H, Parker PJ. The extended protein kinase C superfamily. Biochem J 1998; 332:281-292.
132. Toker A. Signaling through protein kinase C. Frontiers in Bioscience 1998; 3:d1134-1147.
133. Braiman L, Alt A, Kuroki T, Ohba M, Bak A, Tennenbaum T, Sampson SR. Protein kinase Cγ mediates insulin-induced glucose transport in primary cultures of rat skeletal muscle. Mol Endo 1999; 13:2002-2012.
134. Cooper DR, Watson JE, Patel N, Illingworth P, Acevedo-Duncan M, Goodnight J, Chalfant CE, Mischak H. Ectopic expression of protein kinase C-beta II,-delta, and –epsilon, but not -betaI or-zeta, provide for insulin stimulation of glucose uptake in NIH-3T3 cells. Arch Biochem Biophys 1999; 372:69-79.
135. Kotani K, Ogawa W, Matsumoto M, Kitamura T, Sakaue H, Hino Y, Miyake K, Sano W,Akimoto K, Ohno S, Kasuga M Requirement of atypical protein kinase C lambda for insulin stimulation of glucose uptake but not for Akt activation in 3T3-L1 adipocytes. Mol Cell Biol 1998 ;18(12):6971-82.
136. Standaert ML, Bandyopadhyay G, Perez L, Price D, Galloway L, Poklepovic A, SajanMP, Cenni V, Sirri A, Moscat J, Toker A, Farese RV Insulin activates protein kinases C-zeta and C-lambda by an autophosphorylation-dependent mechanism and stimulates their translocation to GLUT4 vesicles and other membrane fractions in rat adipocytes. J Biol Chem 1999 Sep 3;274(36):25308-16
137. Handyopadhyay G, Standaert ML, Kikkawa U, Ono Y, Moscat J, Farese RV. Effects of transiently expressed atypical (ζ, λ), conventional (α,β) and novel (δ,ε) protein kinase C isoforms on insulin-stimulated translocation of epitope-tagged GLUT4 glucose transporters in rat adipocytes: specific interchangeable effects of protein kinases C-ζ and C-λ. Biochem J 1999; 33: 461-470.

138. Etgen GJ, Valasek KM, Broderick CL Miller AR. *In vivo* adenoviral delivery of recombinant human protein kinase C-ζ stimulates glucose transport activity in rat skeletal muscle. J. Biol Chem 1999; 274:22139-22142.
139. Bandyopadhyay G, Standaert ML, Sajan MP, Karnitz LM, Cong L, Quon MJ, Farese RV. Dependence of insulin stimulated glucose transporter 4 translocation on 3-phosphoinositide-dependent protein kinse-1 and its target threonine-410 in the activation loop of protein kinase C-ζ. Mol Endo 1999; 13:1766-1772.
140. Le Good JA, Ziegler WH, Parekh DB, Alessi DR, Cohen P, Parker PJ. Protein kinase C isotypes controlled by phosphoinositide 3-kinase through the protein kinase PDK1. Science. 1998;281:2042-2045.
141. Chou MM, Hou W, Johnson J, Graham LK, Lee MH, Chen CS, Newton AC, Schaffhausen BS, Toker A. Regulation of protein kinase C zeta by PI 3-kinase and PDK-1. Curr. Biol.1998; 8:1069-1077.
142. Dutil EM, Toker A, Newton AC. Regulation of conventional protein kinase C isozymes by phosphoinositide-dependent kinase 1 (PDK-1). Curr. Biol. 1998;8:1366-1375.
143. Behn-Krappa A, Newton AC. The hydrophobic phosphorylation motif of conventional protein kinase C is regulated by autophosphorylation. Curr Biol 1999; 9(14): 728-37.
144. Dutil EM, Newton AC. Dual role of pseudosubstrate in the coordinated regulation of protein kinase C by phosphorylation and diacylglycerol. J Biol Chem 2000; 275(14): 10697-10701.
145. Prekh DB, Ziegler W, Parker PJ. Multiple pathways control protein kinase C phosphorylation. EMBO J 2000; 19: 496-503.
146. Flynn P, Mellor H, Casamassima A, Parker, P. Rho GTPase Control of Protein Kinase C-related Protein Kinase Activation by 3-Phosphoinositide-dependent Protein Kinase. J Biol Chem 2000; 275: 11064-11070.
147. Nakanishi H, Brewer KA, Exton JH. Activation of the zeta isozyme of protein kinase C by phosphatidylinositol 3,4,5-trisphosphate. J Biol Chem 1993;268:13-16.
148. Toker A, Meyer M, Reddy KK, Falck JR, Aneja R, Aneja S, Parra A, Burns DJ, Ballas LM, Cantley LC. Activation of protein kinase C family members by the novel polyphosphoinositides PtdIns-3,4-P2 and PtdIns-3,4,5-P3. J Biol Chem 1994;269:32358-32368.
149. Akimoto K, Takahashi R, Moriya S, Nishioka N, Takayanagi J, Kimura K, Fukui Y, Osada S-i, Mizuno K, Hirai S-i, Kazlauskas A, Ohno S. EGF or PDGF receptors activate atypical PKC through phosphatidylinositol 3-kinase. EMBO J. 1996;15:788-798.
150. Moriya S, Kazlauskas A, Akimoto K, Hirai S, Mizuno K, Takenawa T, Fukui Y, Watanabe Y, Ozaki S, Ohno S. Platelet-derived growth factor activates protein kinase C epsilon through redundant and independent signaling pathways involving phospholipase C gamma or phosphatidylinositol 3-kinase. Proc. Natl. Acad. Sci. 1996;9:151-155.
151. Bandyopadhyay G, Standaert ML, Zhao L, Yu B, Avignon A, Galloway L, Karnam P, Moscat J, Farese R. Activation of protein kinase (α,β,and ζ) by insulin in 3T3/LI Cells. J Biol Chem1997; 272:2551-2558.
152. Ohmori S, Shirai Y, Sakai N, Fujii M, Konishi H, Kikkawa U, Saito N. Three distinct mechanisms for translocation and activation of the δ subspecies of protein kinase C. Mol Cell Biol 1998; 18:5263-5271.
153. Mendez R, Kollmorgen G, White MF, Rhoads RE. Requirement of protein kinase C zeta for stimulation of protein synthesis by insulin. Mol Cell Biol1997;17:5184-92.
154. Pessin J, Thurmond D, Elmendorf J, Coker K, Okada S. Molecular basis of insulin-stimulated GLUT4 vesicle trafficking. J Biol Chem 1999; 274:2593-2596.
155. Czech M, Corvera S. Signaling mechanisms that regulate glucose transport J Biol Chem 1999; 274: 1865-1868.

156. Whitehead JP, Clark SF, Urso B, James DE. Signaling through the insulin receptor. Curr Opin Cell Biol. 2000 Apr;12:222-228.
157. Moss J, Vaughan M. Molecules in the ARF Orbit. J Biol Chem 1998;273:21431-21434.
158. Springer, S, Spang A, Schekman R. A Primer on Vesicle Budding. Cell 1999; 97: 145-148.
159. Novick P, Zerial, M. The diversity of Rab proteins in vesicle transport. Curr Opin Biol 1997; 496-504.
160. Schimmoller F, Simon I, Pfeffer, S. Rab GTPases, directors of vesicle docking J Biol Chem 1998; 273: 22161-22164.
161. Pfeffer, S. Transport-vesicle targeting: tethers before SNAREs. Nature Cell Biology 1999; E17-E22.
162. Hay J, Scheller, R. SNAREs and NSF in targeted membrane fusion. Curr Opin Cell Biol 1997; 9:505-512.
163. Bock JB, Scheller RH. SNARE proteins mediate lipid bilayer fusion. Proc Natl Acad Sci 1999; 96:1227-12229.
164. Kawanishi M, Tamori Y, Okazawa H, Araki A, Shinoda H, Kasuga M. Role of SNAP23 in insulin-induced translocation of GLUT4 in 3T3-L1 adipocytes. J Biol Chem 2000; 275:8240-8247.
165. Min J, Okada S, Kanzaki M, Elmendorf JS, Coker KH, Ceresa BP, Syu L-J, Noda Y, Saltiel AR, Pessin JE. Synip: A novel insulin-regulated syntaxin 4-binding protein mediating GLUT4 translocation in adipocytes. Mol Cell 1999; 3:751-760.
166. Klarlund JK, Guilherme A, Holik JJ, Virbasius JV, Chawla A, Czech MP. Signaling by phosphoinositide-3,4,5-tirsphosphate through proteins containing pleckstrin and Sec7 homology domains. Science 1997; 275:1927-1930.
167. Emoto M, Klarlund JK, Waters SB, Hu V, Buxton JM, Chawla A, Czech MP. The role for phospholipase D in GLUT4 glucose transporter translocation. J Biol Chem 2000; 275:7144-7151.
168. Kao AW, Ceresa BP, Santeler SR, Pessin JE. Expression of a dominant interfering dynamin mutant in 3T3L1 adipocytes inhibits GLUT4 endoyctosis without affecting insulin signaling. J Biol Chem 1998; 273:25450-25457.
169. Hausdorff SF, Fingar DC, Morioka K, Garza LA, Whiteman EL, Summers SA, Birnbaum MJ. Identification of wortmannin-sensitive targets in 3T3-L1 adipocytes. J Biol Chem 1999; 274:24677-24684.
170. Mackay DJG, Hall A. Rho GTPases. J Biol Chem 1998; 273: 20685-20688.
171. Sweeney G, Somwar R, Ramlal T, Volchuk A, Ueyama A, Klip A. An inhibitor of p38 mitogen-activated protein kinase prevents insulin-stimulated glucose transporter translocation in 3T3-L1 adipocytes and L6 myotubes. J Biol Chem 1999; 274:10071-10078.
172. Geiger D, Carpentier JL, Gorden P, Orci L. Down-regulation of insulin receptors is related to insulin internalization. Exp Cell Res 1989;185:33-40.
173. Backer JM, Shoelson SE, Haring E, White MF. Insulin receptors internalize by a rapid saturable pathway requiring receptor autophosphorylation and an intact juxtamembrane region. J Cell Biol 1991;115:1535-1545.
174. Carpentier JL, Paccaud JP, Backer J, Gilbert A, Orci L, Kahn CR, Baecker J. Two steps of insulin receptor internalization depend on different domains of the beta-subunit. J Cell Biol 1993;122:1243-1252.
175. Carpentier JL, Paccaud JP, Gorden P, Rutter WJ, Orci L. Insulin-induced surface redistribution regulates internalization of the insulin receptor and requires its autophosphorylation. Proc Natl Acad Sci 1992; 89:162-166.
176. Joazeiro CA, Wing SS, Huang H, Leverson JD, Hunter T, Liu YC. The tyrosine kinase negative regulator c-Cbl is a RING –type, E2 –dependent ubiquitin-protein ligase. Science 1999;286:309-312.

177. Levkowitz G, Waterman H, Ettenberg SA, Katz M, Tsygankov AY, Alroy I, Lavi S, Iwai K, Reiss Y, Ciechanover A, Lipkowitz, Yarden Y. Ubiquitin ligase activity and tyrosine phosphorylation underlie suppression of growth factor signaling by c-Cbl/Sli-1. Mol Cell 1999;4:1029-1040.
178. Clark SF, Molero JC, James DE. Release of insulin receptor substrate proteins from an intracellular complex coincides with the development of insulin resistance. J Biol Chem 2000; 275:3819-3826.
179. Freidenberg GR, Suter SL, Henry RR, Reichart D, Olefsky JM. In vivo stimulation of the insulin receptor kinase in human skeletal muscle. Correlation with insulin-stimulated glucose disposal during euglycemic clamp studies. J Clin Invest 1991; 87:2222-2229.
180. Thies RS, Molina JM, Ciaraldi TP, Friedenberg GR, Olefsky JM. Insulin-receptor autophosphorylation and endogenous substrate phosphorylation in human adipocytes from control, obese, and NIDDM subjects. Diabetes 1990;39:250-259.
181. Goldfine AB, Simonson DC, Folli F, Patti ME, Kahn CR. In vivo and in vitro studies of vanadate in human and rodent diabetes mellitus. Mol Cell Biochem 1995; 153:217-231.
182. Di Guglielmo GM, Drake PG, Baass PC, Authier F, Posner BI, Bergeron JJM. Insulin receptor internalization and signaling. Mol Cell Biochem 1998; 182:59-63.
183. Calera MR, Vallega G, Pilch PF. Dynamics of protein-tyrosine phosphates in rat adipocytes. J Biol Chem 2000;275:6308-6312.
184. Goldstein BJ, Ahmad F, Ding W, Li PM, Zhang WR. Regulation of the insulin signaling pathway by cellular protein-tyrosine phosphatases. Mol Cell Biochem 1998; 182:91-99.
185. Walchli S, Churchod M-L, Pescini Gobert R, Arkinstall S, Hooft van Huijsduijnen. Identification of tyrosine phosphatases that dephosphorylate the insulin receptor. 2000; 275:9792-9796.
186. Kenner KA, Anyanwu W, Olefsky JM, Kusari J. Protein-tyrosine phosphatase 1B is a negative regulator of insulin-and insulin-like growth factor-I-stimulated signaling. J Biol Chem 1996; 19810-19816.
187. Chen H, Wertheimer SJ, Lin CH, Katz SL, Amrein KE, Burn P, Quon MJ. Protein-tyrosine phosphatases PTP1B and Syp are modulators of insulin-stimulated translocation of GLUT4 in transfected rat adipose cells. J Biol Chem 1997; 272:8026-8031.
188. Arnott CH, Sale EM, Miller J, Sale GJ. Use of an antisense strategy to dissect the signaling role of protein-tyrosine phosphatase alpha. J Biol Chem 1999;274:26105-26112.
189. Bleyle LA, Peng Y, Ellis C, Mooney RA. Dissociation of PTPase levels from their modulation of insulin receptor signal transduction. Cell Signal 1999; 11:719-725.
190. Ren JM, Li PM, Zhang WR, Sweet LJ, Gline G, Shulman GI, Livingston JN, Goldstein BJ. Transgenic mice deficient in the LAR protein-tyrosine phosphatase exhibit profound defects in glucose homeostasis. Diabetes 1998;47:493-497.
191. Bandyopadhyay D, Kusari A, Kenner KA, Liu F, Chernoff J, Gustafson TA, Kusari J. Protein-tyrosine phosphatase 1B complexes with the insulin receptor in vivo and is tyrosine-phosphorylated in the presence of insulin. J Biol Chem. 1997; 272:1639-1645.
192. Elchebly M., Payette P, Michaliszyn E, Cromlish W, Collins S, Loy AL, Normandin D, Cheng A, Himms-Hagen J, Chan CC, Ramachandran C, Gresser MJ, Tremblay ML, Kennedy BP. Increased insulin sensitivity and obesity resistance in mice lacking the protein tyrosine phosphatase-1B gene Science 1999; 283:1544-1548.
193. Moxham CM, Malbon CC, Insulin action impaired by deficiency of the G-protein subunit G ialpha2. Nature 1996; 379:840-844.
194. Vasquez F, Sellers WR. The PTEN tumor suppressor protein: an antagonist of phosphoinositide 3-kinase signaling. Biochim et Biophy Acta 2000;1470:M21-M35.

195. Maehama T, Dizon JE. PTEN: a tumour suppressor that functions as a phospholipid phosphatase. Trends Cell Biol 1999; 9:125-128.
196. Goberdhan DC, Paricio N, Goodman EC, Mlodzik M., Wilson C. Drosophila tumor suppressor PTEN controls cell size and number by antagonizing the Chico/PI3-kinase signaling pathway. Genes Dev. 1999; 13:3244-3258.
197. Dunaif A, Xia J, Book CB, Schenker E, Tang Z. Excessive insulin receptor serine phosphorylation in cultured fibroblasts and in skeletal muscle. A potential mechanism for insulin resistance in the polycystic ovary syndrome. J Clin Inv 1995: 96:801-810.
198. Chin JE, Dickens M, Tavare JM, Roth RA. Overexpression of protein kinase C isoenzymes alpha, beta I, gamma, and epsilon in cells overexpressing the insulin receptor. Effects on receptor phosphorylation and signaling. J Biol Chem. 1993 ; 268:6338-6347.
199. Chin JE, Liu F, Roth RA. Activation of protein kinase Cα inhibits insulin-stimulated tyrosine phosphorylation of insulin receptor substrate-1. Mol Endo 1994; 8:51-58.
200. De Fea K, Roth RA. Protein kinase C modulation of insulin receptor substrate-1 tyrosine phosphorylation requires serine 612. Biochem 1997; 36:12939-12947.
201. De Fea K, Roth RA. Modulation of insulin receptor substrate-1 tyrosine phosphorylation and function by mitogen-activated protein kinase. J Biol Chem. 1997; 272:31400-31406.
202. Li J, DeFea K, Roth RA. Modulation of insulin receptor asubstarte-1 tyrosine phosphorylation by an Akt/phosphatidylinositol 3 kinase pathway. J Biol Chem 1999; 274:9351-9356.
203. Delahaye L, Mothe-Satney I, Myers MG, White MF, Van Obberghen E. Interaction of insulin receptor substrate-1(IRS-1) with phosphatidylinositol 3-kinase: effect of substitution of alanine for serine in potential IRS-1 serine phosphorylation sites. Endocrinology 1998 139:4911-4919.
204. Peraldi P, Spiegelman B. TNF-α and insulin resistance: Summary and future prospects. Mol Cell Bichem 1998; 182:169-175.
205. Hotamisligil GS. Mechanisms of TNF-alpha-induced insulin resistance. Exp Clin Endocrinol Diabetes 1999; 107:119-125.
206. Aguirre V, Uchida T, Yenush L, Davis R, White MF. The c-Jun NH(2)-terminal kinase promotes insulin resistance during association with insulin receptor substrate-1 and phosphorylation of Ser J Biol Chem 2000; 275:9047-9054.
207. Paz K, Hemi R, LeRoith D, Karasik A, Elhanany E, Kanety H, Zick Y. A molecular basis for insulin resistance. Elevated serine/threonine phosphorylation of IRS-1 and IRS-2 inhibits their binding to the juxtamembrane region of the insulin receptor and impairs their ability to undergo insulin-induced tyrosine phosphorylation. J Biol Chem 1997; 272:29911-29918.
208. Pickup JC, Crook MA. Is type II diabetes mellitus a disease of the innate immune system? Diabetologia 1998; 41: 1241-1248.
209. Fernandez-Real JM, Ricart W. Insulin resistance and inflammation in an evolutionary perspective: the contribution of cytokine genotype/phenotype to thriftiness. Diabetologia 1999; 42:1367-1374.
210. Uysal KT, Wiesbrock SM., Marino MW, Hotamisligil GS. Protection from obesity-induced insulin resistance in mice lacking TNF-alpha function. Nature 1997; 389:610-614.
211. Schreyer SA, Chua SC Jr., LeBoeuf RC. Obesity and diabetes in TNF-alpha receptor-deficient mice. J Clin Invest 1998; 102:402-411.
212. Paquot N, Castillo MJ, Lefebvre PJ, Scheen AJ. No increased insulin sensitivity after a single intravenous administration of a recombinant human tumor necrosis factor receptor: Fc fusion protein in obese insulin-resistant patients. J Clin Endocrinol Metab 2000; 85:1316-1319.

213. Paz K, Liu YF, Shorer H, Hemi R, LeRoith D, Quan M. Kanety H, Seger R, Zick Y. Phosphorylation of insulin receptor substrate-1 (IRS-1) by protein kinase B positively regulates IRS-1 function. J Biol Chem 1999; 274:28816-228822.
214. Eldar-Finkelman H, Krebs EG. Phosphorylation of insulin receptor substrate 1 by glycogen synthase kinase 3 impairs insulin action. Proc Natl Acad Sci 1997; 94:9660-9664.
215. Eldar-Finkelman H, Schreyer SA, Shinohara MM, LeBoeuf RC, Krebs EG. Increased glycogen sythase kinase-3 activity in diabetes- and obesity- prone C57BL/6J mice. Diabetes 1999; 48:1662-1666.
216. Cengel KA, Kason RE, Freund GG. Phosphatidylinositol 3'-kinase associates with an insulin receptor substrate-1 serine kinase distinct from its intrinsic serine kinase. Biochem J 1998; 335:397-404.
217. Qiao LY, Goldberg JL, Russell JC, Sun XJ. Identification of enhanced serine kinase activity in insulin resistance. J Biol Chem 1999; 274:10625-10632.
218. Craparo A, Freund R, Gustafson TA. 14-3-3 (epsilon) interacts with the insulin-like growth factor I receptor and insulin receptor substrate I in a phosphoserine-dependent manner. J Biol Chem 1997; 272:11663-11669.
219. Ogihara T, Isobe T, Ichimura T, Taoka M, Funaki M, Sakoda H, Onishi Y, Inukai K, Anai M, Fukushima Y, Kikuchi M, Yazaki Y, Oka Y.Asano T. 14-3-3 protein binds to insulin receptor substrate-1, one of the binding sites of which is in the phosphotyrosine binding domain. J Biol Chem 1997; 272:25267-25274.
220. Kosaki A, Yamada K, Suga J, Otaka A, Kuzuya H. 14-3-3beta protein associates with insulin receptor substrate 1 and decreases insulin-stimulated phosphatidylinositol 3'-kinase activity in 3T3L1 adipocytes. J Biol Chem 1998; 273:940-944.
221. Willson TM, Brown PJ, Sternbach DD, Henke BR. The PPARs: from orphan receptors to drug discovery. J Med Chem 2000; 43:527-550.
222. Barroso I, Gurnell M., Crowley VE, Agostini M, Schwabe JW, Soos MA, Maslen GL, Williams TD, Lewis H, Schafer AJ, Chatterjee VK, O'Rahilly S. Dominant negative mutations in human PPAR gamma associated with severe insulin resistance, diabetes mellitus and hypertension Nature 1999; 402:880-883.
223. Ristow M, Muller-Wieland D, Pfeiffer A, Krone W, Kahn CR. Obesity associated with a mutation in a genetic regulator of adipocyte differentiation. N Engl J Med 1998; 339:953-959.
224. Kubota N, Terauchi Y, Miki H, Tamemoto H, Yamauchi T, Komeda K, Satoh S, Nakano R, Ishii C, Sugiyama T, Eto K, Tsubamoto Y, Okuno A, Murakami K, Sekihara H, Hasegawa G, Naito M, Toyoshima Y, Tanaka S, Shiota K, Kitamura T, Fujita T, Ezaki O, Aizawa S, Kadowaki T. PPAR γ mediates high-fat diet-induced adipocyte hypertrophy and insulin resistance. Mol Cell 1999; 4:597-609.
225. Miles PDG, Barak Y, He W, Evans RM, Olefsky JM. Improved insulin-sensitivity in mice heterozygous for PPAR-gamma deficiency. J Clin Invest 2000;105:287-292.
226. Deeb SS, Fajas L, Nemoto M., Pihlajamaki J, Mykkanen L, Kuusisto J, Laakso M, Fujimoto W, Auwerx J. A Pro12Ala substitution in PPARgamma2 associated with decreased receptor activity, lower body mass index and improved insulin sensitivity. Nat Genet 1998 20:284-287.
227. Masugi J, Tamori Y, Mori H, Koike T, Kasuga M. Inhibitory effect of a proline-to-alanine substitution at codon 12 of peroxisome proliferator-activated receptor-gamma 2 on thiazolidinedione-induced adipogenesis. Biochem Biophys Res Commun 2000;268:178-182
228. Chen D, Garg A. Monogenic disorders of obesity and body fat distribution. J Lipid Res 1999; 40:1735-1746.
229. Shimomura I, Hammer RE, Richardson JA, Ikemoto S, Bashmakov Y, Goldstein JL, Brown MS. Insulin resistance and diabetes mellitus in transgenic mice expressing nuclear SREBP-1c in adipose tissue: model for congenital generalized lipodystrophy. Genes Dev 1998; 12:3182-314.

230. Shimomura I, Hammer RE, Ikemoto S, Brown MS, Goldstein JL. Leptin reverses insulin resistance anddiabetes mellitus in mice with congenital lipodystrophy. Nature 1999; 401:73-76.
231. Moitra J, Mason MM, Olive M, Krylov D, Gavrilova O, Marcus-Samuels B, Feigenbaum L, Lee E, Aoyama T, Eckhaus M., Reitman ML, Vinson C. Life without white fat: a transgenic mouse. Genes & Development. 1998; 12:3168-3181.
232. Gavrilova O, Marcus-Samuels B, Leon LR, Vinson C, Teitman ML. Leptin and diabetes in lipoatrophic mice. Nature 2000; 24:850-851.
233. Gavrilova O, Marcus-Samuels B, Graham D, Kim JK, Shulman GI, Castle AL, Vinson C, Eckhaus M, Reitman ML. Surgical implantation of adipose tissue reverses diabetes in lipoatrophic mice. J Clin Invest 2000; 105:271-278.
234. Kim JK, Gavrilova O, Chen Y, Reitman ML, Shulman GI Mechanisms of insulin resistance in A-ZIP/F-1 fatless mice. J Biol Chem 2000; 275:8456-8460.
235. Hotamisligil GS, Johnson RS, Distel RJ, Ellis R, Papaioannou VE. Spiegelman BM. Uncoupling of obesity from insulin resistance through a targeted mutation in aP2, the adipocyte fatty acid binding protein. Science 1996; 274:1377-1379.
236. Marshall S, Garvey WT, Traxinger RR. New insights into the metabolic regulation of insulin action and insulin resistance: role of glucose and amino acids. FASEB J 1991; 5:3031-3036.
237. Hawkins M., Barzilai N, Liu R, Hu M,. Chen W, Rossetti L. Role of the glucosamine pathway in fat-induced insulin resistance. J Clin Invest 1997 ; 99:2173-2182.
238. Hebert LF Jr, Daniels MC, Zhou J, Crook ED, Turner RL, Simmons ST, Neidigh JL, Zhu JS, Baron AD, McClain DA. Overexpression of glutamine: fructose-6-phosphate amidotransferase in transgenic mice leads to insulin resistance. J Clin Invest 1996; 98:930-936.
239. Wang J, Liu R, Hawkins M, Barzilai N, Rossetti L. A. nutrient-sensing pathway regulates leptin gene expression in muscle and fat. Nature 1998; 393:684-688.
240. Liu F, Roth RA. Binding of SH2 containing proteins to the insulin receptor: a new way for modulating insulin signaling. Mol Cell Biochem 182:73-78.
241. He W, Rose DW, Olefsky JM., Gustafson TA. Grb10 interacts differentially with the insulin receptor, insulin-like growth factor I receptor, and epidermal growth factor receptor via the Grb10 Src homology 2(SH2) domain and a second novel domain located between the pleckstrin homology and SH2 domains. J Biol Chem 1998; 273:6860-6867.
242. Maddux BA, Sbraccia P, Kumakura S, Sasson S, Youngren J, Fisher A, Spencer S, Grupe A, Henzel W, Stewart TA, Reaven GM, Goldfine IR. Membrane glycoprotein PC-1 and insulin resistance in non-insulin-dependent diabetes mellitus Nature. 1995; 373:448-451
243. Sakoda H, Ogihara T, Anai M, Funaki M, Inukai K, Katagiri H, Fukushima Y, Onishi Y, Ono H, YazakiY, Kikuchi M, Oka Y, Asano T. No correlation of plasma cell 1 overexpression with insulin resistance in diabetic rats and 3T3-L1 adipocytes. Diabetes 1999; 48:1365-1371.
244. Condorelli G, Vigliotta G, Iavarone C, Caruso M,. Tocchetti CG,. Andreozzi F, Cafieri A, Tecce MF, Formisano P, Beguinot L, Beguinot F. PED/PEA-15 gene controls glucose transport and is overexpressed in type2 diabetes mellitus. EMBO J 1998; 17:3858-3866.
245. DeFronzo RA, Tobin JD, Andres R Glucose clamp technique: a method for quantifying insulin secretion and resistance. Am J Physiol 1979; 237:E214-223
246. Matsuda M, DeFronzo RA. Insulin sensitivity indices obtained from oral glucose tolerance testing: comparison with the euglycemic insulin clamp. Diabetes Care. 1999; 22:1462-7140.
247. Soop M, Nygren J, Brismar K, Thorell A, Ljungqvist O. The hyperinsulinaemic-euglycaemic glucose clamp: reproducibility and metabolic effects of prolonged insulin infusion in healthy subjects. Clin Sci 2000; 98:367-374.

248. Hanson RL, Pratley RE, Bogardus C, Venkat Narayan KM, Roumain JM, Imperatore G,Fagot-Campagna A, Pettitt DJ, Bennett PH, Knowler WC Evaluation of simple indices of insulin sensitivity and insulin secretion for use in epidemiologic studies. Am J Epidemiol 2000; 151:190-198
249. Rizza RA, Mandarino LJ, Gerich JE. Dose-response characteristics for effects of insulin on production and utilization of glucose in man. Amer J Physiol 1981; 240(6):E630-639.
250. Frayn KN. Calculation of substrate oxidation rates in vivo from gaseous exchange J Appl Physiol 1983; 55:628-634..
251. Shulman GI, Rothman DL, Jue T, Stein P, DeFronzo RA, Shulman RG. Quantitation of muscle glycogen synthesis in normal subjects and subjects with non-insulin-dependent diabetes by 13C nuclear magnetic resonance spectroscopy N Engl J Med 1990; 322:223-238.
252. Petersen KF, Hendler R, Price T, Perseghin G, Rothman DL, Held N, Amatruda JM, Shulman GI. 13C/31P NMR studies on the mechanism of insulin resistance in obesity. Diabetes 1998; 47:381-386
253. Olefsky JM, Kolterman OG, Scarlett JA Insulin action and resistance in obesity and noninsulin-dependent type II diabetes mellitus. Am J Physiol 1982; 243:E15-30.
254. Kolterman OG, Insel J, Saekow M, Olefsky JM. Mechanisms of insulin resistance in human obesity: evidence for receptor and postreceptor defects. J Clin Invest. 1980;65:1272-1284.
255. Kolterman OG, Gray RS, Griffin J, Burstein P, Insel J, Scarlett JA, Olefsky JM. Receptor and postreceptor defects contribute to the insulin resistance in noninsulin-dependent diabetes mellitus. J Clin Invest. 1981; 68:957-969.
256. Baron AD, Clark MG. Role of blood flow in the regulation of muscle glucose uptake. Annu Rev Nutr. 1997;17:487-499.
257. Laakso M., Edelman SV, Brechtel G, Baron AD. Decreased effect of insulin to stimulate skeletal muscle blood flow in obese man. A novel mechanism for insulin resistance. J Clin Invest 1990; 85:1844-1852.
258. Laakso M, Edelman SV, Brechtel G, Baron AD. Impaired insulin-mediated skeletal muscle blood flow in patients with NIDDM. Diabetes 1992; 41:1076-1083.
259. Steinberg HO, Chaker H, Leaming R, Johnson A, Brechtel G, Baron AD. Obesity/insulin resistance is associated with endothelial dysfunction. Implications for the syndrome of insulin resistance. J Clin Invest 1996; 97:2601-2610.
260. Rothman DL, Shulman RG, Shulman GI. 31P nuclear magnetic resonance measurements of muscleglucose-6-phosphate. Evidence for reduced insulin-dependent muscle glucose transport or phosphorylation activity in non-insulin-dependent diabetes mellitus. J Clin Invest 1992; 89:1069-1075.
261. Cline GW, Magnusson I, Rothman DL, Petersen KF, Laurent D, Shulman GI. Mechanism of impaired insulin-stimulated muscle glucose metabolism in subjects with insulin-dependent diabetes mellitus. J Clin Invest 1997; 99:2219-2224.
262. Cline GW, Jucker BM, Trajanoski Z, Rennings AJ, Shulman GI. A novel 13C NMR method to assess intracellular glucose concentration in muscle, in vivo. Amer J Physiol Soc 1998; 274:E381-389.
263. Cline GW, Petersen KF, Krssak M, Shen J, Hundal RS, Trajanoski Z, Inzucchi S, Dresner A, Rothman DL, Shulman GI. Impaired glucose transport as a cause of decreased insulin-stimulated muscle glycogen synthesis in type 2 diabetes. N Engl J Med 1999; 341:240-246.
264. Jucker BM, Barucci N, Shulman GI. Metabolic control analysis of insulin-stimulated glucose disposal in rat skeletal muscle. Am J Physiol 1999; 277:E505-512.
265. Levine R and Goldstein M. On the mechanism of action of insulin. Recent Progress Hormone Research. 1955;11:343-380.
266. Goodyear LJ, Kahn BB. Exercise, glucose transport, and insulin sensitivity. Ann Rev Med 1998; 49:235-261.

267. Shepherd PR, Kahn BB. Glucose transporters and insulin action – implications for insulin resistance and diabetes mellitus. N Engl J Med 1999; 341:248-257.
268. Beck-Nielsen H, Groop LC. Metabolic and genetic characterization of prediabetic states. J Clin Invest 1994; 94:1714-1721.
269. Groop LC. Early metabolic defects in persons at increased risk for non-insulin-dependent diabetes mellitus. N Engl J Med 1989; 321:337-343.
270. Kim YB, Nikoulina SE, Ciaraldi TP, Henry RR, Kahn BB. Normal insulin-dependent activation of Akt/protein kinase B, with diminished activation of phosphoinositide 3-kinase, in muscle in type 2 diabetes J Clin Invest 1999; 104:733-471.
271. Cusi K, Maezono K, Osman A, Pendergrass M, Patti MEk Pratipanawatr T, DeFronzo RA, Kahn CR, Mandarino LJ. .Insulin resistance differentially affects the PI 3-kinase- and MAP kinase-mediated signaling in human muscle. J Clin Invest 2000; 105:311-320.
272. Dresner A, Laurent D, Marcucci M, Griffin ME, Dufour S, Cline GW, Slezak LA, Andersen DK, Hundal RS, Rothman DL, Petersen KF, Shulman GI. Effects of free fatty acids on glucose transport and IRS-1-associated phosphatidylinositol 3-kinase activity. J Clin Invest 1999; 103:253-259.
273. Boden G. Free fatty acids, insulin resistance, and Type 2 diabetes mellitus. Proc Assoc Am Physicians 1999; 111:241-248.
274. Randle PJ, Garland PB, Hales CN, Newsholme EA. The glucose fatty-acid cycle: Its role in insulin sensitivity and the metabolic disturbances of diabetes mellitus. Lancet í: 1963;785-789.
275. Griffin ME, Marcucci MJ, Cline GW, Bell K, Barucci N, Lee D, Goodyear LJ, Kraegen EW, White MF, Shulman GI. Free fatty acid-induced insulin resistance is associated with activation of protein kinase C theta and alterations in the insulin signaling cascade. Diabetes. 1999; 48:1270-1274.

9
MOUSE MODELS OF TYPE 2 DIABETES

Domenico Accili, M.D. and Byung-Chul Park, Ph.D.
Dept. of Medicine, Columbia University, New York, NY 10032, USA

INTRODUCTION

Type 2 diabetes is characterized by genetically determined insulin resistance and impaired insulin secretion. Although insulin resistance is generally recognized to precede beta cell dysfunction, a decreased capacity of the beta cell to compensate for increased insulin production can be demonstrated in healthy first degree relatives of diabetic patients, consistent with a genetic etiology of both defects. Both traits are inherited in a non-Mendelian fashion. Thus, simple genetic models, such as those based on studies of candidate genes, have failed to identify common susceptibility alleles for the two major metabolic abnormalities in type 2 diabetes. This could be explained by their genetic heterogeneity, and also by a polygenic or an oligogenic pathogenesis. To dissect the complex genetics of insulin resistance and beta cell dysfunction, investigators have generated transgenic and knock-out mice bearing various mutations in genes required for insulin action and/or insulin secretion. This chapter reviews recent progress in the field and analyzes outstanding questions.

MUTATIONS AFFECTING INSULIN SIGNALING

Insulin Receptor

Mice nullizygous at the insulin receptor (IR) locus show modest developmental delay, resulting in a 10% weight reduction at birth (1). Lack of IRs results in death from diabetic ketoacidosis. This suggests that IRs are necessary and sufficient to mediate the metabolic actions of insulin in post-natal life (2, 3). The early post-natal death caused by inactivation of the IR gene indicates that fetal metabolism is unaffected by the lack of IRs, and that the functional maturation of a fuel sensing apparatus in rodents occurs in the perinatal period, rather than during the late phase of gestation, as in humans (4). Like IR-deficient mice, humans homozygous for null IR mutations are born alive, albeit with significant metabolic abnormalities (5-8). Moreover, they develop a characteristic fasting hypoglycemia that is not seen in mice (9, 10) (Table 1). The pathophysiologic basis has been extensively reviewed in previous publications (11, 12).

Table 1. Phenotypic differences between humans and mice lacking insulin receptors

	Humans	Mice
Fetal growth	<10%	~90%
Appearance	Dysmorphic	Normal
Glucose	Low	High
Insulin (fold increase)	>100	2-3
Ketosis	Transient	Constant
Hepatic Steatosis	Severe	Massive

Insulin-Like Growth Factor-1 Receptor

Lack of IGF-1 receptors (IGF1Rs) is lethal in the immediate post-natal period. Nullizygous animals are born with the expected Mendelian frequency, suggesting that IGF-1Rs are not required for successful completion of gestation. The cause of death is unclear. Efstratiadis has attributed it to respiratory failure caused by hypoplasia of intercostal muscles (13). More recently, Withers et al. have reported an increase in glucose levels associated with beta cell hypoplasia (14). However, it is unlikely that the magnitude of the hyperglycemia would be sufficient to cause relatively sudden death, considering that even insulin-deficient mice survive a few days postnatally (15). The weight of IGF1R null mice is about 45% of normal, and the mice are born with multiple abnormalities, including hypoplastic muscles, delayed bone development and thin epidermis (16).

Role of IGF1R in metabolic control

Insulin and IGF receptors are structurally very similar (17, 18). In addition to binding each other's ligand with low affinity, they both bind IGF-2 with high affinity (19, 20). Moreover, they form hybrid heterodimeric receptors in many tissues where they are co-expressed (21). Finally, their signaling pathways are similar (see Chapter 8) (22). Thus, one would expect that a certain degree of compensation by the cognate receptor would occur in mice lacking IR or IGF1R. However, compensation occurs only under certain conditions. For example, IGF1R can compensate for the growth-promoting actions of IR in mid-gestation (1), but does not compensate for the metabolic actions of IR post-natally, even when adequate IGF1 is supplied (23). In contrast, IR can virtually replace IGF1R in mice lacking both IGF1R and IGF2R. This is probably due to increased levels of IGF2 (24). Thus, the emerging paradigm is that IR can compensate for the growth-promoting actions of IGF1R, but IGF1R cannot fully compensate for the metabolic actions of IR. *In vitro* studies with hepatocytes derived from IR-deficient mice have begun to provide some mechanistic insight into this phenomenon. These experiments suggest that there are intrinsic signaling differences between IRs and IGF1Rs that make IR intrinsically more suited to metabolic signaling than IGF1R (25-28). An additional metabolic role for IGF1R has been proposed recently. Withers and colleagues have suggested that IGF1R is the beta cell growth factor receptor (14). This interesting hypothesis is still awaiting further clarification.

Insulin Receptor Substrate-1

Insulin receptor substrate (IRS) proteins play an important role in mediating the actions of insulin (22). IRS-1 was the first member of this family to be identified and to be ablated in mice using gene knockouts (29, 30). The main consequence of IRS-1 inactivation in mice is growth retardation (both intrauterine and post-natal). Moreover, mice lacking IRS-1 develop mild insulin resistance without overt diabetes (29, 30). However, lack of IRS-1 impairs insulin secretion in beta cells (31), suggesting that insulin/IGF-1 signaling through IRS-1 is required for proper beta cell function. Together, the above findings suggest that IRS-1 is primarily a mediator of the growth promoting actions of IGF1R. In fact, it is apparent that lack of IRS-1 impacts more on IGF-1 than on insulin signaling. However, the role of IRS-1 in metabolic signaling is highlighted by a different series of experiments, in which mice bearing IRS-1 null mutations have been bred mice bearing the IR null allele (32, 33). These experiments are reviewed below.

IRS-2

Lack of IRS-2 is associated with a normal size at birth. However, within a few weeks mice develop fasting hyperglycemia, followed by insulin deficiency and, in males, death from non-ketotic hyperosmolar coma (34). These findings recapitulate the natural history of type 2 diabetes, and have led to the suggestion that IRS-2 may represent a diabetes susceptibility gene, a conclusion that has not been borne out by the genetic analyses carried out thus far in humans (35). These data are consistent with an important role of IRS-2 in fuel homeostasis, but also underline the conclusion that multiple substrates are required to mediate insulin action, since the phenotype due to lack of IRs is substantially more severe than that due to lack of IRS-2.

IRS-3

IRS-3 was originally identified as a small IRS in adipose tissue. While further analyses have shown that it is widely distributed (36, 37), it represents the most abundant IRS protein in adipocytes (38, 39). Interestingly, lack of IRS-3 has no apparent effect on mouse development and metabolism, or on insulin-dependent glucose uptake in isolated adipose cells (40). It remains to be seen whether this is due to the compensatory actions of other IRSs.

IRS-4

The last member of the IRS family to be cloned was IRS-4 (41). To date, data on the tissue expression of this protein are incomplete, but suggest a broader distribution than originally described. Nevertheless, ablation of the IRS-4 gene results in a mild phenotype with reduced growth, impaired glucose tolerance and reproductive abnormalities (42). This phenotype is reminiscent of the IRS-1 phenotype, albeit considerably milder. It remains to be seen whether this subtle phenotype is due to compensation by other family members.

Combined Mutations of IRS-1 and IRS-2

Withers and colleagues have attempted to generate mice lacking IRS-1 and IRS-2, and have failed to recover embryos even at the pre-implantation stage (14). This is one of the most dramatic embryonic lethal phenotypes observed in mice with targeted gene mutations to date. Interestingly, this phenotype is substantially more severe than the phenotype due to combined lack of IR and IGF1R, suggesting that IRS proteins play additional roles to mediate the actions of other receptors, as predicted by studies of cytokine receptor signaling (43). On the other hand, the metabolic phenotype of IRS-1$^{-/-}$/IRS-2$^{+/-}$ mice, bearing the minimum number of IRS-1 and IRS-2 alleles compatible with live birth, is significantly milder than the IR knockout phenotype, suggesting that the metabolic actions of insulin may require more than IRS-1 and IRS-2 signaling (14).

Combined IR, IRS-1 and/or IRS-2 Mutations

The different roles of IRS-1 and IRS-2 in insulin signaling have been analyzed by generating mice with combined heterozygous null mutations in IR, IRS-1 and/or IRS-2 (32, 33). IR$^{+/-}$ mice are insulin resistant, and a small fraction (5-10%) develops diabetes. Combined heterozygosity for IR/IRS-1$^{+/-}$ and IR/IRS-2$^{+/-}$ results in a similarly higher number of diabetic mice (20% and 17%, respectively), compared to single IR$^{+/-}$ mice. However, the underlying pathophysiology differs in the two strains. IR/IRS-1$^{+/-}$ mice are primarily insulin resistant in skeletal muscle, whereas IR/IRS-2$^{+/-}$ mice are primarily insulin resistant in liver. Triple heterozygotes are severely insulin resistant in both organs (33). These data suggest that different IRS proteins play tissue-specific roles to mediate insulin action, with IRS-1 being important in skeletal muscle and IRS-2 in liver. The notion that IRS proteins play different roles in different tissues are confirmed by *in vitro* studies on hepatocytes (25) and isolated muscle (44) lacking IRS proteins.

PI 3-Kinase Regulatory Subunit

It is generally agreed that insulin signaling requires the lipid kinase activity of the enzyme phosphatidylinositol-3-kinase (22). Nevertheless, it remains unclear whether PI 3-kinase is both necessary and sufficient for insulin action (45). To address this question, Terauchi *et al.* generated mice lacking the regulatory p85 subunit of this enzyme (46). p85-deficient mice showed increased insulin sensitivity and hypoglycemia due to increased glucose transport in skeletal muscle and adipocytes. This unexpected phenotype was associated with a compensatory increase in insulin-dependent association between IRS proteins and the products of alternative splicing of the P85 gene (especially P50 alpha). This experiment provides evidence for a role of PI 3-kinase in insulin action. The mechanism by which p85 affects PI 3-kinase activity remains unclear, but these data suggest that the regulatory subunit behaves as an inhibitor of PI 3-kinase activity under basal conditions, with insulin acting to remove this inhibition via IRS proteins.

GLUT4

The insulin-sensitive glucose transporter mediates insulin-dependent glucose uptake in muscle and adipose tissue by translocating from an intracellular compartment to the plasma membrane (22). Mice lacking GLUT4 show growth-retardation, cardiac hypertrophy and hypotrophy of adipose tissues. Plasma glucose levels are in the diabetic range in fed males, but not in females or in fasted animals of either sex. However, all mice develop moderate insulin resistance (47). Somewhat surprisingly, heterozygous males develop insulin-resistant diabetes, without obesity (48). It is not clear why heterozygotes are more severely affected than homozygotes.

Heart-Specific GLUT4 Ablation

To determine whether the cardiac abnormalities seen in GLUT4-deficient mice are the result of a primary role of GLUT4 in the heart, or a consequence of metabolic abnormalities, Abel et al. (49) have used cre-loxP recombination to generate mice lacking GLUT4 expression in the heart. These mice develop modest cardiac hypertrophy associated with increased myocyte size and preserved contractile function.

Peroxisome Proliferator-Activated Receptor-γ

Activation of peroxisome proliferator-activated receptor γ (PPAR-γ) by, among other ligands, the anti-diabetic thiazolidinedione agents, is associated with increased insulin sensitivity. Lack of PPARγ results in embryonic lethality (50, 51). Surprisingly, two groups have reported that heterozygous PPARγ-deficient mice are more insulin sensitive than normal controls (50, 52). The mechanism is unclear, but may be related to smaller adipocyte size and increased leptin secretion (50).

TISSUE-SPECIFIC INSULIN RECEPTOR KNOCKOUTS

In diabetic subjects, insulin resistance affects all target tissues of insulin action. However, this is partly a result of chronic tissue exposure to elevated insulin and glucose concentrations. It is not clear whether insulin resistance is initially restricted to certain organs, and what the relative contributions of each organ to the pathophysiology of the disease are. This analysis of insulin action in selected organs cannot be accomplished using "classic" gene targeting strategies. However, using various additional techniques, including dominant negative mutants (53) and tissue-specific recombination (54), this functional dissection has begun.

Muscle-specific IR knockout

Using cre/loxP-based recombination, Kahn and associates have generated various tissue-specific deletions of the insulin receptor gene (54, 55). Ablation of insulin receptors in skeletal muscle resulted in dyslipidemia, without overt insulin resistance. The lack of even a mild elevation in insulin concentrations was totally unexpected, since skeletal muscle is thought to be the primary site of insulin resistance in humans. On the other hand, the lack of overt diabetes in these mice was not unexpected, since in humans only about 20% of genetically-predisposed insulin resistant individuals will develop diabetes. Despite the absence of overt insulin resistance, these mice provide an extremely useful model to study the metabolic abnormalities associated with impaired glucose utilization in skeletal muscle, including the role of alternative pathways to mediate glucose uptake (56).

Muscle- and fat-specific functional IR knockout

Lauro et al. (53) used a slightly different approach to address a similar question. It has been argued that insulin resistance in muscle and adipose tissue causes type 2 diabetes through a direct effect on glucose uptake and an indirect effect mediated by free fatty acids on glucose oxidation and insulin secretion. Selective insulin resistance in skeletal muscle and fat is associated with impaired glucose tolerance and insulin resistance, without overt type 2 diabetes (53). These findings challenge the idea that insulin resistance in the adipose cell and muscle is sufficient to set in motion the complex chain of events leading to type 2 diabetes by impairing glucose utilization and beta cell function. Based on these findings, it has to be concluded that, in mice, compensation by the liver for the impairment of insulin action in muscle and fat protects against the development of diabetes. Nevertheless, it has to be pointed out that the liver accounts for a much larger fraction of glucose storage in rodents than it does in humans. Thus, these conclusions should be cautiously applied to humans.

Beta cell-specific IR knockout

Surprisingly, IR inactivation in the beta cell (55), using insulin promoter-Cre transgenic mice, resulted in progressive glucose intolerance due to impaired insulin secretion. The selective loss of glucose-dependent insulin secretion observed in these mice is reminiscent of the defect seen in type 2 diabetic patients (57). The impairment of beta cell function observed in various models of defective insulin signaling (beta cell-specific IR knockout, IRS-1 and IRS-2 knockouts) (34), raises the possibility that insulin signaling plays a physiologic role in insulin secretion. This is a new concept in the pathogenesis of type 2 diabetes, which implies that defective insulin signaling may account for both metabolic abnormalities of diabetes, namely peripheral insulin resistance and impaired beta cell function. However, this hypothesis awaits further clarification.

MUTATIONS AFFECTING INSULIN SECRETION

GLUT2

GLUT2 is the low-affinity glucose transporter of beta cells, liver, kidney and intestine. It has been suggested that beta cell GLUT2 participates in the regulation of glucose-stimulated insulin secretion. Loss of GLUT2 expression in beta cells is a sign of glucose toxicity and is observed in many different models of diabetes. Mice lacking GLUT2 develop hypoinsulinemia and are hyperglycemic. Isolated beta cells from these animals show a loss of insulin gene expression and absence of first phase insulin secretion, with preserved second phase. Post-natal development of pancreatic islets is profoundly affected, with alpha cells outnumbering beta cells (58). Similar results have been obtained using anti-sense GLUT2 mRNA targeted to beta cells by the insulin promoter to inhibit GLUT2 expression (59).

MODY Genes

HNF4-α

Mutations of the transcription factor hepatocyte nuclear factor (HNF)-4α cause MODY1 by impairing HNF-1α expression (60, 61). However, mice lacking HNF-4α show a complex phenotype, including defective hepatocyte differentiation during embryogenesis (62). Thus, HNF-4α could potentially affect metabolism in several ways.

Table 2. Summary of phenotypes associated with targeted gene knockouts in insulin signaling and insulin secretion pathways.

Gene	Phenotype	Ref.
Insulin Receptor (IR)	Ketoacidotic diabetes	(2, 3)
Muscle/fat-specific IR	Impaired glucose tolerance	(53)
Muscle-specific IR	Dyslipidemia	(54)
Beta cell-specific IR	Impaired glucose tolerance	(55)
IGF1 receptor	Impaired beta cell growth	(14)
IRS-1	Growth retardation, insulin resistance	(29, 30)
IRS-2	Beta cell dysfunction	(34)
IRS-3	None apparent	(40)
IRS-4	Modest growth retardation and insulin resistance	(42)
PI 3-kinase (P85α)	Hypoglycemia	(46)
GLUT2	Impaired insulin secretion, diabetes	(58)
GLUT4	Cardiac hypertrophy,	(47)
GLUT4 (heterozygous)	Insulin resistance, diabetes	(48)
GLUT4 (heart-specific)	Cardiac hypertrophy	(49)
HNF1-α	Impaired insulin secretion	(64)
HNF4-α	Impaired hepatic differentiation, HNF1α transcription	(61, 62)
Glucokinase	Impaired insulin secretion	(71, 72)
IPF1/PDX1	Impaired insulin gene expression	(70)
PPARγ (heterozygous)	Increased insulin sensitivity	(50, 52)

HNF1-α

Mutations of the gene encoding HNF1-α cause MODY 3 (63). Studies of mice lacking HNF1-α show that these mice develop hyperglycemia and impaired insulin secretory responses to glucose and arginine in perfused pancreas and islets (64). These defects appear to be due to defective beta cell glycolytic signaling (65) and support the view that HNF1-α is required for maintenance of normal beta cell function.

IPF1/PDX1

Homozygous null mutations of the homeodomain transcription factor IPF1/PDX1 have been associated with pancreatic agenesis (66), whereas haploinsufficiency causes MODY4 (63) or early-onset type 2 diabetes (67-69). Indeed, beta cell-specific disruption of the IPF1/PDX1 gene results in diabetes as a consequence of impaired expression of several genes required for proper beta cell function, including insulin, GLUT2 and amyloid polypeptide (70).

Glucokinase

Glucokinase acts as the beta cell glucose sensor by coupling glucose metabolism to insulin secretion. Mutations of glucokinase are associated with impaired insulin secretion in humans (63). Mouse models of glucokinase gene defects include both ubiquitous null mutations (71) and tissue-specific inactivation (72). Combined mutations of glucokinase and IRS-1 give rise to a polygenic form of type 2 diabetes due to combined defects in insulin action and secretion (73).

MOUSE MODELS SUGGEST AN OLIGOGENIC AND GENETICALLY HETEROGENEOUS PATHOGENESIS OF INSULIN RESISTANCE

Combined null mutations of IR and IRS-1 or IRS-2 in mice have a synergistic effect to impair insulin action and increase the prevalence of diabetes. These observations are consistent with an oligogenic model for the inheritance of type 2 diabetes, in which the genetic component of the susceptibility to type 2 diabetes can be accounted for by the interaction among few (in this case, two) susceptibility alleles (32, 33). Interestingly, the relative risk of diabetes (λ_s in table 3) in siblings of IR/IRS-1$^{+/-}$ mice is about as high as the relative risk observed in first degree relatives of type 2 diabetics. These data provide initial evidence for genetic epistasis as a mechanism for complex diseases (74, 75).

Table 3. Effect of combined mutations of IR and IRS-1 on the development of diabetes in mice.

Genotype	Insulin (ng/ml)	Glucose (mg/dl)	%Diabetic	λ_s
WT	1.5	156	5	-
IR$^{+/-}$	7.1	168	10	2.0
IR/IRS-1 $^{+/-}$	21.0	250	40	4.0

Moreover, the different pathophysiology of insulin resistance observed in diabetic IR/IRS-1 and IR/IRS-2 mice illustrates the genetic heterogeneity of the interactions leading to diabetes (33), and provides a sober reminder that different patients may benefit from different therapeutic options aimed at ameliorating insulin action in different organs.

Genetic Modifiers of Insulin Resistance

It is certainly surprising that, even when three different mutations are introduced in important genes of the insulin signaling cascade (IR, IRS-1, IRS-2), only about half of the mice develops diabetes (33). Why don't all mice become diabetic? To answer this question, it should be remembered that different mutations have different phenotypic consequences on different genetic backgrounds. The best illustration of this is provided by the IR mutation. The effect of this mutation is modified by the genetic background. On the genetic background of B6 mice, the IR null mutation causes mild hyperinsulinemia. In contrast, on the genetic background of 129/Sv mice, the same mutation causes severe hyperinsulinemia, suggesting that the 129/Sv strain harbors alleles that interact with the IR mutation and predispose to insulin resistance. The identification of these predisposing alleles has an important role to play in the ongoing quest for diabetes susceptibility genes. Using an F2 intercross between IR mutant mice on different backgrounds and a genome-wide scan with polymorphic markers, we have identified several loci that show significant evidence for linkage to plasma insulin levels as a quantitative trait and are likely to harbor susceptibility genes for insulin resistance (76).

CONCLUSIONS

Mutagenesis in mice has provided a useful tool to analyze the genetic predisposition to type 2 diabetes. In addition to defining the role of various signaling proteins in insulin action, crosses among the various mutant mice have provided important clues as to the mechanisms of oligogenic inheritance and genetic heterogeneity. Moreover, our understanding of the pathophysiology of insulin resistance has radically changed as a result of tissue-specific mutations. Finally, we have begun to make inroads into the identification of novel susceptibility loci using inter-strain differences in the susceptibility to insulin resistance and diabetes. The mouse, with significant limitations due to species-specific metabolic differences, has proved to be a versatile and informative model system for diabetes investigators.

REFERENCES

1. Louvi, A., D. Accili, and A. Efstratiadis. 1997. Growth-promoting interaction of IGF-II with the insulin receptor during mouse embryonic development. *Dev. Biol.* 189:33-48.
2. Accili, D., J. Drago, E.J. Lee, M.D. Johnson, M.H. Cool, P. Salvatore, L.D. Asico, P.A. Jose, S.I. Taylor, and H. Westphal. 1996. Early neonatal death in mice homozygous for a null allele of the insulin receptor gene. *Nature Genet.* 12:106-109.

3. Joshi, R.L., B. Lamothe, N. Cordonnier, K. Mesbah, E. Monthioux, J. Jami, and D. Bucchini. 1996. Targeted disruption of the insulin receptor gene in the mouse results in neonatal lethality. *EMBO J.* 15:1542-1547.
4. Girard, J.R., A. Kervan, E. Soufflet, and R. Assan. 1973. Factors affecting the secretion of insulin and glucagon by the rat fetus. *Diabetes.* 23:310-317.
5. Wertheimer, E., S.P. Lu, P.F. Backeljauw, M.L. Davenport, and S.I. Taylor. 1993. Homozygous deletion of the human insulin receptor gene results in leprechaunism. *Nat Genet.* 5:71-73.
6. Psiachou, H., S. Mitton, Z.J. Alaghband, J. Hone, S.I. Taylor, and L. Sinclair. 1993. Leprechaunism and homozygous nonsense mutation in the insulin receptor gene. *Lancet.* 1:342.
7. Krook, A., L. Brueton, and S. O'Rahilly. 1993. Homozygous nonsense mutation in the insulin receptor gene in infant with leprechaunism. *Lancet.* 342:277-278.
8. Jospe, N., P.B. Kaplowitz, and R.W. Furlanetto. 1996. Homozygous nonsense mutation in the insulin receptor gene of a patient with severe congenital insulin resistance: leprechaunism and the role of the insulin-like growth factor receptor. *Clin Endocrinol.* 45:229-235.
9. Accili, D. 1995. Molecular defects of the insulin receptor gene. *Diabetes Metab Rev.* 11:47-62.
10. Taylor, S.I., A. Cama, D. Accili, F. Barbetti, M.J. Quon, M. Sierra, Y. Suzuki, E. Koller, T.R. Levy, E. Wertheimer, and T. Kadowaki. 1992. Mutations in the insulin receptor gene. *Endocr Rev.* 13:566-595.
11. Accili, D. 1997. Insulin receptor knock-out mice. *Trends Endocrinol Metab.* 8:101-104.
12. Accili, D., J. Nakae, J.J. Kim, B.C. Park, and K.I. Rother. 1999. Targeted gene mutations define the roles of insulin and IGF-I receptors in mouse embryonic development. *J Pediatr Endocrinol Metab.* 12:475-485.
13. Efstratiadis, A. 1998. Genetics of mouse growth. *Int J Dev Biol.* 42:955-976.
14. Withers, D.J., D.J. Burks, H.H. Towery, S.L. Altamuro, C.L. Flint, and M.F. White. 1999. Irs-2 coordinates Igf-1 receptor-mediated beta-cell development and peripheral insulin signalling. *Nat Genet.* 23:32-40.
15. Duvillie, B., N. Cordonnier, L. Deltour, F. Dandoy-Dron, J.M. Itier, E. Monthioux, J. Jami, R.L. Joshi, and D. Bucchini. 1997. Phenotypic alterations in insulin-deficient mutant mice. *Proc Natl Acad Sci U S A.* 94:5137-5140.
16. Liu, J.P., J. Baker, A.S. Perkins, E.J. Robertson, and A. Efstratiadis. 1993. Mice carrying null mutations of the genes encoding insulin-like growth factor I (Igf-1) and type 1 IGF receptor (Igf1r). *Cell.* 75:59-72.
17. Ullrich, A., J.R. Bell, E.Y. Chen, R. Herrera, L.M. Petruzzelli, T.J. Dull, A. Gray, L. Coussens, Y.C. Liao, M. Tsubokawa, and a.l. et. 1985. Human insulin receptor and its relationship to the tyrosine kinase family of oncogenes. *Nature.* 313:756-761.
18. Ullrich, A., A. Gray, A.W. Tam, F.T. Yang, M. Tsubokawa, C. Collins, W. Henzel, B.T. Le, S. Kathuria, E. Chen, and a.l. et. 1986. Insulin-like growth factor I receptor primary structure: comparison with insulin receptor suggests structural determinants that define functional specificity. *EMBO J.* 5:2503-2512.
19. Morrione, A., B. Valentinis, S.Q. Xu, G. Yumet, A. Louvi, A. Efstratiadis, and R. Baserga. 1997. Insulin-like growth factor II stimulates cell proliferation through the insulin receptor. *Proc Natl Acad Sci U S A.* 94:3777-3782.
20. Frasca, F., G. Pandini, P. Scalia, L. Sciacca, R. Mineo, A. Costantino, I.D. Goldfine, A. Belfiore, and R. Vigneri. 1999. Insulin receptor isoform A, a newly recognized, high-affinity insulin- like growth factor II receptor in fetal and cancer cells. *Mol Cell Biol.* 19:3278-3288.
21. Lauro, D., Y. Kido, H. Hayashi, Y. Ebina, and D. Accili. 1999. Expression of kinase-inactive mutant insulin receptors does not rescue insulin receptor-deficient mice from perinatal death. *Diabetologia.* 42:1441-1442.

22. Nakae, J., and D. Accili. 1999. The mechanism of insulin action. *J Pediatr Endocrinol Metab.* 12 (Suppl 3):721-731.
23. Di Cola, G., M.H. Cool, and D. Accili. 1997. Hypoglycemic effect of insulin-like growth factor-1 in mice lacking insulin receptors. *J. Clin. Invest.* 99:2538-2544.
24. Ludwig, T., J. Eggenschwiler, P. Fisher, A.J. D'Ercole, M.L. Davenport, and A. Efstratiadis. 1996. Mouse mutants lacking the type 2 IGF receptor (IGF2R) are rescued from perinatal lethality in Igf2 and Igf1r null backgrounds. *Dev Biol.* 177:517-535.
25. Rother, K.I., Y. Imai, M. Caruso, F. Beguinot, P. Formisano, and D. Accili. 1998. Evidence that IRS-2 phosphorylation is required for insulin action in hepatocytes. *J. Biol. Chem.* 273:17491-17497.
26. Park, B.C., Y. Kido, and D. Accili. 1999. Differential Signaling of Insulin and IGF-1 Receptors to Glycogen Synthesis in Murine Hepatocytes. *Biochemistry.* 38:7517-7523.
27. Nakae, J., V. Barr, and D. Accili. 2000. Differential regulation of gene expression by insulin and IGF-1 receptors correlates with phosphorylation of a single amino acid residue in the forkhead transcription factor FKHR. *EMBO J.* 19:989-996.
28. Kim, J.J., B.C. Park, and D. Accili. 1999. Expression of IGF-1 receptors in insulin receptor-deficient hepatocytes restores mitogenic, but not metabolic responses. *Diabetes.* 48 (Suppl. 1):0041 (abstract).
29. Araki, E., M.A. Lipes, M.E. Patti, J.C. Bruning, B.r. Haag, R.S. Johnson, and C.R. Kahn. 1994. Alternative pathway of insulin signalling in mice with targeted disruption of the IRS-1 gene. *Nature.* 372:186-190.
30. Tamemoto, H., T. Kadowaki, K. Tobe, T. Yagi, H. Sakura, T. Hayakawa, Y. Terauchi, K. Ueki, Y. Kaburagi, S. Satoh, H. Sekihara, S. Yoshioka, H. Horikoshi, Y. Furuta, Y. Ikawa, M. Kasuga, Y. Yazaki, and S. Aizawa. 1994. Insulin resistance and growth retardation in mice lacking insulin receptor substrate-1. *Nature.* 372:182-186.
31. Kulkarni, R.N., J.N. Winnay, M. Daniels, J.C. Bruning, S.N. Flier, D. Hanahan, and C.R. Kahn. 1999. Altered function of insulin receptor substrate-1-deficient mouse islets and cultured beta-cell lines. *J Clin Invest.* 104:R69-75.
32. Bruning, J.C., J. Winnay, W.S. Bonner, S.I. Taylor, D. Accili, and C.R. Kahn. 1997. Development of a novel polygenic model of NIDDM in mice heterozygous for IR and IRS-1 null alleles. *Cell.* 88:561-572.
33. Kido, Y., D.J. Burks, D. Withers, J.C. Bruning, C.R. Kahn, M.F. White, and D. Accili. 2000. Tissue-specific insulin resistance in mice with combined mutations of Insulin Receptor, IRS-1 and IRS-2. *J. Clin. Invest.* 105:199-205.
34. Withers, D.J., J. Sanchez-Gutierrez, H. Towery, D.J. Burks, J.-M. Ren, S. Previs, Y. Zhang, D. Bernal, S. Pons, G.I. Shulman, S. Bonner-Weir, and M.F. White. 1998. Disruption of IRS-2 causes type 2 diabetes in mice. *Nature.* 391:900-904.
35. Bernal, D., K. Almind, L. Yenush, M. Ayoub, Y. Zhang, L. Rosshani, C. Larsson, O. Pedersen, and M.F. White. 1998. Insulin receptor substrate-2 amino acid polymorphisms are not associated with random type 2 diabetes among Caucasians. *Diabetes.* 47:976-979.
36. Lavan, B.E., W.S. Lane, and G.E. Lienhard. 1997. The 60-kDa phosphotyrosine protein in insulin-treated adipocytes is a new member of the insulin receptor substrate family. *J Biol Chem.* 272:11439-11443.
37. Sciacchitano, S., and S.I. Taylor. 1997. Cloning, Tissue expression, and chromosomal localization of the mouse IRS-3 gene. *Endocrinology.* 138:4931-4940.
38. Smith-Hall, J., S. Pons, M.E. Patti, D.J. Burks, L. Yenush, X.J. Sun, C.R. Kahn, and M.F. White. 1997. The 60 kDa insulin receptor substrate functions like an IRS protein (pp60IRS3) in adipose cells. *Biochemistry.* 36:8304-8310.
39. Xu, P., A.R. Jacobs, and S.I. Taylor. 1999. Interaction of insulin receptor substrate 3 with insulin receptor, insulin receptor-related receptor, insulin-like growth factor-1 receptor, and downstream signaling proteins. *J Biol Chem.* 274:15262-15270.
40. Liu, S.C.H., Q. Wang, G.E. Lienhard, and S.R. Keller. 1999. Insulin receptor substrate 3 is not essential for growth or glucose homeostasis. *J. Biol. Chem.* 274:18093-18099.

41. Lavan, B.E., V.R. Fantin, E.T. Chang, W.S. Lane, S.R. Keller, and G.E. Lienhard. 1997. A novel 160-kDa phosphotyrosine protein in insulin-treated embryonic kidney cells is a new member of the insulin receptor substrate family. *J. Biol. Chem.* 272:21403-21407.
42. Fantin, V.R., Q. Wang, G.E. Lienhard, and S.R. Keller. 2000. Mice lacking insulin receptor substrate 4 exhibit mild defects in growth, reproduction, and glucose homeostasis. *Am J Physiol Endocrinol Metab.* 278:E127-E133.
43. White, M.F. 1998. The IRS-signalling system: a network of docking proteins that mediate insulin and interleukin signalling. *Mol. Cell. Biochem.* 182:3-11.
44. Higaki, Y., J.F. Wojtaszewski, M.F. Hirshman, D.J. Withers, H. Towery, M.F. White, and L.J. Goodyear. 1999. Insulin receptor substrate-2 is not necessary for insulin- and exercise-stimulated glucose transport in skeletal muscle. *J Biol Chem.* 274:20791-20795.
45. Isakoff, S.J., C. Taha, E. Rose, J. Marcusohn, A. Klip, and E.Y. Skolnik. 1995. The inability of phosphatidylinositol 3-kinase activation to stimulate GLUT4 translocation indicates additional signaling pathways are required for insulin-stimulated glucose uptake. *Proc Natl Acad Sci U S A.* 92:10247-10251.
46. Terauchi, Y., Y. Tsuji, S. Satoh, H. Minoura, K. Murakami, A. Okuno, K. Inukai, T. Asano, Y. Kaburagi, K. Ueki, H. Nakajima, T. Hanafusa, Y. Matsuzawa, H. Sekihara, Y. Yin, J.C. Barrett, H. Oda, T. Ishikawa, Y. Akanuma, I. Komuro, M. Suzuki, K. Yamamura, T. Kodama, H. Suzuki, T. Kadowaki, and et al. 1999. Increased insulin sensitivity and hypoglycaemia in mice lacking the p85 alpha subunit of phosphoinositide 3-kinase. *Nat Genet.* 21:230-235.
47. Katz, E.B., A.E. Stenbit, K. Hatton, R. DePinho, and M.J. Charron. 1995. Cardiac and adipose tissue abnormalities but not diabetes in mice deficient in GLUT4. *Nature.* 377:151-155.
48. Stenbit, A.E., T.S. Tsao, J. Li, R. Burcelin, D.L. Geenen, S.M. Factor, K. Houseknecht, E.B. Katz, and M.J. Charron. 1997. GLUT4 heterozygous knockout mice develop muscle insulin resistance and diabetes. *Nat Med.* 3:1096-1101.
49. Abel, E.D., H.C. Kaulbach, R. Tian, J.C. Hopkins, J. Duffy, T. Doetschman, T. Minnemann, M.E. Boers, E. Hadro, C. Oberste-Berghaus, W. Quist, B.B. Lowell, J.S. Ingwall, and B.B. Kahn. 1999. Cardiac hypertrophy with preserved contractile function after selective deletion of GLUT4 from the heart. *J Clin Invest.* 104:1703-1714.
50. Kubota, N., Y. Terauchi, H. Miki, H. Tamemoto, T. Yamauchi, K. Komeda, S. Satoh, R. Nakano, C. Ishii, T. Sugiyama, K. Eto, Y. Tsubamoto, A. Okuno, K. Murakami, H. Sekihara, G. Hasegawa, M. Naito, Y. Toyoshima, S. Tanaka, K. Shiota, T. Kitamura, T. Fujita, O. Ezaki, S. Aizawa, and T. Kadowaki. 1999. PPAR gamma mediates high-fat diet-induced adipocyte hypertrophy and insulin resistance. *Mol Cell.* 4:597-609.
51. Barak, Y., M.C. Nelson, E.S. Ong, Y.Z. Jones, P. Ruiz-Lozano, K.R. Chien, A. Koder, and R.M. Evans. 1999. PPAR gamma is required for placental, cardiac, and adipose tissue development. *Mol Cell.* 4:585-595.
52. Miles, P.D., Y. Barak, W. He, R.M. Evans, and J.M. Olefsky. 2000. Improved insulin-sensitivity in mice heterozygous for PPAR-gamma deficiency. *J Clin Invest.* 105:287-292.
53. Lauro, D., Y. Kido, A.L. Castle, M.J. Zarnowski, H. Hayashi, Y. Ebina, and D. Accili. 1998. Impaired glucose tolerance in mice with a targeted impairment of insulin action in muscle and adipose tissue. *Nature Genet.* 20:294-298.
54. Bruning, J.C., M.D. Michael, J.N. Winnay, T. Hayashi, D. Horsch, D. Accili, L.J. Goodyear, and C.R. Kahn. 1998. A muscle-specific insulin receptor knockout exhibits features of the metabolic syndrome of NIDDM without altering glucose tolerance. *Mol Cell.* 2:559-569.
55. Kulkarni, R.N., J.C. Bruning, J.N. Winnay, C. Postic, M.A. Magnuson, and C.R. Kahn. 1999. Tissue-specific knockout of the insulin receptor in pancreatic beta cells creates an insulin secretory defect similar to that in type 2 diabetes. *Cell.* 96:329-339.
56. Wojtaszewski, J.F., Y. Higaki, M.F. Hirshman, M.D. Michael, S.D. Dufresne, C.R. Kahn, and L.J. Goodyear. 1999. Exercise modulates postreceptor insulin signaling and glucose transport in muscle-specific insulin receptor knockout mice. *J Clin Invest.* 104:1257-1264.

57. Polonsky, K.S., J. Sturis, and G.I. Bell. 1996. Non-insulin-dependent diabetes mellitus - a genetically programmed failure of the beta cell to compensate for insulin resistance. *N. Engl. J. Med.* 334:777-783.
58. Guillam, M.T., E. Hummler, E. Schaerer, J.I. Yeh, M.J. Birnbaum, F. Beermann, A. Schmidt, N. Deriaz, B. Thorens, and J.Y. Wu. 1997. Early diabetes and abnormal postnatal pancreatic islet development in mice lacking Glut-2. *Nat Genet.* 17:327-330.
59. Valera, A., G. Solanes, A.J. Fernandez, A. Pujol, J. Ferrer, G. Asins, R. Gomis, and F. Bosch. 1994. Expression of GLUT-2 antisense RNA in beta cells of transgenic mice leads to diabetes. *J Biol Chem.* 269:28543-28546.
60. Yamagata, K., H. Furuta, N. Oda, P.J. Kaisaki, S. Menzel, N.J. Cox, S.S. Fajans, S. Signorini, M. Stoffel, and G.I. Bell. 1996. Mutations in the hepatocyte nuclear factor-4alpha gene in maturity-onset diabetes of the young (MODY1). *Nature.* 384:458-460.
61. Duncan, S.A., M.A. Navas, D. Dufort, J. Rossant, and M. Stoffel. 1998. Regulation of a transcription factor network required for differentiation and metabolism. *Science.* 281:692-695.
62. Li, J., G. Ning, and S.A. Duncan. 2000. Mammalian hepatocyte differentiation requires the transcription factor HNF-4alpha. *Genes Dev.* 14:464-474.
63. Froguel, P., and G. Velho. 1999. Molecular Genetics of Maturity-onset Diabetes of the Young. *Trends Endocrinol Metab.* 10:142-146.
64. Pontoglio, M., S. Sreenan, M. Roe, W. Pugh, D. Ostrega, A. Doyen, A.J. Pick, A. Baldwin, G. Velho, P. Froguel, M. Levisetti, S. Bonner-Weir, G.I. Bell, M. Yaniv, and K.S. Polonsky. 1998. Defective insulin secretion in hepatocyte nuclear factor 1alpha- deficient mice. *J Clin Invest.* 101:2215-2222.
65. Dukes, I.D., S. Sreenan, M.W. Roe, M. Levisetti, Y.P. Zhou, D. Ostrega, G.I. Bell, M. Pontoglio, M. Yaniv, L. Philipson, and K.S. Polonsky. 1998. Defective pancreatic beta-cell glycolytic signaling in hepatocyte nuclear factor-1alpha-deficient mice. *J Biol Chem.* 273:24457-24464.
66. Stoffers, D.A., N.T. Zinkin, V. Stanojevic, W.L. Clarke, and J.F. Habener. 1997. Pancreatic agenesis attributable to a single nucleotide deletion in the human IPF1 gene coding sequence. *Nat Genet.* 15:106-110.
67. Stoffers, D.A., J. Ferrer, W.L. Clarke, and J.F. Habener. 1997. Early-onset type-II diabetes mellitus (MODY4) linked to IPF1 [letter]. *Nat Genet.* 17:138-139.
68. Hani, E.H., D.A. Stoffers, J.C. Chevre, E. Durand, V. Stanojevic, C. Dina, J.F. Habener, and P. Froguel. 1999. Defective mutations in the insulin promoter factor-1 (IPF-1) gene in late-onset type 2 diabetes mellitus. *J Clin Invest.* 104:R41-R48.
69. Macfarlane, W.M., T.M. Frayling, S. Ellard, J.C. Evans, L.I. Allen, M.P. Bulman, S. Ayres, M. Shepherd, P. Clark, A. Millward, A. Demaine, T. Wilkin, K. Docherty, and A.T. Hattersley. 1999. Missense mutations in the insulin promoter factor-1 gene predispose to type 2 diabetes. *J Clin Invest.* 104:R33-R39.
70. Ahlgren, U., J. Jonsson, L. Jonsson, K. Simu, and H. Edlund. 1998. beta-cell-specific inactivation of the mouse Ipf1/Pdx1 gene results in loss of the beta-cell phenotype and maturity onset diabetes. *Genes Dev.* 12:1763-1768.
71. Grupe, A., B. Hultgren, A. Ryan, Y.H. Ma, M. Bauer, and T.A. Stewart. 1995. Transgenic knockouts reveal a critical requirement for pancreatic beta cell glucokinase in maintaining glucose homeostasis. *Cell.* 83:69-78.
72. Postic, C., M. Shiota, K.D. Niswender, T.L. Jetton, Y. Chen, J.M. Moates, K.D. Shelton, J. Lindner, A.D. Cherrington, and M.A. Magnuson. 1999. Dual roles for glucokinase in glucose homeostasis as determined by liver and pancreatic beta cell-specific gene knock-outs using Cre recombinase. *J Biol Chem.* 274:305-315.
73. Terauchi, Y., K. Iwamoto, H. Tamemoto, K. Komeda, C. Ishii, Y. Kanazawa, N. Asanuma, T. Aizawa, Y. Akanuma, K. Yasuda, T. Kodama, K. Tobe, Y. Yazaki, and T. Kadowaki. 1997. Development of non-insulin-dependent diabetes mellitus in the double knockout mice with disruption of insulin receptor substrate-1 and beta cell glucokinase genes. Genetic reconstitution of diabetes as a polygenic disease. *J Clin Invest.* 99:861-866.

74. Cox, N.J., M. Frigge, D.L. Nicolae, P. Concannon, C.L. Hanis, G.I. Bell, and A. Kong. 1999. Loci on chromosomes 2 (NIDDM1) and 15 interact to increase susceptibility to diabetes in Mexican Americans. *Nat Genet*. 21:213-215.
75. Ghosh, S., and F.S. Collins. 1996. The geneticist's approach to complex disease. *Annu Rev Med*. 47:333-353.
76. Kido, Y., N. Philippe, A.A. Schaeffer, and D. Accili. 2000. Genetic modifiers of the insulin resistance phenotype. *Diabetes*. 49: 589-596.

10
Candidate Genes for Type 2 Diabetes

William L. Lowe, Jr., M.D.
Northwestern University Medical School, Chicago, IL 60611 USA

INTRODUCTION

The pathogenesis of type 2 diabetes is complex, but is characterized by hyperglycemia secondary to a combination of insulin resistance and pancreatic β-cell dysfunction that is manifest as inadequate insulin secretion in the face of insulin resistance and hyperglycemia (see Chapters 7 and 8) (1,2). Previous studies have established a clear genetic predisposition for type 2 diabetes (3-5). The concordance rate among monozygotic twins is 50 to 90% compared to 25 to 35% for dizygotic twins (6). Similarly ~30% of offspring of affected individuals develop either type 2 diabetes or impaired glucose tolerance (3-5). Together, these data are consistent with a significant genetic contribution to the development of type 2 diabetes, but the lack of 100% concordance among monozygotic twins suggests that environmental influences are also important. Moreover, mathematical modeling has suggested that type 2 diabetes is polygenic, i.e., it is inherited in a non-Mendelian fashion and onset of the disease requires the simultaneous presence of a subset of susceptibility genes whose gene products affect insulin production, secretion or sensitivity (3-5). This has complicated efforts to identify diabetes susceptibility genes for several reasons: (1) the relative contributions of insulin resistance and altered insulin secretion to the pathogenesis of type 2 diabetes probably vary between individuals; (2) because of the above heterogeneity, susceptibility genes likely differ between and within populations; and (3) the effect of any single susceptibility gene on disease risk may be small, making identification of susceptibility genes difficult. Furthermore, environmental factors that still have not been fully defined, but include diet and physical activity, contribute to the development of type 2 diabetes (7-9). Thus, susceptibility genes for type 2 diabetes may be present in unaffected individuals because they lack a required complement of susceptibility genes or needed environmental factors to induce diabetes.

As described in Chapter 1, one approach to defining susceptibility genes for a complex disease is allelic association studies. For these studies, candidate genes are chosen based upon their role in insulin production, secretion, or action, and the frequencies of polymorphic alleles of these genes are compared between a population with type 2 diabetes and a control population. Association is present if the polymorphic allele is present with increased or decreased frequency in the diabetic compared to control population. Polymorphisms associated with type 2 diabetes or a related phenotype may have a direct functional consequence and, thus, confer increased risk, or they may be in linkage disequilibrium with another polymorphism in the same or a nearby gene that is of functional significance. This chapter will address the role of allelic association studies in the identification of susceptibility genes for type 2 diabetes.

CANDIDATE GENES

The potential contribution of a wide variety of candidate genes to diabetes risk or diabetes-related phenotypes has been examined. As will be described below, for most of these genes, studies have either been negative or follow-up studies have failed to replicate initial positive findings. A list of the candidate genes that have been studied to date is provided in Table 1. A detailed discussion of the results obtained for each of these genes is beyond the scope of this chapter. Rather, the results of studies with specific, well-studied candidate genes and/or genes that are important in metabolic or signaling pathways important for type 2 diabetes will be described.

Table 1. Candidate genes examined for association with and/or linkage to type 2 diabetes

Genes that regulate β-cell development or function	**Genes important for insulin action and glucose metabolism**
Hepatocyte nuclear factor-1α	Insulin receptor
Hepatocyte nuclear factor-4α	Insulin receptor substrate-1
Hepatocyte nuclear factor-1β	Insulin receptor substrate-2
Hepatocyte nuclear factor-3β	Insulin receptor substrate-4
Hepatocyte nuclear factor-6	Phosphatidylinositol 3-kinase
IPF-1	Protein kinase B
NeuroD1	Phosphoinositide dependent kinase-1
Islet-brain-1	Glucose transporter 1 (GLUT1)
Islet-1	Glucose transporter 4 (GLUT4)
Caudal-type homeodomain 3 (*CDX3*)	Hexokinase II (*HK2*)
Inwardly rectifying K^+ channel (*KIR6.2*)	Inhibitor 2 of type 1 protein phosphatase (*PP1R2*)
G-protein-coupled muscarinic K^+ channel (*KCNJ3*)	Protein targeting to glycogen (PTG) (*PP1R5*)

G-protein-coupled inwardly rectifying K^+ channel 2 (*KCNJ7*)
Sulfonylurea receptor (*SUR1*)
Glucagon
Glucagon receptor
Glucagon-like peptide-1 receptor
Gastric inhibitory polypeptide receptor
Glucokinase
Glucokinase regulatory protein
Amylin
Prohormone convertase 1
Prohormone convertase 2 (*PCSK2*)
Carboxypeptidase E
Glucose transporter 2 (*GLUT2*)
Mitochondrial FAD-linked glycerol-phosphate dehydrogenase (*GPD2*)
Pyruvate kinase (*PKM*)
Hexokinase I (*HK1*)
Insulin (*INS*)
Sarcoplasmic reticulum Ca^{2+}-transport ATPase 3 (*SERCA3*)
CD38
Presenilin 2
Frataxin (*FRDA1*)

Genes that inhibit insulin action
Growth hormone
Rad (*RAD1*)
Tumor necrosis factor-α
Tumor necrosis factor-β

Glycogen-targeting subunit of type 1 protein phosphatase 1 (*PPP1R3*)
Glycogen synthase (*GSY1*)
Glycogen synthase (*GSY2*)
Glycogen synthase kinase-α, -β
Protein phosphatase 1-α, -β, -γ
Peroxisome proliferator-activated receptor-γ (*PPARγ*)
Fructose 1,6-bisphosphatase
Hepatic phosphofructokinase
Phosphoenolpyruvate carboxykinase
Glucose-6-phosphatase

Genes important for metabolism
β3-adrenergic receptor
Fatty acid binding protein 2 (FABP2)
Uncoupling protein 2 (UCP2)
Uncoupling protein 1 (UCP1)
Hormone sensitive lipase
Lipoprotein lipase
Hepatic triglyceride lipase
Very low density lipoprotein receptor
Apolipoprotein CII
Apolipoprotein A_2
Apolipoprotein B
Apolipoprotein D
Cholesterol ester-transfer protein
Vitamin D receptor
Vitamin D binding protein
Paraoxonase (*PON*)
Paraoxonase-2 (*PON2*)
Leptin (*ob*)
Tubby (*TUB*)
Cholecystokinin receptor B
Insulin-like growth factor-I
Insulin-like growth factor-I receptor

Candidate Genes for Type 2 Diabetes with an Effect on β-Cell Function

Given the contribution β-cell dysfunction to type 2 diabetes, genes that express proteins important for β-cell development and insulin production and secretion represent an important class of potential candidate genes. Mutations in transcription factors important for β-cell development and insulin production have been identified, and, in some cases, cause a monogenic form of obesity, maturity onset diabetes of the young (MODY) (see Chapter 5). NeuroD1 is a helix-loop-helix transcription factor that is important for development of pancreatic islets and regulation of insulin gene expression (10,11). Sequencing this gene in members of large families in which type 2 diabetes segregates as an autosomal dominant disorder revealed four sequence variants (12). Two of these variants, a G to T substitution that resulted in an Arg to Leu change at codon 111 and insertion of a cytosine residue in a poly C tract at codon 206 which introduced a premature stop codon, cosegregated with diabetes. Moreover, both mutations altered transactivation of the insulin gene by NeuroD1. How important these or other mutations are for typical "late-onset" type 2 diabetes is less clear. In French Caucasians with type 2 diabetes, the NeuroD1 locus was not linked with type 2 diabetes, the above mutations were not found, and other polymorphisms in the NeuroD1 gene were not associated with type 2 diabetes (13).

Insulin promoter factor-1 (IPF-1) is another transcription factor that plays a critical role in pancreatic development and insulin gene expression. A mutation in the *IPF-1* gene that results in premature termination of translation causes pancreatic agenesis in the homozygous state and MODY in the heterozygous state (see Chapter 5) (14,15). Additional missense mutations in the *IPF-1* gene (substitution of cysteine by arginine at codon 18, glutamine by leucine at codon 59, aspartic acid by asparagine at codon 76, and arginine by histidine at codon 197, as well as an in-frame proline insertion at codon 243) have been identified in Caucasian subjects with type 2 diabetes and, with the exception of the codon 76 missense mutation, have not been identified in control populations (16,17). These mutations alter IPF-1 function and, although rare, appear to increase susceptibility to type 2 diabetes. The role of the Asn^{76} allele as a susceptibility gene is less clear, however, given the recent finding that it is not associated with type 2 diabetes in a population of Danish Caucasians (18). Sequence analysis of the islet brain 1 (*IB1*) gene, which encodes a transcription factor important for expression of the β-cell- and hepatocyte-specific glucose transporter, GLUT2, identified a missense mutation in one family (of 149 total) with type 2 diabetes (19). This missense mutation, substitution of asparagine for serine at codon 59, altered protein function and co-segregated with diabetes. Thus, transcription factors important for pancreas development and insulin gene expression are important for MODY and may contribute to susceptibility to type 2 diabetes.

Another potential susceptibility gene for type 2 diabetes is the insulin gene itself. As described in Chapter 4, a variable number of tandem repeats (VNTR) polymorphism is present in the 5'-flanking region of the insulin gene (20). The VNTR consists of a 14- to 15-base pair core sequence that is repeated a variable number of times. Three different alleles have been identified based upon the number of repeats that are present, the class I (23-63 repeats), class II (80 repeats), and class III alleles (141-209 repeats) (21).

The class III allele is associated with decreased insulin gene expression in adult and fetal pancreas (22,23), although its effect on insulin secretion is unclear, since both decreased and no change in insulin secretion have been reported in those with the class III allele (24). When the results of several small studies in Caucasian populations were considered together, type 2 diabetes was associated with the VNTR class III/III homozygous genotype (odds ratio = 1.86) (20). Given the possible association of the insulin VNTR with birth weight and the known association of low birth weight with type 2 diabetes (25,26), a subsequent study which controlled for birth weight and early postnatal growth demonstrated a greater risk for type 2 diabetes (odds ratio = 4.6) in those homozygous for the III/III genotype (27). Finally, a recent study using transmission disequilibrium testing (TDT) analysis, which obviates potential problems with population stratification through the use of family-based controls (28), demonstrated an excess of paternal, but not maternal, transmissions of the class III allele to offspring affected by type 2 diabetes (29). These data suggest that diabetes susceptibility is limited to paternally-derived alleles and is related to a gene that is maternally imprinted (29). Interestingly, the insulin gene locus is located ~4.5 kb upstream of the *IGF2* gene, which encodes the fetal growth factor insulin-like growth factor-II (IGF-II) and is maternally imprinted. Moreover, the insulin VNTR influences placental expression of the *IGF2* gene (30). These data raise the possibility that the *IGF2* and not the insulin gene is the susceptibility allele for type 2 diabetes at this locus (29).

A common therapy for type 2 diabetes is sulfonylureas, a class of drugs that stimulate insulin secretion. Recently, the molecular mechanisms by which sulfonylureas stimulate insulin secretion have been defined. Sulfonylureas inhibit an ATP-sensitive potassium channel which results in decreased potassium outflow from the cell (31,32). This decrease in potassium outflow causes β-cell depolarization, an influx of calcium, and insulin secretion (31,32). The ATP-sensitive potassium channel in β-cells is composed of two subunits, the sulfonylurea receptor (SUR1) and a member of the inwardly rectifying K^+ channel subfamily 6.0 which is encoded by the *KIR6.2* gene (31,32). Mutations of the *SUR1* and *KIR6.2* genes have been found in some patients with familial persistent hyperinsulinemic hypoglycemia of infancy, suggesting an important role for these gene products in the regulation of insulin secretion (33).

Multiple studies have also examined the potential contribution of these genes to susceptibility to type 2 diabetes. These two genes are located 4.5 kilobase pairs (kbp) apart on chromosome 11p15.1 (34). A previous genome scan demonstrated linkage of this region of chromosome 11 to glucose levels in Mexican Americans (35), although other studies in French Caucasians, Japanese, Mexican-Americans, and non-Hispanic whites have failed to demonstrate linkage of this region to type 2 diabetes (36-41).

Additional studies have identified sequence variants in the *SUR1* gene and examined their association with type 2 diabetes (38,39,42-47). Several missense mutations have been identified, but only one is common (serine to alanine substitution at codon 1369), and it is present with equal frequency in subjects with and without type 2 diabetes (38,39,42,45,47). Other missense mutations are rare, occur with equal frequency in controls and type 2 diabetic subjects, and/or do not segregate with diabetes in affected families (45,47). In contrast, two other polymorphisms, a silent C to T change in exon 18 and an intronic –3 c to t change in intron 15 have been associated with type 2 diabetes in some populations, although these results have not been replicated in other populations. The C to T change in exon 18 was observed with increased frequency in diabetic compared with normoglycemic control Caucasians from the United Kingdom, France, Utah, and Denmark (38,39,45); this association was not observed, however, in Caucasians from Finland and Holland (42,43). The exon 18 C to T change is rare in African Americans and absent in Pimas and Japanese (39,46). The second polymorphism, the intron 15 -3 c to t change, is present with increased frequency in diabetic Caucasians from Finland, Utah, Holland, and the United Kingdom but not in diabetic Caucasians from France and Denmark, African Americans, or Japanese (38,39,42,43,45-47). Haplotype analyses using the sequence variants in exon 18 and intron 15 have not identified a haplotype that clearly confers increased risk (38,39,43,45). Since neither of the above polymorphisms is thought to be of functional significance, one is silent and the other has not been shown to affect splicing of SUR1 mRNA (39), it is likely that they are in linkage disequilibrium with another variant that increases susceptibility to type 2 diabetes. Despite their lack of clear functional significance, the intron 15 –3c/t/exon 18 C/T combination has been associated with decreased tolbutamide- but normal glucose-stimulated insulin and C-peptide release and the intron 15 –3t allele was associated with decreased insulin secretion during a hyperglycemic clamp in Caucasians (45,48). In other Caucasians, however, the intron 15 –3c/t variant was not associated with area under the insulin curve during an intravenous glucose tolerance test or the fasting, one hour, or two hour insulin levels during an oral glucose tolerance test (42).

An additional silent polymorphism in the *SUR1* gene is a G to A change at codon 1273 (R1273R). An increased frequency of the G allele has been observed in diabetic Caucasian subjects, although normoglycemic subjects bearing the G allele did not demonstrate changes in intravenous or oral glucose-induced insulin secretion (42). The R1273R was in linkage disequilibrium with the intron 15 –3c/t change in diabetic but not normoglycemic subjects (42). This same polymorphism has been found in Mexican Americans, although, in this population, nondiabetic subjects homozygous for the A allele exhibited higher fasting and 2 hr insulin levels during an oral glucose tolerance test (44).

The potential role of genetic variants of the *KIR6.2* gene in type 2 diabetes susceptibility has also been examined. Multiple missense mutations have been identified in Caucasian populations from the United Kingdom, France, USA, and Denmark (49-52), although most are rare and/or show no association with type 2 diabetes. One missense mutation, a glutamic acid to lysine substitution at codon 23 (E23K), was present with increased frequency in the homozygous state in French Caucasians with type 2 diabetes, and a meta-analysis of studies in Caucasians from France, the United Kingdom and Denmark demonstrated a significant association of the E23K variant with type 2 diabetes (50). Importantly, this missense mutation is not in linkage disequilibrium with the intron 15 –3c/t and exon 18 C to T polymorphisms in the *SUR1* gene, suggesting that the association between this polymorphism and type 2 diabetes is independent of the *SUR1* gene (50). *In vitro* functional studies failed to demonstrate an effect of this amino acid change on protein function (49).

In summary, many studies in different ethnic groups have demonstrated association, albeit inconsistent, of various polymorphisms in the *SUR1* or *KIR6.2* genes with type 2 diabetes or related phenotypes. These polymorphisms appear to lack functional significance, suggesting that they are in linkage disequilibrium with other variants of these genes or a nearby gene that increases diabetes susceptibility. In contrast, missense mutations in transcription factors important for insulin production and β-cell development apparently increase diabetes susceptibility, although their importance in the majority of type 2 diabetic subjects is still unclear.

Role of Molecules Involved in Insulin Signaling

As reviewed in Chapter 8, insulin signaling is complex and involves activation of several distinct signaling pathways and molecules which mediate the metabolic effects of insulin. Given the important role of insulin resistance in type 2 diabetes, these signaling pathways represent logical candidate genes for type 2 diabetes.

As the most proximal site of insulin action, the insulin receptor is a logical candidate gene for type 2 diabetes. Mutations in the insulin receptor gene that significantly impact insulin receptor synthesis or processing, insulin binding or receptor tyrosine kinase activity are associated with syndromes of extreme insulin resistance that may result in diabetes mellitus (53). Examples include leprechaunism, Rabson-Mendenhall syndrome, and type A extreme insulin resistance. The role of the insulin receptor gene as a susceptibility gene for type 2 diabetes is not as clear. Sequence analysis of the insulin receptor of patients with type 2 diabetes has failed to reveal a large number of mutations, suggesting that mutations that have a significant impact on receptor function contribute to only 1 to 2% of cases of type 2 diabetes (3). A recent population-based study in Dutch Caucasians identified a polymorphic variant of the insulin receptor in which methionine is substituted for valine at codon 985 in the juxtamembrane region of the β-subunit of the receptor (54). Subjects with the Met^{985} allele present in the heterozygous state had an increased fasting glucose level and prevalence of type 2 diabetes (56.3% vs. 22.3%) compared to subjects homozygous for the wild-type allele (54). Similarly, among subjects with type 2 diabetes, 5.6% were heterozygous for the Met^{985} allele compared to 1.3% of control subjects. Subsequent studies have been performed in Dutch and Danish Caucasians and Tamil Indians (55-57). None of these studies demonstrated a significant increase in the frequency of the Met985 allele in diabetic compared with control subjects, although, when the four studies were considered together, the Met985 allele demonstrated a significant association (odds ratio = 1.87) with type 2 diabetes (55). Functional studies, however, have been unable to demonstrate alterations in the proximal steps in insulin signaling in cells expressing the mutant compared with the wild-type receptor (58), so the role of this receptor polymorphism in susceptibility to type 2 diabetes remains unclear.

Given their fundamental role in insulin signal transduction, members of the insulin receptor substrate family of proteins have also received much attention as potential candidate genes for type 2 diabetes. As described in Chapter 9, in the context of other genetic alterations, decreased or absent expression of insulin receptor substrate-1 (IRS-1) can result in type 2 diabetes in mouse models. In humans, a marked reduction in IRS-1 protein has been demonstrated in adipocytes from subjects with type 2 diabetes, whereas levels of other signaling molecules, including the insulin receptor, p85 subunit of phosphatidylinositol 3-kinase, and the phosphotyrosine phosphatase SH-PTP2/Syp were unaltered (59). Similarly, in obese individuals and nondiabetic lean individuals with a family history of type 2 diabetes, those with a marked reduction in adipocyte IRS-1 protein levels were more insulin resistant as defined by an increasing fasting glucose and insulin level and, when available, glucose infusion rate during a euglycemic, hyperinsulinemic clamp (60). In nondiabetic individuals with decreased IRS-1 protein levels, decreased gene expression appears to account for the decreased protein levels (60), although the mechanism for this is unclear.

Many studies have also screened for polymorphic variants of the *IRS-1* gene. The most common polymorphism in the *IRS-1* gene and the one that has been studied in greatest detail is a point mutation that results in substitution of arginine for glycine at codon 972. This variant has been shown to be associated with altered insulin signaling in some, but not all, *in vitro* studies (61-63) and with altered insulin secretion (63,64). Nondiabetic first degree relatives of patients with type 2 diabetes who bear the Arg^{972} allele have similar insulin secretion and/or insulin sensitivity compared to similar subjects who lack this allele (65-67), whereas in randomly selected subjects, the Arg^{972} allele was associated with decreased insulin sensitivity in obese but not lean individuals (65). Allelic association studies have been similarly inconclusive, with some studies alone or when analyzed in combination with others demonstrating association of the Arg^{972} allele with type 2 diabetes or impaired glucose tolerance (68-71) and others failing to demonstrate a similar association (72-76). Most of the above studies were small and not population-based, increasing the likelihood for false positive or negative findings because of population stratification. More recently, two large population-based studies, one in Dutch Caucasians and the other in African Americans, failed to demonstrate association of the Arg^{972} allele with type 2 diabetes (55,77). Similarly, linkage of the *IRS-1* gene locus on chromosome 2 with type 2 diabetes has not been demonstrated (78). Thus, variants of the *IRS-1* gene, and specifically the Arg^{972} variant of this gene, are unlikely to have a marked effect on susceptibility for type 2 diabetes, but, given the many positive studies, a modest effect of this gene locus on type 2 diabetes susceptibility in some populations remains a possibility.

Other members of the IRS family of proteins (IRS-2-4) were recognized more recently and have not been as intensively studied. Studies in Ashkenazi Jewish families and families with an autosomal dominant pattern of inheritance of early-onset type 2 diabetes failed to demonstrate linkage of the *IRS2* gene region with type 2 diabetes (79,80). Several amino acid substitutions have been identified in IRS-2 which are either rare or not associated with type 2 diabetes (81,82), although one of these variants, Asp^{1057}, when present in the homozygous state, was associated with decreased fasting insulin levels, as well as reductions in insulin levels at 30 and 60 min during an oral glucose tolerance test (81). Amino acid substitutions in IRS-4 have been identified but are not associated with either type 2 diabetes or insulin resistance (83).

An additional signaling molecule that is proximal in the insulin-signaling cascade and important for insulin-stimulated glucose uptake is phosphatidylinositol 3-kinase (PI 3-kinase). Screening studies in Pima Indians, Caucasians, and Japanese revealed a relatively common polymorphism, substitution of isoleucine for methionine at codon 326 of the p85α regulatory subunit of PI 3-kinase (84-86). In the Japanese and Caucasians, the Ile^{326} allele was not associated with diabetes, although in the Caucasian population, subjects homozygous for the variant allele had a decreased insulin sensitivity index, glucose effectiveness and glucose disappearance constant (85,86). In Pima Indians, women bearing the Ile^{326} allele in its homozygous form exhibited a decreased prevalence of type 2 diabetes and an increased acute insulin response to intravenous glucose and a decreased postload 2 hour glucose compared with subjects heterozygous and homozygous for wild-type Met^{326} allele (84). A functional study failed to demonstrate an effect of this amino substitution on insulin-stimulated lipid kinase activity or its ability to form complexes with tyrosine phosphorylated proteins (87).

Role of genes encoding proteins involved in glucose uptake and glycogen synthesis

Twin studies, population-based studies in Pima Indians, and studies in nondiabetic offspring of diabetic probands have all suggested that insulin-stimulated glucose uptake is heritable (88). Moreover, reduced insulin-stimulated peripheral glucose uptake, which is manifest as a reduction in non-oxidative glucose metabolism, is among the early metabolic defects present in nondiabetic offspring of diabetic parents (89-91). Reduced nonoxidative glucose metabolism primarily reflects decreased glycogen synthesis in skeletal muscle, which is secondary to decreased insulin-stimulated glucose transport into skeletal muscle, although additional abnormalities in the glycogen synthesis pathway, some of which may be genetically determined, may also contribute to reduced glycogen synthesis (92,93).

Insulin-responsive glucose transport into skeletal muscle occurs primarily via the insulin-responsive glucose transporter, GLUT4 (94). Previous studies have failed to demonstrate linkage of the GLUT4 locus on chromosome 17 with type 2 diabetes (78,95). Moreover, sequence variations and missense mutations in the *GLUT4* gene are rare and have not been shown to be associated with type 2 diabetes (96-98). Thus, despite the central role of decreased skeletal muscle glucose uptake in type 2 diabetes, there is no evidence that GLUT4 mutations have a major impact on susceptibility to type 2 diabetes.

Genes encoding proteins important in the glycogen synthesis pathway have also been examined as potential diabetes susceptibility genes. Subsequent to glucose transport into skeletal muscle, glucose is phosphorylated by hexokinase 2 (99). Reduced hexokinase 2 activity has been found in subjects with type 2 diabetes and impaired glucose tolerance (100,101), although it is unclear whether the change is due to a primary genetic abnormality or to metabolic perturbations associated with hyperglycemia. The hexokinase 2 (*HK2*) gene is located on chromosome 2p13. Three previous studies have failed to demonstrate linkage of the *HK2* locus to type 2 diabetes (78,102,103). Screening of the *HK2* gene and its promoter for sequence variants identified several silent polymorphisms, one promoter variant that did not alter promoter function, and several missense mutations that were rare (allele frequencies 1% or less) (100,104-109). One missense mutation, substitution of histidine for glutamine at codon 142, is relatively common but does not alter enzyme activity and is present with equal frequencies in type 2 diabetic subjects and controls and is not associated with altered glucose effectiveness or insulin sensitivity (104,108-110).

Both basal and insulin-stimulated glycogen synthase activity are also reduced in type 2 diabetic subjects (1), and numerous studies have examined the role of the glycogen synthase (*GSY1*) gene as a susceptibility gene for type 2 diabetes. Although two studies have failed to demonstrate linkage of markers in or near the *GSY1* locus with type 2 diabetes (111,112), association of polymorphisms in or near the *GSY1* gene with type 2 diabetes have been demonstrated. A dinucleotide repeat within the *GSY1* gene is associated with type 2 diabetes in Japanese and Pima Indians (112,113), and an early study identified a single nucleotide polymorphism in intron 14 (the A2 allele) which was associated with type 2 diabetes in Caucasians (114). In this study, diabetic subjects bearing the A2 allele had decreased insulin-stimulated nonoxidative glucose metabolism and an increased prevalence of hypertension. The increase in hypertension was also observed in nondiabetic subjects bearing the A2 allele. A repeat association study in a similar population confirmed the previously-demonstrated association of the A2 allele with type 2 diabetes, and analysis of sex-matched sibling pairs discordant for the A2 allele demonstrated increased triglyceride and fasting serum insulin levels and decreased high density lipoprotein (HDL) cholesterol levels in sibs bearing the A2 allele (115). Moreover, among male sib pairs, those with the A2 allele had increased systolic and diastolic blood pressure, whereas in sib pairs concordant for diabetes, those with the A2 allele had an earlier age of onset of type 2 diabetes. Subsequent studies in Japanese and another Caucasian population failed to confirm association of the A2 allele with type 2 diabetes (116,117), and, among Northern European Caucasians, there was no evidence for increased sharing of the A2 allele among affected sib pairs (111). In another group of Caucasians, the frequency of the A1 allele was increased in diabetic subjects (118). Thus, despite evidence for association in many studies, consistent association of the A2 allele with type 2 diabetes has not been demonstrated. One possibility is that the A2 allele is in linkage disequilibrium with another variant of the *GSY1* gene or a neighboring gene. To date, only one common missense mutation in the *GSY1* gene has been identified, substitution of valine for methionine at codon 461, but this variant has not been consistently associated with either type 2 diabetes or related phenotypes (96,119-121).

Activation of glycogen synthase requires it to be dephosphorylated, a process which is thought to be mediated by glycogen bound type 1 protein phosphatase (PP1G) (99). PP1G consists of a catalytic subunit as well as a muscle-specific regulatory targeting subunit which is encoded by the *PPP1R3* gene (122). Analysis of the genes encoding the three isoforms of PPIG, PP1G-α, -β, and –γ, in subjects with type 2 diabetes demonstrated only silent mutations and no evidence for linkage of the PPIG-β locus to type 2 diabetes (123,124). Attention has also been focused on the role of polymorphic variants of the *PPP1R3* gene in susceptibility for type 2 diabetes and related phenotypes. A missense mutation, substitution of tyrosine for aspartic acid at codon 905 was identified in Caucasians (125). Although the Tyr^{905} allele was not associated with type 2 diabetes, it was associated with decreased insulin-stimulated non-oxidative glucose metabolism (glycogen synthesis) and an increased rate of basal glucose oxidation in this population (125). Subsequent studies in Guadalupe Indians, Tamil Indians, and Japanese failed to demonstrate association of the Tyr^{905} allele with type 2 diabetes and, in the case of the Tamil Indians, diabetes-related phenotypes (56,126,127). More recently, a polymorphism in the 3'-untranslated region of the *PPP1R3* gene that affects spacing between two ATTTA pentanucleotides has been identified (128). This pentanucleotide is the shortest consensus sequence for an mRNA-destabilizing AT-rich element (ARE) (129). The two polymorphic variants contain either 10 (ARE1 allele) or 2 nucleotides (ARE2 allele) between two ATTTA motifs (128). Messenger RNAs that contain the ARE2 allele demonstrate increased protein binding and a decreased half-life, suggesting that mRNAs transcribed from the ARE2 allele are less stable (128,130). In both Japanese and Pima Indians, the frequency of the ARE2 allele was higher in diabetic compared with control subjects (128,131), and, in Pima Indians, it was associated with an increased fasting insulin level and decreased insulin-mediated glucose uptake (128). In Caucasians, there was a weak trend towards decreasing insulin-mediated glucose uptake in those with an increasing number of ARE2 alleles, although in neither the Caucasian nor Japanese populations was the ARE2 allele associated with an increased fasting insulin level (131,132). Moreover, among Caucasians, the frequency of the ARE2 allele was not increased in type 2 diabetic subjects (132). In aboriginal Canadian Oji-Cree, the ARE2 allele was not associated with type 2 diabetes or impaired glucose tolerance, but subjects with type 2 diabetes or impaired glucose tolerance who were homozygous for the ARE2 allele had a decreased 2 hr glucose level during an oral glucose tolerance test, suggesting that in this population those with the ARE2 allele had increased insulin sensitivity (133). Thus, despite the clear functional significance of this allelic variant, its role as a susceptibility gene is still unclear. Finally, sequence variants of another PPP1 regulatory targeting subunit gene, phosphatase targeting to glycogen (PTG) or regulatory subunit of type 1 phosphatase (*PPP1R5*), which is located on chromosome 10q23-24, a region with evidence for suggestive linkage to insulin action in Pima Indians, do not make a significant contribution to insulin resistance n Pima Indians (134).

Other studies have examined the potential role of other molecules important in glycogen synthesis. As described, glycogen synthase is activated by dephosphorylation (99). The sites on glycogen synthase that are dephosphorylated in response to insulin are phosphorylated by glycogen synthase kinase-3 (GSK3). GSK-3 activity, in turn, is inhibited by insulin via a signaling cascade that involves activation of PI 3-kinase, phosphoinositide-dependent kinase-1 (PDK-1), and subsequently protein kinase B (PKB). The above genes have been studied as possible candidate genes for type 2 diabetes. Except for silent mutations, sequence variants of the genes encoding PDK-1, two isoforms of PKB, PKB-α and $-\beta$, and two isoforms of GSK3, GSK-3α and -3β, have not been found (99,124,135,136). Moreover, sequence variations of potentially functional importance have not been identified in either of the two inhibitors of PP1G (136,137).

Role of the gene encoding peroxisome proliferator-activated receptor-γ

With the recognition that the effect of a new class of insulin-sensitizing agents, the thiazolidinediones, is mediated by a transcription factor, PPAR-γ (138), increased attention has been focused on the role of the *PPARγ* gene as a potential susceptibility gene for type 2 diabetes. In humans, three PPARγ mRNA isoforms are present, although two of these, PPARγ1 and PPARγ3, encode the same protein (138). The third mRNA encodes PPARγ2, a protein that has an additional 28 amino acids at the amino terminus (138). PPARγ1 is expressed in a wide range of tissues, whereas PPARγ2 is expressed to an appreciable degree only in adipose tissue (138).

An important role for PPARγ in insulin action was confirmed by the identification of mutations in the *PPARγ* gene that resulted in severe insulin resistance and type 2 diabetes (139). Two different missense mutations in the ligand binding domain which interfere with ligand-induced transactivation, substitution of leucine for proline at codon 467 and methionine for valine at codon 290, have been identified in patients. Interestingly, neither of the probands with these mutations were obese and both exhibited early-onset hypertension, hypertriglyceridemia, and low HDL cholesterol levels. Since these mutations were present in the heterozygous state, they presumably act in a dominant negative fashion.

Screening of the *PPARγ* gene in subjects with type 2 diabetes identified a missense mutation, substitution of alanine for proline at codon 12 of PPAR-γ2 (140,141). This missense mutation was relatively frequent in Caucasian populations (~12%) and Mexican Americans (10%) but less so in African Americans, Chinese, and Japanese (1-3%) (141,142). Transfection studies and gel shift analyses demonstrated that the Ala^{12} isoform bound with decreased affinity to the PPARγ DNA binding site and exhibited decreased ligand-induced transactivation, although the effect of the Pro12Ala substitution was not as dramatic as that demonstrated by the mutations described above (140).

The potential role of this polymorphism in susceptibility to type 2 diabetes and obesity has also been examined. Studies in Japanese Americans and Japanese have demonstrated decreased frequency of the Ala^{12} allele in subjects with type 2 diabetes and impaired glucose tolerance compared with normal controls (140,143), although in a specific subset of Oji-Cree women, the Ala^{12} allele was present with increased frequency in those with type 2 diabetes (144). Subsequent studies in Koreans and several Caucasian populations demonstrated a similar frequency of the Ala^{12} allele in type 2 diabetic subjects and controls, although in many studies there was a trend towards a decreased frequency of the Ala^{12} allele in those with diabetes (145-149). Consistent with the above trend, a more recent study, which analyzed over 3,000 Caucasian individuals, demonstrated that the more common Pro^{12} allele is associated with a 1.25-fold increase in diabetes risk (150). The functional differences between the proteins encoded by the Ala^{12} and Pro^{12} alleles suggest that this variation accounts for the difference in risk, although it can be ruled out that this polymorphism is in linkage disequilibrium with another causal variant (150).

In Caucasians and Japanese Americans, increased insulin sensitivity in subjects bearing the Ala^{12} allele has been reported (140), whereas increased insulin sensitivity in a different Caucasian population was observed only in subjects with a BMI > 30 (151). A trend towards increased insulin sensitivity in Caucasian women bearing the Ala^{12} allele has also been reported (152). In contrast, several studies have demonstrated no change in insulin sensitivity in Caucasian or Japanese subjects bearing the Ala^{12} allele (142,146,150,153). Similar discrepant findings have been reported for the effect of the Ala^{12} allele on body weight; it has been associated with either increased (147,152,153), decreased (140), or no change (146,150,151) in body weight in different Caucasian populations.

CONCLUSIONS

To date, with the exception of the *PPARγ* and, possibly, the insulin (*INS*) genes, the candidate gene approach has failed to clearly identify susceptibility genes that are important in the majority of type 2 diabetic subjects. There are many potential reasons for this lack of apparent progress. (1) It is still unclear whether there are two or three major variants of type 2 diabetes or whether it is truly heterogeneous with multiple variants, each of which accounts for a small percentage of affected individuals (3). If the latter is the case, susceptibility genes are likely to differ between different ethnic groups and populations with different founders, which would account for positive and negative studies with the same susceptibility gene in different ethnic groups and populations. (2) In a polygenic disease like type 2 diabetes, the effect of any gene on disease risk may be small. Thus, many studies may lack sufficient power to definitively demonstrate or exclude association with disease. The recent findings with the Pro12Ala variant of the *PPARγ* gene exemplify this problem. Several studies with a relatively modest sample size failed to replicate an initial positive finding (although most showed a trend similar to the initial positive finding), but the initial finding was subsequently replicated through the use of family-based controls and a large population sample (150). (3) As described, the contribution of diet and physical activity to disease risk suggests that gene x environment interactions will be important for disease susceptibility, and, in a polygenic disease, gene x gene interactions also may contribute to disease risk. These interactions add additional layers of complexity to the genetic analyses. (4) The majority of candidate gene analyses were performed in the context of case-control studies. These types of studies are susceptible to the confounding effect of type I and II errors (i.e., false positive and negative studies) related to unrecognized population stratification and other problems.

A promising approach for the future will be to perform analyses similar to those described above for positional candidate genes. As will be described in Chapter 11, chromosomal loci that segregate with type 2 diabetes or related phenotypes are starting to be identified. With completion of the Human Genome Project, genes within these loci have and will be identified. Based upon the known function of these genes, positional candidate genes can be identified and studied. By using both linkage data and gene function in the choice of candidates, identification of true susceptibility genes should be facilitated.

REFERENCES

1. DeFronzo RA. 1997. Pathogenesis of type diabetes: metabolic and molecular implications for identifying diabetes genes. *Diabetes Rev* 5:177-269.
2. Gerich JE. 1998. The genetic basis of type 2 diabetes mellitus: impaired insulin secretion versus impaired insulin sensitivity. *Endocr Rev* 19:491-503.
3. Kahn CR, Vicent D, Doria A. 1996. Genetics of non-insulin-dependent (type-II) diabetes mellitus. *Annu Rev Med* 47:509-31.
4. Lowe WL, Jr. Diabetes Mellitus. In: Jameson JL, editor. Principles of Molecular Medicine. Totowa: Humana Press; 1998. p 433-442.
5. Permutt MA, Chiu K, Ferrer J, Glaser B, Inoue H, Nestorowicz A, Stanley CA, Tanizawa Y. 1998. Genetics of type II diabetes. *Recent Prog Horm Res* 53:201-16.
6. Hawkes CH. 1997. Twin studies in diabetes mellitus. *Diabet Med* 14:347-52.
7. Howard BV. 1997. Dietary fatty acids, insulin resistance, and diabetes. *Ann N Y Acad Sci* 827:215-20.
8. Storlien LH, Baur LA, Kriketos AD, Pan DA, Cooney GJ, Jenkins AB, Calvert GD, Campbell LV. 1996. Dietary fats and insulin action. *Diabetologia* 39:621-31.
9. Eriksson J, Taimela S, Koivisto VA. 1997. Exercise and the metabolic syndrome. *Diabetologia* 40:125-35.
10. Naya FJ, Huang HP, Qiu Y, Mutoh H, DeMayo FJ, Leiter AB, Tsai MJ. 1997. Diabetes, defective pancreatic morphogenesis, and abnormal enteroendocrine differentiation in BETA2/neuroD-deficient mice. *Genes Dev* 11:2323-34.
11. Naya FJ, Stellrecht CM, Tsai MJ. 1995. Tissue-specific regulation of the insulin gene by a novel basic helix- loop-helix transcription factor. *Genes Dev* 9:1009-19.
12. Malecki MT, Jhala US, Antonellis A, Fields L, Doria A, Orban T, Saad M, Warram JH, Montminy M, Krolewski AS. 1999. Mutations in NEUROD1 are associated with the development of type 2 diabetes mellitus. *Nat Genet* 23:323-8.
13. Dupont S, Vionnet N, Chevre JC, Gallina S, Dina C, Seino Y, Yamada Y, Froguel P. 1999. No evidence of linkage or diabetes-associated mutations in the transcription factors BETA2/NEUROD1 and PAX4 in Type II diabetes in France. *Diabetologia* 42:480-4.
14. Stoffers DA, Ferrer J, Clarke WL, Habener JF. 1997. Early-onset type-II diabetes mellitus (MODY4) linked to IPF1. *Nat Genet* 17:138-9.

15. Stoffers DA, Zinkin NT, Stanojevic V, Clarke WL, Habener JF. 1997. Pancreatic agenesis attributable to a single nucleotide deletion in the human IPF1 gene coding sequence. *Nat Genet* 15:106-10.
16. Hani EH, Stoffers DA, Chevre JC, Durand E, Stanojevic V, Dina C, Habener JF, Froguel P. 1999. Defective mutations in the insulin promoter factor-1 (IPF-1) gene in late-onset type 2 diabetes mellitus. *J Clin Invest* 104:R41-8.
17. Macfarlane WM, Frayling TM, Ellard S, Evans JC, Allen LI, Bulman MP, Ayres S, Shepherd M, Clark P, Millward A and others. 1999. Missense mutations in the insulin promoter factor-1 gene predispose to type 2 diabetes. *J Clin Invest* 104:R33-9.
18. Hansen L, Urioste S, Petersen HV, Jensen JN, Eiberg H, Barbetti F, Serup P, Hansen T, Pedersen O. 2000. Missense mutations in the human insulin promoter factor-1 gene and their relation to maturity-onset diabetes of the young and late-onset type 2 diabetes mellitus in caucasians. *J Clin Endocrinol Metab* 85:1323-6.
19. Waeber G, Delplanque J, Bonny C, Mooser V, Steinmann M, Widmann C, Maillard A, Miklossy J, Dina C, Hani EH and others. 2000. The gene MAPK8IP1, encoding islet-brain-1, is a candidate for type 2 diabetes. *Nat Genet* 24:291-5.
20. Bennett ST, Todd JA. 1996. Human type 1 diabetes and the insulin gene: principles of mapping polygenes. *Annu Rev Genet* 30:343-70.
21. Bell GI, Selby MJ, Rutter WJ. 1982. The highly polymorphic region near the human insulin gene is composed of simple tandemly repeating sequences. *Nature* 295:31-5.
22. Vafiadis P, Bennett ST, Colle E, Grabs R, Goodyer CG, Polychronakos C. 1996. Imprinted and genotype-specific expression of genes at the IDDM2 locus in pancreas and leucocytes. *J Autoimmun* 9:397-403.
23. Bennett ST, Wilson AJ, Cucca F, Nerup J, Pociot F, McKinney PA, Barnett AH, Bain SC, Todd JA. 1996. IDDM2-VNTR-encoded susceptibility to type 1 diabetes: dominant protection and parental transmission of alleles of the insulin gene- linked minisatellite locus. *J Autoimmun* 9:415-21.
24. Ahmed S, Bennett ST, Huxtable SJ, Todd JA, Matthews DR, Gough SC. 1999. INS VNTR allelic variation and dynamic insulin secretion in healthy adult non-diabetic Caucasian subjects. *Diabet Med* 16:910-7.
25. Dunger DB, Ong KK, Huxtable SJ, Sherriff A, Woods KA, Ahmed ML, Golding J, Pembrey ME, Ring S, Bennett ST and others. 1998. Association of the INS VNTR with size at birth. ALSPAC Study Team. Avon Longitudinal Study of Pregnancy and Childhood. *Nat Genet* 19:98-100.
26. Hales CN, Barker DJ, Clark PM, Cox LJ, Fall C, Osmond C, Winter PD. 1991. Fetal and infant growth and impaired glucose tolerance at age 64. *BMJ* 303:1019-22.
27. Ong KK, Phillips DI, Fall C, Poulton J, Bennett ST, Golding J, Todd JA, Dunger DB. 1999. The insulin gene VNTR, type 2 diabetes and birth weight. *Nat Genet* 21:262-3.
28. Spielman RS, Ewens WJ. 1996. The TDT and other family-based tests for linkage disequilibrium and association. *Am J Hum Genet* 59:983-9.
29. Huxtable SJ, Saker PJ, Haddad L, Walker M, Frayling TM, Levy JC, Hitman GA, O'Rahilly S, Hattersley AT, McCarthy MI. 2000. Analysis of parent-offspring trios provides evidence for linkage and association between the insulin gene and type 2 diabetes mediated exclusively through paternally transmitted class III variable number tandem repeat alleles. *Diabetes* 49:126-30.
30. Paquette J, Giannoukakis N, Polychronakos C, Vafiadis P, Deal C. 1998. The INS 5' variable number of tandem repeats is associated with IGF2 expression in humans. *J Biol Chem* 273:14158-64.
31. Miki T, Nagashima K, Seino S. 1999. The structure and function of the ATP-sensitive K+ channel in insulin- secreting pancreatic beta-cells. *J Mol Endocrinol* 22:113-23.
32. Aguilar-Bryan L, Bryan J. 1999. Molecular biology of adenosine triphosphate-sensitive potassium channels. *Endocr Rev* 20:101-35.

33. Meissner T, Beinbrech B, Mayatepek E. 1999. Congenital hyperinsulinism: molecular basis of a heterogeneous disease. *Hum Mutat* 13:351-61.
34. Inagaki N, Gonoi T, Clement JPt, Namba N, Inazawa J, Gonzalez G, Aguilar-Bryan L, Seino S, Bryan J. 1995. Reconstitution of IKATP: an inward rectifier subunit plus the sulfonylurea receptor. *Science* 270:1166-70.
35. Stern MP, Duggirala R, Mitchell BD, Reinhardt OC, Benavides E, Blangero J, P. OC. 1996. Evidence for linkage of regions on chromosomes 6 and 11 to plasma glucose concentrations in Mexican Americans. *Genome Res* 6:724-734.
36. Elbein SC, Bragg KL, Hoffman MD, Mayorga RA, Leppert MF. 1996. Linkage studies of NIDDM with 23 chromosome 11 markers in a sample of whites of northern European descent. *Diabetes* 45:370-5.
37. Lindner T, Gragnoli C, Schulze J, Rietzsch H, Petzold C, Schroder HE, Cox NJ, Bell GI. 1997. The 31-cM region of chromosome 11 including the obesity gene tubby and ATP-sensitive potassium channel genes, SUR1 and Kir6.2, does not contain a major susceptibility locus for NIDDM in 127 non-Hispanic white affected sibships. *Diabetes* 46:1227-9.
38. Hani EH, Clement K, Velho G, Vionnet N, Hager J, Philippi A, Dina C, Inoue H, Permutt MA, Basdevant A and others. 1997. Genetic studies of the sulfonylurea receptor gene locus in NIDDM and in morbid obesity among French Caucasians. *Diabetes* 46:688-94.
39. Inoue H, Ferrer J, Welling CM, Elbein SC, Hoffman M, Mayorga R, Warren-Perry M, Zhang Y, Millns H, Turner R and others. 1996. Sequence variants in the sulfonylurea receptor (SUR) gene are associated with NIDDM in Caucasians. *Diabetes* 45:825-31.
40. Stirling B, Cox NJ, Bell GI, Hanis CL, Spielman RS, Concannon P. 1995. Linkage studies in NIDDM with markers near the sulphonylurea receptor gene. *Diabetologia* 38:1479-81.
41. Iwasaki N, Kawamura M, Yamagata K, Cox NJ, Karibe S, Ohgawara H, Inagaki N, Seino S, Bell GI, Omori Y. 1996. Identification of microsatellite markers near the human genes encoding the beta-cell ATP-sensitive K+ channel and linkage studies with NIDDM in Japanese. *Diabetes* 45:267-9.
42. Rissanen J, Markkanen A, Karkkainen P, Kekalainen J, Mykkanen L, Kuusisto J, Karhapaa P, Niskanen L, Laakso M. 2000. Sulfonylurea receptor 1 gene variants are associated with gestational diabetes and type 2 diabetes but not with altered secretion of insulin. *Diabetes Care* 23:70-73.
43. t Hart LM, de Knijff P, Dekker JM, Stolk RP, Nijpels G, van der Does FE, Ruige JB, Grobbee DE, Heine RJ, Maassen JA. 1999. Variants in the sulphonylurea receptor gene: association of the exon 16- 3t variant with Type II diabetes mellitus in Dutch Caucasians. *Diabetologia* 42:617-20.
44. Goksel DL, Fischbach K, Duggirala R, Mitchell BD, Aguilar-Bryan L, Blangero J, Stern MP, O'Connell P. 1998. Variant in sulfonylurea receptor-1 gene is associated with high insulin concentrations in non-diabetic Mexican Americans: SUR-1 gene variant and hyperinsulinemia. *Hum Genet* 103:280-5.
45. Hansen T, Echwald SM, Hansen L, Moller AM, Almind K, Clausen JO, Urhammer SA, Inoue H, Ferrer J, Bryan J and others. 1998. Decreased tolbutamide-stimulated insulin secretion in healthy subjects with sequence variants in the high-affinity sulfonylurea receptor gene. *Diabetes* 47:598-605.
46. Ishiyama-Shigemoto S, Yamada K, Yuan X, Koyama W, Nonaka K. 1998. Clinical characterization of polymorphisms in the sulphonylurea receptor 1 gene in Japanese subjects with Type 2 diabetes mellitus. *Diabet Med* 15:826-9.
47. Ohta Y, Tanizawa Y, Inoue H, Hosaka T, Ueda K, Matsutani A, Repunte VP, Yamada M, Kurachi Y, Bryan J and others. 1998. Identification and functional analysis of sulfonylurea receptor 1 variants in Japanese patients with NIDDM. *Diabetes* 47:476-81.

48. t Hart LM, Dekker JM, van Haeften TW, Ruige JB, Stehouwer CD, Erkelens DW, Heine RJ, Maassen JA. 2000. Reduced second phase insulin secretion in carriers of a sulphonylurea receptor gene variant associating with Type II diabetes mellitus [In Process Citation]. *Diabetologia* 43:515-9.

49. Sakura H, Wat N, Horton V, Millns H, Turner RC, Ashcroft FM. 1996. Sequence variations in the human Kir6.2 gene, a subunit of the beta- cell ATP-sensitive K-channel: no association with NIDDM in while Caucasian subjects or evidence of abnormal function when expressed in vitro. *Diabetologia* 39:1233-6.

50. Hani EH, Boutin P, Durand E, Inoue H, Permutt MA, Velho G, Froguel P. 1998. Missense mutations in the pancreatic islet beta cell inwardly rectifying K+ channel gene (KIR6.2/BIR): a meta-analysis suggests a role in the polygenic basis of Type II diabetes mellitus in Caucasians. *Diabetologia* 41:1511-5.

51. Hansen L, Echwald SM, Hansen T, Urhammer SA, Clausen JO, Pedersen O. 1997. Amino acid polymorphisms in the ATP-regulatable inward rectifier Kir6.2 and their relationships to glucose- and tolbutamide-induced insulin secretion, the insulin sensitivity index, and NIDDM. *Diabetes* 46:508-12.

52. Inoue H, Ferrer J, Warren-Perry M, Zhang Y, Millns H, Turner RC, Elbein SC, Hampe CL, Suarez BK, Inagaki N and others. 1997. Sequence variants in the pancreatic islet beta-cell inwardly rectifying K+ channel Kir6.2 (Bir) gene: identification and lack of role in Caucasian patients with NIDDM. *Diabetes* 46:502-7.

53. Taylor SI. 1992. Lilly Lecture: molecular mechanisms of insulin resistance. Lessons from patients with mutations in the insulin-receptor gene. *Diabetes* 41:1473-90.

54. t Hart LM, Stolk RP, Heine RJ, Grobbee DE, van der Does FE, Maassen JA. 1996. Association of the insulin-receptor variant Met-985 with hyperglycemia and non-insulin-dependent diabetes mellitus in the Netherlands: a population-based study. *Am J Hum Genet* 59:1119-25.

55. t Hart LM, Stolk RP, Dekker JM, Nijpels G, Grobbee DE, Heine RJ, Maassen JA. 1999. Prevalence of variants in candidate genes for type 2 diabetes mellitus in The Netherlands: the Rotterdam study and the Hoorn study. *J Clin Endocrinol Metab* 84:1002-6.

56. Lepretre F, Vionnet N, Budhan S, Dina C, Powell KL, Genin E, Das AK, Nallam V, Passa P, Froguel P. 1998. Genetic studies of polymorphisms in ten non-insulin-dependent diabetes mellitus candidate genes in Tamil Indians from Pondichery. *Diabetes Metab* 24:244-50.

57. Hansen L, Hansen T, Clausen JO, Echwald SM, Urhammer SA, Rasmussen SK, Pedersen O. 1997. The Val985Met insulin-receptor variant in the Danish Caucasian population: lack of associations with non-insulin-dependent diabetes mellitus or insulin resistance. *Am J Hum Genet* 60:1532-5.

58. Strack V, Bossenmaier B, Stoyanov B, Mushack J, Haring HU. 1997. A 973 valine to methionine mutation of the human insulin receptor: interaction with insulin-receptor substrate-1 and Shc in HEK 293 cells. *Diabetologia* 40:1135-40.

59. Rondinone CM, Wang LM, Lonnroth P, Wesslau C, Pierce JH, Smith U. 1997. Insulin receptor substrate (IRS) 1 is reduced and IRS-2 is the main docking protein for phosphatidylinositol 3-kinase in adipocytes from subjects with non-insulin-dependent diabetes mellitus. *Proc Natl Acad Sci U S A* 94:4171-5.

60. Carvalho E, Jansson PA, Axelsen M, Eriksson JW, Huang X, Groop L, Rondinone C, Sjostrom L, Smith U. 1999. Low cellular IRS 1 gene and protein expression predict insulin resistance and NIDDM. *FASEB J* 13:2173-8.

61. Imai Y, Philippe N, Sesti G, Accili D, Taylor SI. 1997. Expression of variant forms of insulin receptor substrate-1 identified in patients with noninsulin-dependent diabetes mellitus. *J Clin Endocrinol Metab* 82:4201-7.

62. Almind K, Inoue G, Pedersen O, Kahn CR. 1996. A common amino acid polymorphism in insulin receptor substrate-1 causes impaired insulin signaling. Evidence from transfection studies. *J Clin Invest* 97:2569-75.
63. Porzio O, Federici M, Hribal ML, Lauro D, Accili D, Lauro R, Borboni P, Sesti G. 1999. The Gly972-->Arg amino acid polymorphism in IRS-1 impairs insulin secretion in pancreatic beta cells. *J Clin Invest* 104:357-64.
64. Kulkarni RN, Winnay JN, Daniels M, Bruning JC, Flier SN, Hanahan D, Kahn CR. 1999. Altered function of insulin receptor substrate-1-deficient mouse islets and cultured beta-cell lines. *J Clin Invest* 104:R69-75.
65. Armstrong M, Haldane F, Avery PJ, Mitcheson J, Stewart MW, Turnbull DM, Walker M. 1996. Relationship between insulin sensitivity and insulin receptor substrate-1 mutations in non-diabetic relatives of NIDDM families. *Diabet Med* 13:341-5.
66. Koch M, Rett K, Volk A, Maerker E, Haist K, Deninger M, Renn W, Haring HU. 1999. Amino acid polymorphism Gly 972 Arg in IRS-1 is not associated to lower clamp-derived insulin sensitivity in young healthy first degree relatives of patients with type 2 diabetes. *Exp Clin Endocrinol Diabetes* 107:318-22.
67. Laakso M, Malkki M, Kekalainen P, Kuusisto J, Deeb SS. 1994. Insulin receptor substrate-1 variants in non-insulin-dependent diabetes. *J Clin Invest* 94:1141-6.
68. Yamada K, Yuan X, Ishiyama S, Shoji S, Kohno S, Koyama K, Koyanagi A, Koyama W, Nonaka K. 1998. Codon 972 polymorphism of the insulin receptor substrate-1 gene in impaired glucose tolerance and late-onset NIDDM. *Diabetes Care* 21:753-6.
69. Zhang Y, Wat N, Stratton IM, Warren-Perry MG, Orho M, Groop L, Turner RC. 1996. UKPDS 19: heterogeneity in NIDDM: separate contributions of IRS-1 and beta 3-adrenergic-receptor mutations to insulin resistance and obesity respectively with no evidence for glycogen synthase gene mutations. UK Prospective Diabetes Study. *Diabetologia* 39:1505-11.
70. Sigal RJ, Doria A, Warram JH, Krolewski AS. 1996. Codon 972 polymorphism in the insulin receptor substrate-1 gene, obesity, and risk of noninsulin-dependent diabetes mellitus. *J Clin Endocrinol Metab* 81:1657-9.
71. Baroni MG, D'Andrea MP, Montali A, Pannitteri G, Barilla F, Campagna F, Mazzei E, Lovari S, Seccareccia F, Campa PP and others. 1999. A common mutation of the insulin receptor substrate-1 gene is a risk factor for coronary artery disease. *Arterioscler Thromb Vasc Biol* 19:2975-80.
72. Mori H, Hashiramoto M, Kishimoto M, Kasuga M. 1995. Amino acid polymorphisms of the insulin receptor substrate-1 in Japanese noninsulin-dependent diabetes mellitus. *J Clin Endocrinol Metab* 80:2822-6.
73. Celi FS, Silver K, Walston J, Knowler WC, Bogardus C, Shuldiner AR. 1995. Lack of IRS-1 codon 513 and 972 polymorphism in Pima Indians. *J Clin Endocrinol Metab* 80:2827-9.
74. Chuang LM, Lai CS, Yeh JI, Wu HP, Tai TY, Lin BJ. 1996. No association between the Gly971Arg variant of the insulin receptor substrate 1 gene and NIDDM in the Taiwanese population. *Diabetes Care* 19:446-9.
75. Shimokawa K, Kadowaki H, Sakura H, Otabe S, Hagura R, Kosaka K, Yazaki Y, Akanuma Y, Kadowaki T. 1994. Molecular scanning of the glycogen synthase and insulin receptor substrate-1 genes in Japanese subjects with non-insulin-dependent diabetes mellitus. *Biochem Biophys Res Commun* 202:463-9.
76. Ura S, Araki E, Kishikawa H, Shirotani T, Todaka M, Isami S, Shimoda S, Yoshimura R, Matsuda K, Motoyoshi S and others. 1996. Molecular scanning of the insulin receptor substrate-1 (IRS-1) gene in Japanese patients with NIDDM: identification of five novel polymorphisms. *Diabetologia* 39:600-8.
77. Lei HH, Coresh J, Shuldiner AR, Boerwinkle E, Brancati FL. 1999. Variants of the insulin receptor substrate-1 and fatty acid binding protein 2 genes and the risk of type

2 diabetes, obesity, and hyperinsulinemia in African-Americans: the Atherosclerosis Risk in Communities Study. *Diabetes* 48:1868-72.

78. Elbein SC, Chiu KC, Hoffman MD, Mayorga RA, Bragg KL, Leppert MF. 1995. Linkage analysis of 19 candidate regions for insulin resistance in familial NIDDM. *Diabetes* 44:1259-65.

79. Kalidas K, Wasson J, Glaser B, Meyer JM, Duprat LJ, White MF, Permutt MA. 1998. Mapping of the human insulin receptor substrate-2 gene, identification of a linked polymorphic marker and linkage analysis in families with Type II diabetes: no evidence for a major susceptibility role. *Diabetologia* 41:1389-91.

80. Bektas A, Warram JH, White MF, Krolewski AS, Doria A. 1999. Exclusion of insulin receptor substrate 2 (IRS-2) as a major locus for early-onset autosomal dominant type 2 diabetes. *Diabetes* 48:640-2.

81. Almind K, Frederiksen SK, Bernal D, Hansen T, Ambye L, Urhammer S, Ekstrom CT, Berglund L, Reneland R, Lithell H and others. 1999. Search for variants of the gene-promoter and the potential phosphotyrosine encoding sequence of the insulin receptor substrate-2 gene: evaluation of their relation with alterations in insulin secretion and insulin sensitivity. *Diabetologia* 42:1244-9.

82. Bernal D, Almind K, Yenush L, Ayoub M, Zhang Y, Rosshani L, Larsson C, Pedersen O, White MF. 1998. Insulin receptor substrate-2 amino acid polymorphisms are not associated with random type 2 diabetes among Caucasians. *Diabetes* 47:976-9.

83. Almind K, Frederiksen SK, Ahlgren MG, Urhammer S, Hansen T, Clausen JO, Pedersen O. 1998. Common amino acid substitutions in insulin receptor substrate-4 are not associated with Type II diabetes mellitus or insulin resistance. *Diabetologia* 41:969-74.

84. Baier LJ, Wiedrich C, Hanson RL, Bogardus C. 1998. Variant in the regulatory subunit of phosphatidylinositol 3-kinase (p85alpha): preliminary evidence indicates a potential role of this variant in the acute insulin response and type 2 diabetes in Pima women. *Diabetes* 47:973-5.

85. Hansen T, Andersen CB, Echwald SM, Urhammer SA, Clausen JO, Vestergaard H, Owens D, Hansen L, Pedersen O. 1997. Identification of a common amino acid polymorphism in the p85alpha regulatory subunit of phosphatidylinositol 3-kinase: effects on glucose disappearance constant, glucose effectiveness, and the insulin sensitivity index. *Diabetes* 46:494-501.

86. Kawanishi M, Tamori Y, Masugi J, Mori H, Ito C, Hansen T, Andersen CB, Pedersen O, Kasuga M. 1997. Prevalence of a polymorphism of the phosphatidylinositol 3-kinase p85 alpha regulatory subunit (codon 326 Met-->Ile) in Japanese NIDDM patients [letter]. *Diabetes Care* 20:1043.

87. Baynes KCR, Beeton CA, Panayotou G, Stein R, Soos M, Hansen T, Simpson H, O'Rahilly S, Shepherd PR, Whitehead JP. 2000. Natural variants of human p85α phosphoinositide 3-kinase in severe insulin resistance: a novel variant with impaired insulin-stimulated lipid kinase activity. *Diabetologia* 43:321-331.

88. Lehtovirta M, Kaprio J, Forsblom C, Eriksson J, Tuomilehto J, Groop L. 2000. Insulin sensitivity and insulin secretion in monozygotic and dizygotic twins [In Process Citation]. *Diabetologia* 43:285-93.

89. Gulli G, Ferrannini E, Stern M, Haffner S, DeFronzo RA. 1992. The metabolic profile of NIDDM is fully established in glucose-tolerant offspring of two Mexican-American NIDDM parents. *Diabetes* 41:1575-86.

90. Eriksson J, Franssila-Kallunki A, Ekstrand A, Saloranta C, Widen E, Schalin C, Groop L. 1989. Early metabolic defects in persons at increased risk for non-insulin-dependent diabetes mellitus. *N Engl J Med* 321:337-43.

91. Vauhkonen I, Niskanen L, Vanninen E, Kainulainen S, Uusitupa M, Laakso M. 1998. Defects in insulin secretion and insulin action in non-insulin- dependent diabetes

mellitus are inherited. Metabolic studies on offspring of diabetic probands. *J Clin Invest* 101:86-96.

92. Cline GW, Petersen KF, Krssak M, Shen J, Hundal RS, Trajanoski Z, Inzucchi S, Dresner A, Rothman DL, Shulman GI. 1999. Impaired glucose transport as a cause of decreased insulin-stimulated muscle glycogen synthesis in type 2 diabetes. *N Engl J Med* 341:240-6.
93. Roden M, Shulman GI. 1999. Applications of NMR spectroscopy to study muscle glycogen metabolism in man. *Annu Rev Med* 50:277-90.
94. Shepherd PR, Kahn BB. 1999. Glucose transporters and insulin action--implications for insulin resistance and diabetes mellitus. *N Engl J Med* 341:248-57.
95. Lesage S, Zouali H, Vionnet N, Philippi A, Velho G, Serradas P, Passa P, Demenais F, Froguel P. 1997. Genetic analyses of glucose transporter genes in French non-insulin-dependent diabetic families. *Diabetes Metab* 23:137-42.
96. Bjorbaek C, Echwald SM, Hubricht P, Vestergaard H, Hansen T, Zierath J, Pedersen O. 1994. Genetic variants in promoters and coding regions of the muscle glycogen synthase and the insulin-responsive GLUT4 genes in NIDDM. *Diabetes* 43:976-83.
97. Buse JB, Yasuda K, Lay TP, Seo TS, Olson AL, Pessin JE, Karam JH, Seino S, Bell GI. 1992. Human GLUT4/muscle-fat glucose-transporter gene. Characterization and genetic variation. *Diabetes* 41:1436-45.
98. Krook A, Stratton IM, O'Rahilly S. 1992. Rapid and simultaneous detection of multiple mutations by pooled and multiplex single nucleotide primer extension: application to the study of insulin-responsive glucose transporter and insulin receptor mutations in non-insulin-dependent diabetes. *Hum Mol Genet* 1:391-5.
99. Lawrence JC, Jr., Roach PJ. 1997. New insights into the role and mechanism of glycogen synthase activation by insulin. *Diabetes* 46:541-7.
100. Lehto M, Huang X, Davis EM, Le Beau MM, Laurila E, Eriksson KF, Bell GI, Groop L. 1995. Human hexokinase II gene: exon-intron organization, mutation screening in NIDDM, and its relationship to muscle hexokinase activity. *Diabetologia* 38:1466-74.
101. Vestergaard H, Bjorbaek C, Hansen T, Larsen FS, Granner DK, Pedersen O. 1995. Impaired activity and gene expression of hexokinase II in muscle from non-insulin-dependent diabetes mellitus patients. *J Clin Invest* 96:2639-45.
102. Vionnet N, Hani EH, Lesage S, Philippi A, Hager J, Varret M, Stoffel M, Tanizawa Y, Chiu KC, Glaser B and others. 1997. Genetics of NIDDM in France: studies with 19 candidate genes in affected sib pairs. *Diabetes* 46:1062-8.
103. Ardehali H, Tiller GE, Printz RL, Mochizuki H, Prochazka M, Granner DK. 1996. A novel (TA)n polymorphism in the hexokinase II gene: application to noninsulin-dependent diabetes mellitus in the Pima Indians. *Hum Genet* 97:482-5.
104. Echwald SM, Bjorbaek C, Hansen T, Clausen JO, Vestergaard H, Zierath JR, Printz RL, Granner DK, Pedersen O. 1995. Identification of four amino acid substitutions in hexokinase II and studies of relationships to NIDDM, glucose effectiveness, and insulin sensitivity. *Diabetes* 44:347-53.
105. Laakso M, Malkki M, Kekalainen P, Kuusisto J, Deeb SS. 1995. Polymorphisms of the human hexokinase II gene: lack of association with NIDDM and insulin resistance. *Diabetologia* 38:617-22.
106. Laakso M, Malkki M, Deeb SS. 1995. Amino acid substitutions in hexokinase II among patients with NIDDM. *Diabetes* 44:330-4.
107. Malkki M, Laakso M, Deeb SS. 1997. The human hexokinase II gene promoter: functional characterization and detection of variants among patients with NIDDM. *Diabetologia* 40:1461-9.
108. Taylor RW, Printz RL, Armstrong M, Granner DK, Alberti KG, Turnbull DM, Walker M. 1996. Variant sequences of the Hexokinase II gene in familial NIDDM. *Diabetologia* 39:322-8.

109. Vidal-Puig A, Printz RL, Stratton IM, Granner DK, Moller DE. 1995. Analysis of the hexokinase II gene in subjects with insulin resistance and NIDDM and detection of a Gln142-->His substitution. *Diabetes* 44:340-6.
110. Malkki M, Laakso M, Deeb SS. 1998. Functional consequences of naturally occurring variants of human hexokinase II. *Diabetologia* 41:1205-9.
111. Elbein SC, Hoffman M, Ridinger D, Otterud B, Leppert M. 1994. Description of a second microsatellite marker and linkage analysis of the muscle glycogen synthase locus in familial NIDDM. *Diabetes* 43:1061-5.
112. Majer M, Mott DM, Mochizuki H, Rowles JC, Pedersen O, Knowler WC, Bogardus C, Prochazka M. 1996. Association of the glycogen synthase locus on 19q13 with NIDDM in Pima Indians. *Diabetologia* 39:314-21.
113. Kuroyama H, Sanke T, Ohagi S, Furuta M, Furuta H, Nanjo K. 1994. Simple tandem repeat DNA polymorphism in the human glycogen synthase gene is associated with NIDDM in Japanese subjects. *Diabetologia* 37:536-9.
114. Groop LC, Kankuri M, Schalin-Jantti C, Ekstrand A, Nikula-Ijas P, Widen E, Kuismanen E, Eriksson J, Franssila-Kallunki A, Saloranta C and others. 1993. Association between polymorphism of the glycogen synthase gene and non-insulin-dependent diabetes mellitus. *N Engl J Med* 328:10-4.
115. Orho-Melander M, Almgren P, Kanninen T, Forsblom C, Groop LC. 1999. A paired-sibling analysis of the XbaI polymorphism in the muscle glycogen synthase gene. *Diabetologia* 42:1138-45.
116. Kadowaki T, Kadowaki H, Yazaki Y. 1993. Polymorphism of the glycogen synthase gene and non-insulin-dependent diabetes mellitus. *N Engl J Med* 328:1568-9.
117. Babadjanova G, Allolio B, Beuschlein F, Chuchalin A, Reincke M. 1997. Polymorphism of the glycogen synthase gene and non-insulin-dependent diabetes mellitus in the Russian population. *Metabolism* 46:121-2.
118. Zouali H, Velho G, Froguel P. 1993. Polymorphism of the glycogen synthase gene and non-insulin-dependent diabetes mellitus. *N Engl J Med* 328:1568.
119. Orho-Melander M, Shimomura H, Sanke T, Rasmussen SK, Nanjo K, Pedersen O, Groop LC. 1999. Expression of naturally occurring variants in the muscle glycogen synthase gene. *Diabetes* 48:918-20.
120. Rissanen J, Pihlajamaki J, Heikkinen S, Kekalainen P, Mykkanen L, Kuusisto J, Kolle A, Laakso M. 1997. New variants in the glycogen synthase gene (Gln71His, Met416Val) in patients with NIDDM from eastern Finland. *Diabetologia* 40:1313-9.
121. Shimomura H, Sanke T, Ueda K, Hanabusa T, Sakagashira S, Nanjo K. 1997. A missense mutation of the muscle glycogen synthase gene (M416V) is associated with insulin resistance in the Japanese population. *Diabetologia* 40:947-52.
122. Chen YH, Hansen L, Chen MX, Bjorbaek C, Vestergaard H, Hansen T, Cohen PT, Pedersen O. 1994. Sequence of the human glycogen-associated regulatory subunit of type 1 protein phosphatase and analysis of its coding region and mRNA level in muscle from patients with NIDDM. *Diabetes* 43:1234-41.
123. Bjorbaek C, Vik TA, Echwald SM, Yang PY, Vestergaard H, Wang JP, Webb GC, Richmond K, Hansen T, Erikson RL and others. 1995. Cloning of a human insulin-stimulated protein kinase (ISPK-1) gene and analysis of coding regions and mRNA levels of the ISPK-1 and the protein phosphatase-1 genes in muscle from NIDDM patients. *Diabetes* 44:90-7.
124. Prochazka M, Mochizuki H, Baier LJ, Cohen PT, Bogardus C. 1995. Molecular and linkage analysis of type-1 protein phosphatase catalytic beta-subunit gene: lack of evidence for its major role in insulin resistance in Pima Indians. *Diabetologia* 38:461-6.
125. Hansen L, Hansen T, Vestergaard H, Bjorbaek C, Echwald SM, Clausen JO, Chen YH, Chen MX, Cohen PT, Pedersen O. 1995. A widespread amino acid polymorphism at codon 905 of the glycogen-associated regulatory subunit of protein

phosphatase-1 is associated with insulin resistance and hypersecretion of insulin. *Hum Mol Genet* 4:1313-20.

126. Shen GQ, Ikegami H, Kawaguchi Y, Fujisawa T, Hamada Y, Ueda H, Shintani M, Nojima K, Kawabata Y, Yamada K and others. 1998. Asp905Tyr polymorphism of the gene for the skeletal muscle-specific glycogen-targeting subunit of protein phosphatase 1 in NIDDM. *Diabetes Care* 21:1086-9.
127. Boullu-Sanchis S, Lepretre F, Hedelin G, Donnet JP, Schaffer P, Froguel P, Pinget M. 1999. Type 2 diabetes mellitus: association study of five candidate genes in an Indian population of Guadeloupe, genetic contribution of FABP2 polymorphism. *Diabetes Metab* 25:150-6.
128. Xia J, Scherer SW, Cohen PT, Majer M, Xi T, Norman RA, Knowler WC, Bogardus C, Prochazka M. 1998. A common variant in PPP1R3 associated with insulin resistance and type 2 diabetes. *Diabetes* 47:1519-24.
129. Ross J. 1996. Control of messenger RNA stability in higher eukaryotes. *Trends Genet* 12:171-5.
130. Xia J, Bogardus C, Prochazka M. 1999. A type 2 diabetes-associated polymorphic ARE motif affecting expression of PPP1R3 is involved in RNA-protein interactions. *Mol Genet Metab* 68:48-55.
131. Maegawa H, Shi K, Hidaka H, Iwai N, Nishio Y, Egawa K, Kojima H, Haneda M, Yasuda H, Nakamura Y and others. 1999. The 3'-untranslated region polymorphism of the gene for skeletal muscle-specific glycogen-targeting subunit of protein phosphatase 1 in the type 2 diabetic Japanese population. *Diabetes* 48:1469-72.
132. Hansen L, Reneland R, Berglund L, Rasmussen SK, Hansen T, Lithell H, Pedersen O. 2000. Polymorphism in the glycogen-associated regulatory subunit of type 1 protein phosphatase (PP1R3) gene and insulin sensitivity. *Diabetes* 49:298-301.
133. Hegele RA, Harris SB, Zinman B, Wang J, Cao H, Hanley AJ, Tsui LC, Scherer SW. 1998. Variation in the AU(AT)-rich element within the 3'-untranslated region of PPP1R3 is associated with variation in plasma glucose in aboriginal Canadians. *J Clin Endocrinol Metab* 83:3980-3.
134. Permana PA, Luczy-Bachman G, Bogardus C. 1999. Protein targeting to glycogen/PPP1R5: screening of coding and flanking genomic regions for polymorphisms and association analysis with insulin action in Pima Indians. *Biochem Biophys Res Commun* 258:184-6.
135. Hansen L, Arden KC, Rasmussen SB, Viars CS, Vestergaard H, Hansen T, Moller AM, Woodgett JR, Pedersen O. 1997. Chromosomal mapping and mutational analysis of the coding region of the glycogen synthase kinase-3alpha and beta isoforms in patients with NIDDM. *Diabetologia* 40:940-6.
136. Hansen L, Fjordvang H, Rasmussen SK, Vestergaard H, Echwald SM, Hansen T, Alessi D, Shenolikar S, Saltiel AR, Barbetti F and others. 1999. Mutational analysis of the coding regions of the genes encoding protein kinase B-alpha and -beta, phosphoinositide-dependent protein kinase-1, phosphatase targeting to glycogen, protein phosphatase inhibitor-1, and glycogenin: lessons from a search for genetic variability of the insulin-stimulated glycogen synthesis pathway of skeletal muscle in NIDDM patients. *Diabetes* 48:403-7.
137. Permana PA, Mott DM. 1997. Genetic analysis of human type 1 protein phosphatase inhibitor 2 in insulin-resistant Pima Indians. *Genomics* 41:110-4.
138. Auwerx J. 1999. PPARgamma, the ultimate thrifty gene. *Diabetologia* 42:1033-49.
139. Barroso I, Gurnell M, Crowley VE, Agostini M, Schwabe JW, Soos MA, Maslen GL, Williams TD, Lewis H, Schafer AJ and others. 1999. Dominant negative mutations in human PPARgamma associated with severe insulin resistance, diabetes mellitus and hypertension. *Nature* 402:880-3.
140. Deeb SS, Fajas L, Nemoto M, Pihlajamaki J, Mykkanen L, Kuusisto J, Laakso M, Fujimoto W, Auwerx J. 1998. A Pro12Ala substitution in PPARgamma2 associated

with decreased receptor activity, lower body mass index and improved insulin sensitivity. *Nat Genet* 20:284-7.

141. Yen CJ, Beamer BA, Negri C, Silver K, Brown KA, Yarnall DP, Burns DK, Roth J, Shuldiner AR. 1997. Molecular scanning of the human peroxisome proliferator activated receptor gamma (hPPAR gamma) gene in diabetic Caucasians: identification of a Pro12Ala PPAR gamma 2 missense mutation. *Biochem Biophys Res Commun* 241:270-4.

142. Mori Y, Kim-Motoyama H, Katakura T, Yasuda K, Kadowaki H, Beamer BA, Shuldiner AR, Akanuma Y, Yazaki Y, Kadowaki T. 1998. Effect of the Pro12Ala variant of the human peroxisome proliferator- activated receptor gamma 2 gene on adiposity, fat distribution, and insulin sensitivity in Japanese men. *Biochem Biophys Res Commun* 251:195-8.

143. Hara K, Okada T, Tobe K, Yasuda K, Mori Y, Kadowaki H, Hagura R, Akanuma Y, Kimura S, Ito C and others. 2000. The Pro12Ala polymorphism in PPAR gamma2 may confer resistance to type 2 diabetes. *Biochem Biophys Res Commun* 271:212-6.

144. Hegele RA, Cao H, Harris SB, Zinman B, Hanley AJG, Anderson CM. 2000. Peroxisome-proliferator-activated receptor-g2 P12A and type 2 diabetes in Canadian Oji-Cree. *J Clin Endocrinol Metab* 85:2014-2019.

145. Oh EY, Min KM, Chung JH, Min Y-K, Lee M-S, Kim K-W, Lee M-K. 2000. Significance of Pro^{12}Ala mutation in peroxisome proliferator-activated receptor-γ2 in Korean diabetic and obese subjects. *J Clin Endocrinol Metab* 85:1801-1804.

146. Mancini FP, Vaccaro O, Sabatino L, Tufano A, Rivellese AA, Riccardi G, Colantuoni V. 1999. Pro12Ala substitution in the peroxisome proliferator-activated receptor- gamma2 is not associated with type 2 diabetes. *Diabetes* 48:1466-8.

147. Meirhaeghe A, Fajas L, Helbecque N, Cottel D, Auwerx J, Deeb SS, Amouyel P. 2000. Impact of the peroxisome proliferator activated receptor gamma2 Pro12Ala polymorphism on adiposity, lipids and non-insulin-dependent diabetes mellitus. *Int J Obes Relat Metab Disord* 24:195-9.

148. Ringel J, Engeli S, Distler A, Sharma AM. 1999. Pro12Ala missense mutation of the peroxisome proliferator activated receptor gamma and diabetes mellitus. *Biochem Biophys Res Commun* 254:450-3.

149. Clement K, Hercberg S, Passinge B, Galan P, Varroud-Vial M, Shuldiner AR, Beamer BA, Charpentier G, Guy-Grand B, Froguel P and others. 2000. The Pro115Gln and Pro12Ala PPAR gamma gene mutations in obesity and type 2 diabetes. *Int J Obes Relat Metab Disord* 24:391-3.

150. Altshuler D, Hirschhorn JN, Klannemark M, Lindgren CM, Vohl M-C, Nemesh J, Lane CR, Schaffner SF, Bolk S, Brewer C and others. 2000. The common PPARγ Pro12Ala polymorphism is associated with decreased risk of type 2 diabetes. *Nat Genet* 26.

151. Koch M, Rett K, Maerker E, Volk A, Haist K, Deninger M, Renn W, Haring HU. 1999. The PPARgamma2 amino acid polymorphism Pro 12 Ala is prevalent in offspring of Type II diabetic patients and is associated to increased insulin sensitivity in a subgroup of obese subjects. *Diabetologia* 42:758-62.

152. Beamer BA, Yen CJ, Andersen RE, Muller D, Elahi D, Cheskin LJ, Andres R, Roth J, Shuldiner AR. 1998. Association of the Pro12Ala variant in the peroxisome proliferator- activated receptor-gamma2 gene with obesity in two Caucasian populations. *Diabetes* 47:1806-8.

153. Valve R, Sivenius K, Miettinen R, Pihlajamaki J, Rissanen A, Deeb SS, Auwerx J, Uusitupa M, Laakso M. 1999. Two polymorphisms in the peroxisome proliferator-activated receptor- gamma gene are associated with severe overweight among obese women. *J Clin Endocrinol Metab* 84:3708-12.

11
USE OF GENOME SCANS TO IDENTIFY SUSCEPTIBILITY GENES FOR TYPE 2 DIABETES

Wen-Chi Hsueh, Ph.D., Braxton D. Mitchell, Ph.D.
Southwest Foundation for Biomedical Research, San Antonio, TX 78227 USA

Alan R. Shuldiner, M.D.
University of Maryland School of Medicine, Baltimore, MD 21201 USA

Introduction

Heredity has long been regarded as a risk factor for type 2 diabetes. Familial aggregation of type 2 diabetes is consistently observed across populations worldwide. The concordance rates for diabetes in monozygotic twins are 50% or higher, whereas those for dizygotic twins are substantially lower, at 10 to 17% (1-3). It is estimated that siblings of diabetic individuals are 1.2 to 3 times more likely to have diabetes compared to the population, depending on the background prevalence of diabetes in the population (4-7).

Segregation analysis studies have suggested that, at least in some populations, the transmission of diabetes through families may be consistent with the presence of a co-segregating major gene (8-10), although such a pattern has not been observed in many other populations. Detection of major gene effects by purely statistical methods has been complicated greatly by the profound increase in diabetes prevalence worldwide (11) and by the likelihood that mutations in multiple genes are involved, many of which may be expressed differentially, depending on the genetic and/or environmental background of the individual.

Within the last several years, progress has been made in identifying susceptibility genes for monogenic forms of diabetes, including maturity-onset diabetes of the young (MODY) [genes for glucokinase, hepatocyte nuclear factors (HNF-4-α, HNF-1-α, HNF-1-α), insulin promoter factor (IPF-1)] (See Chapter 5) (12-16), type A syndrome of extreme of extreme insulin resistance (insulin receptor gene) (17), insulinopathies (18), and maternally-inherited diabetes and deafness (mitochondrial DNA) (see Chapter 6) (19), which in aggregate may account for approximately 5 - 10% of all type 2 diabetes (20). However, despite considerable evidence for genetic influence, identification of genes that increase susceptibility to typical forms of type 2 diabetes has been slow. This is likely due to the oligo- or polygenic nature of typical type 2 diabetes, and the important influences of environmental provocations (i.e., caloric excess and physical inactivity) and age.

Efforts to identify susceptibility genes for type 2 diabetes initially concentrated on candidate genes chosen based upon their presumed relevance to glucose metabolism. To date, numerous candidate genes have been identified and analyzed, but with the possible exception of the Pro12Ala PPARγ2 variant (21-23), none so far have been shown to confer substantial risk on the common forms of type 2 diabetes (see Chapter 10 and reference (24)). The emerging availability of large-scale genotyping technologies and more sophisticated statistical models has led in recent years to the genome-wide linkage approach (genome scan). Genome scans involve the use of highly polymorphic genetic markers (typically 300 – 500 markers) that are dispersed throughout the genome in known locations, so that linkage analyses may be conducted in a very systematic way to identify chromosomal regions harboring disease susceptibility genes. Because coverage of the entire genome is complete, the analysis proceeds without an *a priori* hypothesis regarding the location, function, or number of susceptibility gene(s).

Although this approach appears straightforward for early onset, single-gene defects for which environmental provocations are minimal (i.e., Mendelian diseases), genome-wide linkage analysis for complex diseases such as type 2 diabetes may face particular challenges. Genome scans are based on family collections, and thus the first major challenge is to recruit sufficient numbers of families for analysis. Family collections may be difficult for type 2 diabetes (and other late onset diseases) because, very often, one or both parents of the index cases are not available and/or the children of affected individuals may be too young to develop the disease. An additional challenge is that on a genetic level, type 2 diabetes is probably a manifestation of many distinct susceptibility alleles (i.e., it is genetically heterogeneous). Thus, it may be preferable to select families with a more homogeneous ethnic background in hopes of reducing the number and complexity of the genes involved. Finally, potential interactions among genes and between genes and non-genetic factors may result in pedigree members with one or more diabetes susceptibility genes but who do not manifest the disease, or alternatively some members who have the disease but not the segregating susceptibility gene.

Although genome scans may be conducted on a specific disease trait (such as diabetes), there may also be value in conducting such scans on the intermediate metabolic traits that are precursors of the disease endpoint. In the case of type 2 diabetes, such intermediate traits may include glucose, insulin, or C-peptide concentrations, or more sophisticated measures of insulin sensitivity or beta-cell function. Indeed, evidence supports a heritable component to these traits (25-28). These traits are typically continuous traits and exist in all members of the pedigree, both affected and unaffected, necessitating the use of quantitative trait locus (QTL) analysis.

The goal of this chapter is to contrast some of the different approaches that have been used in genome scan studies of type 2 diabetes and to provide a brief synthesis of the major linkages reported to date.

LINKAGE ANALYSIS APPROACHES USED IN GENOME SCAN STUDIES

Once familial aggregation of a trait has been established, linkage analysis is a statistical tool used to evaluate whether alleles at specific loci along the chromosome co-segregate with the trait and can account for the familial correlations in phenotype. Two contrasting approaches to linkage analysis have been used in studies of type 2 diabetes: the traditional parametric, or heavily model-dependent method; and the more recently developed allele-sharing methods, which require far fewer assumptions about the genetic model.

The traditional parametric approach to linkage analysis is based on estimating the number of recombinations between alleles at an observed marker locus and a putative allele at the disease locus, whose presence is inferred. A very specific genetic model must be assumed so that the transmission probabilities of the disease can be inferred conditional on the observed phenotype. The simplest genetic models require knowledge of the penetrance of the disease given the transmitted genotype. One then calculates the likelihood of the pedigree data given linkage (i.e., co-segregation between the disease and marker loci) and compares that to the likelihood of the data assuming no linkage (i.e., no co-segregation). More complex models (e.g., mixed models) allow for residual genetic effects, over and above that of the linked disease locus. When the estimates of model parameters are accurate, parametric methods may provide great statistical power to detect linkage.

The classical penetrance model-based approach has worked well for simple Mendelian diseases for which it is relatively easy to make assumptions about the disease penetrance. However, this approach has, in general, worked less well for complex genetic diseases, such as diabetes, cardiovascular disease, hypertension, and obesity, which are likely to be influenced by multiple genetic loci and have complex modes of inheritance.

Allele-sharing approaches to linkage analysis, in contrast, are much simpler in concept than the parametric-based approaches and are based on the simple idea that under linkage, there will be a correspondence between similarity of the phenotypes and genotypes between related individuals. The similarity in genotypes is assessed by the number of alleles they share at a particular genetic locus. There are essentially two flavors of linkage analysis that utilize this allele-sharing principle: one that is based on analysis of affected pedigree members (APM); and the second which is based on all pedigree members (affected and unaffected). In APM analysis (of which affected sib-pair analysis is a subset), one tests the hypothesis that affected individuals share more alleles with each other than would be expected on the basis of their biological relationship. For example, for an unlinked locus, affected sib-pairs should share 50% of their alleles in common by chance. Allele-sharing at a particular locus that is in excess of 50% would provide evidence for linkage. Analysis of all pedigree members is typically performed either by regression or variance component approaches. Under the latter, one partitions the variance in the trait (measured on either a discrete or quantitative scale) into components attributable to environmental factors, excess allele sharing at a specific genetic locus (e.g., linkage), and residual familial factors. The hypothesis of linkage is tested by evaluating, by likelihood ratio test, whether inclusion of the linkage component significantly improves the likelihood of the data.

Regardless of the linkage method used, evidence for linkage is typically expressed as a LOD score, which corresponds to the odds of the data in support of linkage compared to the odds of the data not supporting linkage, with this ratio expressed as base 10 logarithm. Thus, a LOD score of 3 indicates that support for linkage is 1000 times better than support for no linkage. There continues to be considerable debate regarding what level of LOD score should be required as support of linkage, particularly for complex genetic diseases and in the context of a genome scan since multiple linkage tests are performed. Some experts have argued that for genome scans, LOD scores of 3.6 (corresponding to a p value of 2.2×10^{-5}) be required as evidence for significant linkage, on the basis that one would expect a LOD score this high by chance alone in only 1 out of every 20 genome scans (29).

Although statistical significance is usually expressed by LOD scores, care must be taken when evaluating linkage results across studies using different statistical methods. When computed empirically, the significance values for LOD scores calculated under different analytic models may vary substantially (30). Thus, comparisons between studies are easier to interpret when significance levels are provided empirically and expressed either as p-values, or back-transformed to LOD scores.

Family studies of type 2 diabetes have been carried out in a number of populations, and since 1996, genome scan results from many of these studies have been reported for both discrete and quantitative traits (e.g., glucose and insulin concentrations). The following sections summarize results published to date and attempt to synthesize areas of concordant (and discordant) findings.

GENOME SCANS OF TYPE 2 DIABETES AND RELATED QUANTITATIVE TRAITS

Genome scans of type 2 diabetes and related quantitative traits have been published from family studies representing a number of different ethnic groups, including Mexican Americans, European-descent Caucasians, African Americans, and American Indians. The study designs, recruitment and analytic schemes, and major linkage results of these studies are summarized in Table 1. As indicated in this table, significant or noteworthy linkages have been reported from 14 different chromosomes. This section highlights what we believe are the most interesting results from these studies, emphasizing those regions for which multiple studies have provided evidence for linkage, for which the linkages were particularly strong, or for which the linked chromosome regions contain particularly strong candidate genes. For a comprehensive listing of all linkages reported in these different studies, the reader is referred to Table 1 and Figure 1.

Chromosome 2q

The first genome scan of type 2 diabetes was published in 1996 by Hanis et al. (31). This study was based on affected siblings from Mexican American families in southern Texas, where the prevalence of type 2 diabetes was several-fold higher than that in the general US population. The sample included 330 affected sib pairs. In an affected sib pair (ASP) analysis, significant evidence for linkage was observed on chromosome 2q, near the marker D2S125 (two-point LOD for *D2S125* = 4.1 or $p = 7 \times 10^{-6}$; multipoint LOD = 2.6 or $p = 0.0003$). Moreover, suggestive evidence for linkage was obtained to this very same region in a second set of Mexican American families (LOD = 0.74), although no evidence for linkage was apparent in additional sets of families analyzed from Japan, Germany, or US whites.

Following the report of the chromosome 2q linkage by Hanis et al., several chromosomal scans were undertaken to evaluate evidence for linkage in other populations. Although no evidence for linkage was detected in a large set of Finnish families (49), modest support for linkage was obtained in an analysis of French families in which the outcome was abnormal glucose levels. Using ASP analysis, Hani et al. (50) reported excess allele sharing among affected individuals for marker *D2S140* ($p = 0.005$ without weighting adjustment, $p = 0.04$ with weighting adjustment), which maps approximately 3 cM from *D2S125*.

Table 1. Results of published genome and chromosomal scans for type 2 diabetes and its related quantitative traits.

Population	Family recruitment strategy (study acronym[†]) (reference no.)	Sample size / Analytic scheme	Marker density (cM)	Trait	LOD (p value)	Peak marker	Note
Mexican American	≥ 1 ASP[a] of diabetes in the family Age at diabetes onset > 30 yrs (31)	440 ASPs from 246 sibships / ASP analysis	9	Diabetes	4.10 (7×10^{-6})	D2S125	
Mexican American	Random sampling through diabetic probands (SAFDS) (32)	440 subjects from 27 extended families / VC[b]	13	Diabetes	2.88 (0.0001)	D10S587	
				Diabetes	2.67 (0.0002)	D3S1566	
				Diabetes	2.38 (0.0005)	D9S288/ D9S925	
				Diabetes	1.99 (0.001)	D4S1615	
				Age at diabetes onset	3.75 (2×10^{-5})	D10S587	
				Age at diabetes onset	2.51 (0.0003)	D3S1566	
				Age at diabetes onset	2.06 (0.001)	D9S288/ D9S925	
	Same as above (SAFDS) (33)	103 sibships from 32 extended families / VC	10-15	Fasting glucose	3.14 (7×10^{-5})	D6S1035	
				2-hr glucose	3.37 (4×10^{-5})	D11S899/ D11S1324	
	Same as above (SAFDS) (34)	403 subjects from 28 extended families / Sibpair analysis	8	2-hr insulin	2.80 (0.0001)	D4S424	Data on chr[c] 4q only
Mexican American	Random sampling through diabetic probands (SAFHS) (35)	391 subjects from 28 extended families / VC	10	Fasting insulin	3.07 ($<10^{-4}$)[d]	D3S1600	
Mexican American	≥ 1ASP and > 3 1st degree relatives of proband (GENNID) (36)	365 ASPs from 53 families / ASP analysis	9	Diabetes or IGH[e]	3.91 (10^{-5})	D3S2432	
Finnish	≥ 3 diabetes cases in the family, with ≥ 2 cases with onset < 60 yrs, and another < 65 yrs (Botnia) (37)	217 subjects from 26 extended families / APM[f] analysis	10	Diabetes	3.65 (2×10^{-5})	D12S1349	Linkage present only in families with low insulin secretion

Table 1. Results of published genome and chromosomal scans for type 2 diabetes and its related quantitative traits (continued).

Population	Family recruitment strategy (study acronym, reference no.)	Sample size / Analytic scheme	Marker density (cM)	Trait	LOD (p value)	Peak marker	Note
Finnish	Proband with age at onset between 35-60 yrs, ≥ 2 diabetes cases and ≥ 1 nondiabetic parent in the family (FUSION) (38)	716 ASPs from 477 families / ASP analysis	3	Diabetes	1.92 (0.013)[d]	D20S905	
				Diabetes	2.06 (0.009)[d]	D20S107	
				Diabetes	2.00 (0.01)[d]	D20S197	
Caucasian	≥ 1 ASP with onset < 65 yrs (39)	405 subjects from 19 extended families / parametric, APM	< 15	Diabetes	N/A (0.001)[d]	D11S935	Data on chr 11 only
	Same as above (5)	468 subjects from 19 extended families / APM	8	Diabetes	4.30 (0.01)[d,h]	CRP/ APOA2 (chr 1)	Linkage was not replicated in 20 more families
Caucasian	Diabetic proband with onset 30-60 yrs, ≥ 1 ASP, and 1 nondiabetic parent (40)	110 ASPs from 29 extended families / ASP analysis	4	Diabetes with onset 50 - 60	N/A (0.009)	D20S197	Data on chr 20q only; autosomal dominant pattern
	Same as above (41)	385 subjects from 26 families / APM	5	Diabetes with early onset	N/A (0.007)	D12S375	Linkage enhanced in families with poor insulin response
Caucasian	Multiple diabetics in the family with history of diabetic nephropathy (42)	53 ASPs from 21 families / ASP analysis	2	Diabetes	1.48 (0.005)	D20S197/ D20S178	Data on chr 12 and 20 only; linkage not seen in African Americans
			3	Diabetes	1.45 (0.005)	D12S349/ D12S86	
Caucasian	≥ 1 ASP and > 3 1st degree relatives of proband (GENNID) (36)	497 ASPs from 77 families / ASP analysis	8	Diabetes or IGH	2.99 (0.0001)	GATA-172D05	On chr X
				Diabetes or IGH	2.81 (0.0002)	D12S853	
				Diabetes or IGH	2.80 (0.0002)	D5S1404	
French Canadian	Random sampling (QFS) (43)	105-213 sib-pairs from 152 families / sib-pair analysis	5	Fasting insulin	N/A[f] (0.0005)	MC3R (chr 20)	Data on chr 20q only

Table 1. Results of published genome and chromosomal scans for type 2 diabetes and its related quantitative traits (continued).

Population	Family recruitment strategy (study acronym)(reference no.)	Sample size / Analytic scheme	Marker density (cM)	Trait	LOD (p value)	Peak marker	Note
French	≥ 1 ASPs in the family (44)	55 ASPs from 42 families / ASP analysis	8	Diabetes with onset <45 yrs	2.74 (0.0004)[c]	D20S100	Data on chr 20 only
African American	≥ 1 ASP and > 3 1st degree relatives of proband (GENNID) (36)	229 ASPs from 65 families / ASP analysis	8	Diabetes or IGH	2.39 (0.0005)	D10S1412	
Australian	Multiple cases transmitted in an autosomal dominant pattern (45)	1 extended pedigree / parametric linkage analysis	5	Diabetes with late onset	3.65 (2×10^{-5})	D12S321	Data on 4 markers on chr 12 only
Amish	Diabetic proband with onset > 35 yrs (AFDS) (unpublished data)	230 subjects from 17 extended families / APM	10	Diabetes	2.8 (0.0002)	D1S2715	
Oji-Cree	72% of whole population recruited (n=728) (46)	49 ASPs / ASP analysis	20	Diabetes	N/A ($<10^{-4}$)	D6S1056, D16S2616	Only two-point analysis performed
Pima Indian	≥ 2 sibs and ≥ 1 diabetes case in the sibship (47)	1766 sib-pairs from 264 families / VC	6	Age-adjusted diabetes	1.7 (0.003)	D11S4464	Evidence was enhanced in bivariate analysis with BMI on 11q ($p = 2\times10^{-6}$)
		1766 sib-pairs / concordant vs. discordant sib-pair analysis	6	Diabetes	2.5 (0.0004)	D1S1677	
		55 ASPs / ASP analysis		Diabetes with onset < 25 yrs	4.10 (7×10^{-6})	D1S2127	
		551 ASPs / ASP analysis	6	Diabetes with onset < 45 yrs	1.8 (0.002)	D7S1799	
	Same as above (48)	123 sib-pairs / sib-pair analysis	~ 10	Fasting insulin	N/A (0.0004)	FABP2 (chr 4)	Data on chr 4q only
				Maximum insulin action	N/A (0.0005)	ANX5 (chr 4)	

[a] affected sib-pair; [b] variance components method; [c] chromosome; [d] empirical p value based on simulation; [e] impaired glucose homeostasis; [f] affected pedigree member analysis; [g] not available; [h] p value based on genome-wide significance

[†]Acronyms: SAFDS = San Antonio Family Diabetes Study; SAFHS = San Antonio Family Hear Study; GENNID = Genetics of non-insulin dependent diabetes; FUSION = Finland-United States Investigation of NIDDM Genetics; QFS = Quebec Family Study; AFDS = Amish Family Diabetes Study

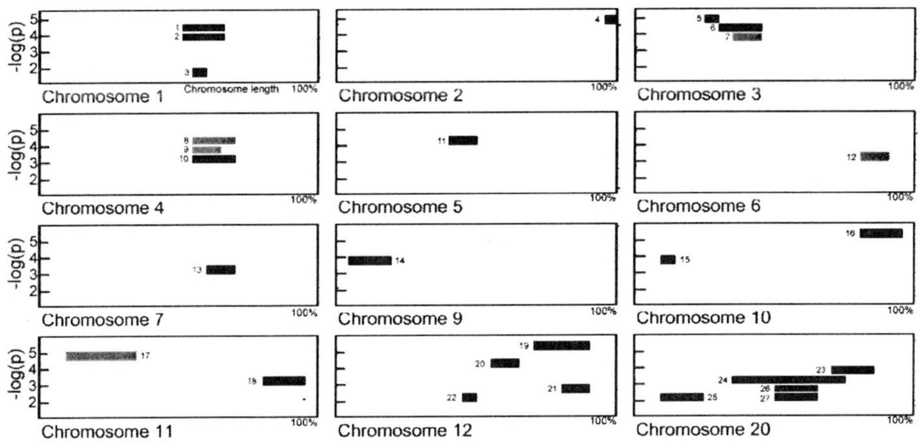

Figure 1. Chromosomal locations†‡ of linkage signals from the literature for discrete (black lines) and quantitative traits (gray lines).

† The unit of the signal location is an approximate percentage (%) of chromosomal length. Marker locations are based on information obtained from the Marshfield Medical Research Foundation website (http://www.mfldclin.edu/). The significance of the linkage peak is expressed as –log (p value). Data on chromosomes 16 and X are not shown.

‡ Number by the signal indicates the source of the information as shown below, including population, trait, and reference number:

1 Amish (DM) (unpublished)	10 Mx Am (DM) (32)	19 Finnish (DM) (37)
2 Pima (DM) (47)	11 Caucasian (DM/IGH) (36)	20 Caucasian (DM)) (36)
3 Caucasian (DM) (5)	12 Mx Am (glucose) (33)	21 Caucasian (DM) (42)
4 Mx Am (DM) (31)	13 Pima (DM) (47)	22 Caucasian (DM) (41)
5 Mx Am (DM/IGH) (36)	14 Mx Am (DM) (32)	23 French (DM) (44)
6 Mx Am (DM) (32)	15 Afr Am (DM/IGH) (36)	24 Finnish (DM) (38)
7 Mx Am (insulin) (35)	16 Mx Am (DM) (32)	25 Finnish (DM) (38)
8 Mx Am (insulin) (34)	17 Mx Am (glucose) (33)	26 Caucasian (DM) (42)
9 Pima (insulin) (48)	18 Pima (DM) (47)	27 Caucasian (DM) (40)

Chromosome 12q

Several groups have observed evidence for linkage to diabetes on chromosome 12q. In 1996, Mahtani *et al.* reported results from their genome scan based on Caucasian families recruited from a relatively homogeneous population in western Finland (37). In the overall sample of 26 families, there was no strong evidence for linkage. However, a separate analysis was then performed using individuals from the 6 families in whom affected individuals had relatively low levels of circulating insulin. In APM analysis, significant evidence for linkage was obtained for markers in a region on chromosome 12 (LOD = 3.65 or $p = 2 \times 10^{-5}$), near *D12S1349*. Interestingly, the *MODY3* locus has been mapped to this chromosomal region (14;51), despite the fact that diabetes in these families resembled typical type 2 diabetes more than MODY. The authors hypothesized that the linkage detected in this analysis could be attributable to previously unknown mutations in *MODY3* (now known to be the HNF1α gene), or to mutations in an altogether different, but closely linked gene.

Two subsequent studies provided further support for the existence of a diabetes susceptibility locus in this region. Bowden et al. (42) showed evidence for linkage with markers in the *MODY3* region in Caucasian sib-pairs affected by diabetic nephropathy, with a p value of 0.02. However, evidence for linkage was not observed in their collection of African American ASPs. Using parametric linkage analysis to analyze data from a single large pedigree from Australia, Shaw et al., reported a multipoint LOD of 3.65 (45). However, diabetic individuals in this pedigree appeared to be insulin resistant and had a relatively late onset of the disease, in contrast to having low insulin secretion and early age of diabetes onset, as observed in the Finnish study reported by Mahtani *et al.* (37). Bektas and colleagues also evaluated evidence for linkage of diabetes to chromosome 12 markers in their collection of Caucasian families from the Joslin Center, and obtained their best evidence for linkage ($p = 0.007$) to a region ~50 cM centromeric to the Finnish signal (41). Families were recruited because they had a form of early-onset autosomal dominant type 2 diabetes. When only those families with low insulin response were used in the analysis (low insulin increment 2 hours after a glucose load in affected subjects), the evidence for linkage increased ($p = 0.002$). Interestingly, the peak of the signal was about 14 cM centromeric from a linkage reported by Ehm et al., in their analysis of Caucasian families from the American Diabetes Association's GENNID (Genetics of NIDDM) collection, where a LOD score of 2.81 ($p = 0.0002$) near *D12S853* was observed for the combined trait diabetes and impaired glucose homeostasis (36).

Chromosome 20

There is substantial evidence for the existence of at least one locus on chromosome 20 that influences susceptibility to diabetes. Two initial studies, published simultaneously, each provided suggestive evidence for linkage of diabetes with markers in the region of *D20S197*. In 14 large Caucasian pedigrees from the Joslin Center, Ji *et al.* reported an NPL score of 3.3 (equivalent to a LOD of 2.4, $p = 0.009$) to this marker (40). Families included in this analysis were selected for having multiple type 2 diabetes cases with age at diabetes diagnosis of 30-60 years. At the same time, Bowden and colleagues published the results of their study of 53 ASPs identified from 21 Caucasian families having at least one member with diabetic nephropathy. These investigators observed a LOD of 1.48 in the *D20S197/D20S178* interval (42). Interestingly, results from two other studies provided modest evidence for linkage to a nearby region, approximately 15 - 25 cM telomeric to the signal reported by Ji *et al.* near marker *D20S197*. Zouali *et al.* analyzed 301 diabetic sib-pairs and found no evidence for linkage with chromosome 20 markers. However, when they restricted the analysis to the 55 ASPs with diabetes onset < 45 years, they observed a multipoint LOD of 2.74 ($p = 0.0004$) in the vicinity of the cytosolic phosphoenolpyruvate gene (*PCK1*)

(44). In a recent study of French Canadian sib-pairs with diabetes, Lembertas *et al.* reported suggestive linkage to fasting insulin near the *MC3R* (melanocortin 3 receptor) gene, which is approximately 25 cM telomeric to marker *D20S197* (43).

Results from the FUSION (Finland-United States Investigation of NIDDM Genetics) Study provide further support for the presence of diabetes susceptibility loci on chromosome 20. In a linkage analysis of markers spanning chromosome 20, Ghosh *et al.* performed an ASP analysis and reported three separate linkage signals (38). These linkages correspond to one region on chromosome 20p near *D20S905* (weighted multipoint LOD = 1.92) and two regions on chromosome 20q, one near *D20S909* (LOD = 2.06) and the other 15-20 cM away near *D20S886* (LOD = 2.0). *P*-values for these LOD scores, computed by simulation, were 0.013, 0.009, 0.01, respectively. A strong candidate gene, associated with MODY1 (now known to be the *HNF4*α gene), is located in one of these regions (near *D20S886*). The investigators identified 17 sequence variations in this gene from 5 families. When these 5 families with *MODY1* variants were removed from analysis, the LOD score for the third peak dropped only from 2.06 to 1.74 under the weighted model, suggesting that these variants were not likely to account for the linkage signal on chromosome 20q.

Chromosome 1q

Several studies have reported evidence for linkage to a region on chromosome 1q. In a genome scan carried out in Pima Indians, Hanson *et al.* compared sib pairs concordant and discordant for diabetes using the sib-pair test and observed moderate evidence for linkage of diabetes to marker *D1S1677* on chromosome 1q (LOD = 2.5 or $p = 0.0004$) (47). Because of the exceptionally high prevalence of diabetes in this population, individuals were considered to be affected if diabetes onset was prior to age 45 years, and unaffected if they were known to be nondiabetic at age 46 (even if they subsequently developed diabetes at a later age). Moreover, when the 55 sib-pairs with age of diabetes onset of ≤ 25 years were analyzed separately in an ASP analysis, very strong evidence for linkage was detected with *D1S2127* (LOD = 4.1 or $p = 7 \times 10^{-6}$), approximately 25 cM telomeric to the peak of the previous signal.

An analysis reported by Elbein and colleagues provides further support for the presence of a locus influencing susceptibility to diabetes to this region on chromosome 1q (5). These analyses were based on 19 extended Utah families of Northern European ancestry. Using parametric analysis, these investigators observed a LOD score of 4.30 in the region of 1q21-1q23; using APM analysis, the LOD score in this region was 2.96. Evidence for linkage peaked at a distance approximately 5 cM away from marker *D1S1677*, previously shown to be linked to diabetes in the Pimas. Empirical *p*-values, generated by simulation, indicated that the true *p*-value for linkage under parametric analysis was likely to fall within a 95% confidence interval ranging from p = 0.0005 - 0.047. Twenty additional smaller Utah families were subsequently analyzed in an attempt to replicate this result, but no evidence for linkage in this region was observed.

Two additional genome scan studies also have reported evidence for linkage to markers in this region. In the Amish Family Diabetes Study, modest evidence for linkage (LOD = 2.88; p = 0.002) was observed at marker *D1S2715* for the trait, diabetes or impaired glucose homeostasis, approximately 10 - 15 cM from the peak signals reported by Elbein and Hanson (St. Jean *et al.*, unpublished data). Evidence for linkage to chromosome 1q has also been reported from a large collection of affected sib-pairs enrolled in the British Diabetic Association (52) close to this same region.

Chromosome 11q

Strong evidence for linkage of a diabetes/obesity trait to a region on chromosome 11q has been reported in Pima Indians (47). Using variance component methods, a LOD of 1.7 (p = 0.003) was observed near *D11S4464* for the trait, diabetes (using an age-adjusted diabetes score). Interestingly, there was very strong evidence for linkage to this same region for the trait, body mass index, a strong risk factor for type 2 diabetes, with a peak LOD of 3.6 ($p = 2.6 \times 10^{-5}$). Upon further analysis, evidence for linkage to chromosome 11q was significantly enhanced when both age of diabetes onset and body mass index were analyzed in a single bivariate model, supporting a contribution of this locus to both traits simultaneously.

Chromosome 3p.

There is some evidence for linkage of diabetes and related traits to a locus on chromosome 3p. Interestingly, these results have all been reported from Mexican American populations. In their analysis of the GENNID study, Ehm *et al.* reported significant evidence for linkage of the trait, diabetes/impaired glucose homeostasis, to *D3S2432* (36). Duggirala *et al.* reported LOD scores of 2.67 and 2.51 for diabetes and age at diabetes onset to markers in a region near marker *D3S2304*, approximately 50 cM centromeric to the region identified by Ehm and colleagues (32). Mitchell *et al.* (53) performed a genome scan of serum insulin levels in 391 nondiabetic subjects from 10 large extended families in the San Antonio Family Heart Study and detected evidence of linkage near markers *D3S1600* and *D3S2406*, a region overlapping considerably with that reported by Duggirala and colleagues. The multipoint LOD was 3.07, and simulations confirmed the corresponding empirical p-value to be < 0.0001. There was no appreciable evidence for linkage to insulin levels elsewhere in the chromosome.

Additional linkages

Linkages to diabetes and/or related traits have been reported at several additional chromosomal regions. On chromosome 11p, Elbein *et al.* reported modest evidence for linkage to marker *D11S935* ($p = 0.001$ by APM analysis) in Caucasian families (39), but could not replicate this finding in a later genome scan based on an overlapping set of families (5). Stern and colleagues analyzed 2-hour glucose levels as a quantitative trait in Mexican American families and reported linkage to markers *D11S899* and *D11S1324* from this same region (LOD = 3.37 or $p = 0.00004$) (33).

Evidence for a locus on chromosome 4q influencing diabetes susceptibility, possibly by influencing insulin sensitivity, has been reported from both Pima Indians and Mexican Americans (34;48). An initial study undertaken in non-diabetic Pima Indians revealed significant linkage between markers in the region of *FABP2*, the gene encoding fatty acid binding protein 2, and clamp-derived measures of insulin sensitivity (48). Subsequently, Mitchell *et al.* used segregation analysis to detect evidence for a major gene influencing serum insulin levels in Mexican Americans, and then later detected evidence for linkage (LOD = 2.80) of this putative major gene using parametric linkage analysis to this region on chromosome 4q (34). A later linkage analysis of these families based on variance components provided modest evidence for linkage to diabetes to this region (LOD = 1.99) (32). Sequencing of the FABP-2 gene revealed a commonly occurring missense mutation (Ala54Thr) that has been shown to be associated with measures of insulin sensitivity in some, but not all studies (24;54-57). Functional studies show that the Ala54Thr substitution results in a two-fold increase in transport of fatty acids, suggesting that this variant may augment intestinal fatty acid absorption and, in so doing, contribute to insulin resistance (57;58).

Regions on chromosomes 5, 6, 7, 9, 10 16 and X have also been identified as being linked to type 2 diabetes or related traits in single studies. The locations of these linkages are shown in Figure 1, and details of these findings are provided in Table 1.

POSITIONAL CLONING OF *NIDDM1*

The positional cloning of genes in regions of linkage are relatively straightforward for monogenic diseases. In general, once compelling evidence for linkage is demonstrated, an effort is made to confirm and narrow the region of linkage by genotyping additional markers (such as STR markers or single nucleotide polymorphisms (SNPs)) within the region of linkage. An advantage of SNP markers over STR markers is that they are much more frequent in the genome (approximately 1 per 1,000 base pairs), thus allowing finer mapping of the region of interest. In addition to providing further evidence for linkage, the dense genotyping of markers also provides the opportunity to construct haplotypes, which may be very useful in further refining the location of the putative susceptibility gene. Typically, this is done by examining the haplotype that is transmitted (or shared) in affected pedigree members in hope of identifying crossover events that might narrow the shared haplotype. Alternatively, shared haplotypes can be compared across several unrelated families in order to narrow the region harboring the putative disease gene. Once the region is narrowed, the arduous task of physically mapping the region, identifying the genes expressed in this region, and DNA sequencing of positional candidate genes usually leads to the identification of the pathogenic mutation. Recent efforts of the Human Genome Project have greatly accelerated this process.

Theory dictates that for complex diseases such as type 2 diabetes, similar methods should be successful for positional cloning of susceptibility genes. However, there are also important caveats that may greatly complicate this general approach. The first successful example of positional cloning of a susceptibility gene for type 2 diabetes identified through a genome scan was recently reported by Horikawa and coworkers (59). As described above, a genome scan in Mexican American ASPs provided evidence for the presence of a diabetes susceptibility locus (designated *NIDDM1*) near the telomere of chromosome 2q (31). Additional genotyping and refinement of the genetic map in the region, coupled with the observation that *NIDDM1* interacted with another susceptibility locus on chromosome 15 (60), localized NIDDM1 to a 7-cM region. A 1.7 Mb contig encompassing most of the region was constructed. The region contained seven known genes and 15 expressed sequence tags (ESTs). Common single nucleotide polymorphisms (SNPs) within the region were identified by DNA sequencing in 10 – 20 unrelated subjects with type 2 diabetes. SNPs were then genotyped, and allele and haplotype frequencies were compared between diabetic cases and a random sample. In addition to testing for association of each SNP with diabetes, tests were performed to determine if a given SNP also accounted for the original linkage that was observed. Several iterations of SNP detection (through extensive DNA sequence analysis), genotyping of SNPs, and association/linkage analyses were performed. The SNPs and SNP haplotypes with the greatest evidence for association that also contributed to the linkage were found to be located within a 66 Kb region. Subsequently, a total of 179 variant sites (mostly SNPs) were identified in this region, many of which were genotyped in larger sets of families. The SNP with the greatest evidence for association and linkage lay within intron 3 (UCSNP-43) of the calpain 10 gene (*CAPN10*), with homozygosity for the G allele (allele frequency 0.80 in Mexican Americans) conferring an increased risk for diabetes.

Further evidence for association was obtained by analysis of haplotypes consisting of three SNPs within *CAPN10*, UCSNP-43, -19 and -63. Interestingly, the haplotype combination 112/121 was associated with a 2.80-fold increased risk of diabetes (95% CI: 1.23 – 6.34), while homozygotes for either of the two haplotypes showed no increased risk of diabetes. These findings suggest that specific combinations of haplotypes are required to confer risk. Similar results were obtained in German and Finnish samples, although the at risk haplotype combination was much less common in these populations than in Mexican Americans. The population attributable risk of variation in *CAPN10* was estimated to be 0.14 in Mexican Americans and 0.04 in the Caucasian populations studied. Although the investigators could not rule out the possibility that other mutations in *CAPN10* or in a gene nearby might be the pathogenic mutation, these data provide reasonable evidence that the identity of *NIDDM1* is *CAPN10*. Several studies reported in abstract form have also shown positive associations between GG homozygosity of UCSNP-43 or haplotypes containing UCSNP-43 and diabetes including studies in African Americans (61;62), while studies in Utah Caucasians suggest that the UCSNP-43 A-allele might confer increased risk in this population (63).

CAPN10 contains 15 exons spanning 31 Kb. Alternative splicing results in mRNA species of several lengths (predicting protein-encoding sequences of differing lengths from 672 to 138 amino acids). *CAPN10* is transcribed in multiple tissues, including heart, brain, liver, skeletal muscle and pancreas. The calpains are calcium-activated neutral proteases that cause activation or inactivation of proteins involved in intracellular signaling, proliferation, and differentiation, including adipocyte differentiation and possibly insulin action and insulin secretion. However, the mechanism by which altered function and/or expression of calpain 10 affects glucose metabolism is presently unknown. Furthermore, since none of the SNPs that determine the at risk haplotype reside in coding regions, it is not readily apparent how these SNPs could be causative. DNA binding studies using nuclear extracts from human pancreatic islets and HepG2 cells suggest that UCSNP-43 may decrease binding of nuclear proteins, and *in vitro* reporter gene studies suggest that UCSNP-43 may decrease transcription. These studies suggest that UCSNP-43 may exert its effects on diabetes risk by decreasing calpain 10 mRNA (and protein) levels. Clearly, further functional studies of calpain 10 are warranted as are studies to investigate genetic variation in this gene in other populations.

CONCLUSION

Genome scans represent a useful first step in the process of gene identification. The approach is particularly attractive for complex genetic diseases since it does not require *a priori* knowledge of gene function or location. A limitation of the genome scan approach, however, is that the statistical power of linkage analysis can be relatively low, especially in diseases like type 2 diabetes for which the penetrance of the disease is highly variable and the phenocopy rate is high. Consequently, most family studies have adequate statistical power to detect relatively large gene effects only. Furthermore, the localization of linkage signals is rather imprecise, since linkage signals may typically extend for 15-20 cM, and regions of this size may contain hundreds of genes.

In recognition that very large samples may be required to detect the effects of mutations that have relatively small effects on susceptibility to diabetes, there is a growing interest among diabetes investigators to pool their resources. As one example of an effort to bring together the resources from major research groups in the field, the International Type 2 Diabetes Linkage Analysis Consortium was formed to pool the samples from 26 different populations in 7 countries, in hope of strengthening the statistical power for linkage analysis (http://www.sph.umich.edu.edu/group/statgen/ consortium/). These types of collaborations, coupled with newer and more powerful statistical approaches, and the availability of the sequences and locations of all human genes as a result of the Human Genome Project, should enhance the ability to find linkages and greatly accelerate positional cloning efforts. Indeed, positional cloning of putative diabetes susceptibility genes on chromosomes 1, 7 and 20 are currently underway. Finally, availability of dense SNP maps also may make possible genome-wide association analyses, which may have the power to detect minor gene effects that would likely escape detection by linkage analysis.

Understanding the genetic basis of type 2 diabetes will help elucidate the molecular mechanisms of this disease and lead to a better appreciation of environmental triggers. These discoveries will provide insights into new preventive and treatment strategies as well as a potential cure for this debilitating and increasingly prevalent disease.

REFERENCES

1. Barnett,A.H., Eff,C., Leslie,R.D., and Pyke,D.A. 1981. Diabetes in identical twins. A study of 200 pairs. *Diabetologia* 20:87-93.
2. Rewers,M. and Hamman,R.F. 1995. Risk factors for non-insulin-dependent diabetes. In Diabetes in America. M.I.Harris, Cowie,C.C., Stern,M.P., Boyko,E.J., Reiber,G.E., and Bennett,P.H., editors. National Institutes of Health, National Institutes of Diabetes and Digestive and Kidney Diseases, Bethesda, MD. 179-220.
3. Newman,B., Selby,J.V., King,M.C., Slemenda,C., Fabsitz,R., and Friedman,G.D. 1987. Concordance for type 2 (non-insulin-dependent) diabetes mellitus in male twins. *Diabetologia* 30:763-768
4. Rich,S.S. 1990. Mapping genes in diabetes. Genetic epidemiological perspective. *Diabetes* 39:1315-1319.
5. Elbein,S.C., Hoffman,M.D., Teng,K., Leppert,M.F., and Hasstedt,S.J. 1999. A genome-wide search for type 2 diabetes susceptibility genes in Utah Caucasians. *Diabetes* 48:1175-1182.
6. Hsueh,W.-C., Mitchell,B.D., Aburomia,R., Pollin,T., Sakul,H., Ehm M.G., Michelsen,B.K., Wagner,M.J., St.Jean,P.L., Knowler,W.C. *et al.* 2000. Diabetes in the Old

Order Amish: characterization and heritability analysis of the Amish Family Diabetes Study . *Diabetes Care* 23:595-601.

7. Hanson,R.L. and Knowler,W.C. 1998. Analytic strategies to detect linkage to a common disorder with genetically determined age of onset: diabetes mellitus in Pima Indians. *Genet. Epidemiol.* 15:299-315.
8. Hanson,R.L., Elston,R.C., Pettitt,D.J., Bennett,P.H., and Knowler,W.C. 1995. Segregation analysis of non-insulin-dependent diabetes mellitus in Pima Indians: evidence for a major-gene effect. *Am.J.Hum.Genet.* 57:160-170.
9. Elston,R.C., Namboodiri,K.K., Nino,H.V., and Pollitzer,W.S. 1974. Studies on blood and urine glucose in Seminole Indians: indications for segregation of a major gene. *Am.J.Hum.Genet.* 26:13-34.
10. Stern,M.P., Mitchell,B.D., Blangero,J., Reinhart,L., Krammerer,C.M., Harrison,C.R., Shipman,P.A., O'Connell,P., Frazier,M.L., and MacCluer,J.W. 1996. Evidence for a major gene for type II diabetes and linkage analyses with selected candidate genes in Mexican-Americans. *Diabetes* 45:563-568.
11. King,H., Aubert,R.E., and Herman,W.H. 1998. Global burden of diabetes, 1995-2025: prevalence, numerical estimates, and projections . *Diabetes Care* 21:1414-1431.
12. Fajans,S.S. 1989. Maturity-onset diabetes of the young (MODY). *Diabetes Metab Rev.* 5:579-606.
13. Yamagata,K., Furuta,H., Oda,N., Kaisaki,P.J., Menzel,S., Cox,N.J., Fajans,S.S., Signorini,S., Stoffel,M., and Bell,G.I. 1996. Mutations in the hepatocyte nuclear factor-4alpha gene in maturity- onset diabetes of the young (MODY1). *Nature* 384:458-460.
14. Yamagata,K., Oda,N., Kaisaki,P.J., Menzel,S., Furuta,H., Vaxillaire,M., Southam,L., Cox,R.D., Lathrop,G.M., Boriraj,V.V. *et al.* 1996. Mutations in the hepatocyte nuclear factor-1alpha gene in maturity- onset diabetes of the young (MODY3). *Nature* 384:455-458.
15. Stoffers,D.A., Stanojevic,V., and Habener,J.F. 1998. Insulin promoter factor-1 gene mutation linked to early-onset type 2 diabetes mellitus directs expression of a dominant negative isoprotein. *J Clin.Invest* 102:232-241.
16. Horikawa,Y., Iwasaki,N., Hara,M., Furuta,H., Hinokio,Y., Cockburn,B.N. , Lindner,T., Yamagata,K., Ogata,M., Tomonaga,O. *et al.* 1997. Mutation in hepatocyte nuclear factor-1 beta gene (TCF2) associated with MODY. *Nat.Genet.* 17:384-385.
17. Taylor,S.I., Kadowaki,T., Kadowaki,H., Accili,D., Cama,A., and McKeon,C. 1990. Mutations in insulin-receptor gene in insulin-resistant patients. *Diabetes Care* 13:257-279.
18. Steiner,D.F., Tager,H.S., Chan,S.J., Nanjo,K., Sanke,T., and Rubenstein,A.H. 1990. Lessons learned from molecular biology of insulin-gene mutations. *Diabetes Care* 13:600-609.
19. Gerbitz,K.D., Gempel,K., and Brdiczka,D. 1996. Mitochondria and diabetes. Genetic, biochemical, and clinical implications of the cellular energy circuit. *Diabetes* 45:113-126.
20. Harris,M.I. 1995. Classification, diagnostic criteria, and screening for diabetes. In Diabetes in America. M.I.Harris, Cowie,C.C., Stern,M.P., Boyko,E.J., Reiber,G.E., and Bennett,P.H., editors. National Institutes of Health, National Institutes of Diabetes and Digestive and Kidney Diseases, Bethesda, MD. 15-36.
21. Yen,C.J., Beamer,B.A., Negri,C., Silver,K., Brown,K.A., Yarnall,D.P., Burns,D.K., Roth,J., and Shuldiner,A.R. 1997. Molecular scanning of the human peroxisome proliferator activated receptor gamma (hPPAR gamma) gene in diabetic Caucasians: identification of a Pro12Ala PPAR gamma 2 missense mutation. *Biochem.Biophys.Res.Commun.* 241:270-274.
22. Deeb,S.S., Fajas,L., Nemoto,M., Pihlajamaki,J., Mykkanen,L., Kuusisto,J., Laakso,M., Fujimoto,W., and Auwerx,J. 1998. A Pro12Ala substitution in PPARgamma2 associated with decreased receptor activity, lower body mass index and improved insulin sensitivity. *Nat.Genet.* 20:284-287.
23. Altshuler,D., Hirschhorn,J.E., Klannemark,M., Lindgren,C.M., Vohl,M.-C., Nemesh,J., Lane,C.R., Schaffner,S.F., Bolk,S., Brewer,C. *et al.* 2000. The common PPARgamma

Pro12Ala polymorphism is associated with decreased risk of type 2 diabetes. *Nat.Genet.* 26:76-80.

24. Silver,K. and Shuldiner,A.R. 1999. Candidate genes for type 2 diabetes mellitus. In Diabetes mellitus: a fundamental and clinical text. D.LeRoith, Olefsky,J.M., and Taylor,S.I., editors. Lippincott Co., Phildelaphia. 565-574.
25. Lillioja,S., Mott,D.M., Zawadzki,J.K., Young,A.A., Abbott,W.G., Knowler,W.C., Bennett,P.H., Moll,P., and Bogardus,C. 1987. In vivo insulin action is familial characteristic in nondiabetic Pima Indians. *Diabetes* 36:1329-1335.
26. Watanabe,R.M., Valle,T., Hauser,E.R., Ghosh,S., Eriksson,J., Kohtamaki,K., Ehnholm,C., Tuomilehto,J. , Collins,F.S., Bergman,R.N. *et al.* 1999. Familiarity of quantitative metabolic traits in Finnish families with non-insulin-dependent diabetes mellitus. Finland-United States Investigation of NIDDM Genetics (FUSION) Study investigators. *Hum.Hered.* 49:159-168.
27. Elbein,S.C., Hasstedt,S.J., Wegner,K., and Kahn,S.E. 1999. Heritability of pancreatic beta-cell function among nondiabetic members of Caucasian familial type 2 diabetic kindreds. *J.Clin.Endocrinol.Metab* 84:1398-1403.
28. Sakul,H., Pratley,R., Cardon,L., Ravussin,E., Mott,D., and Bogardus,C. 1997. Familiality of physical and metabolic characteristics that predict the development of non-insulin-dependent diabetes mellitus in Pima Indians. *Am J Hum Genet.* 60 :651-656.
29. Lander,E. and Kruglyak,L. 1995. Genetic dissection of complex traits: guidelines for interpreting and reporting linkage results. *Nat.Genet.* 11:241-247.
30. Nyholt,D.R. 2000. All LODs are not created equal. *Am J Hum Genet.* 67:282-288.
31. Hanis,C.L., Boerwinkle,E., Chakraborty,R., Ellsworth,D.L., Concannon,P., Stirling,B., Morrison,V.A., Wapelhorst,B., Spielman,R.S., Gogolin-Ewens,K.J. *et al.* 1996. A genome-wide search for human non-insulin-dependent (type 2) diabetes genes reveals a major susceptibility locus on chromosome 2. *Nat.Genet.* 13:161-166.
32. Duggirala,R., Blangero,J., Almasy,L., Dyer,T.D., Williams,K.L., Leach,R.J., O'Connell,P., and Stern,M.P. 1999. Linkage of Type 2 Diabetes Mellitus and of Age at Onset to a Genetic Location on Chromosome 10q in Mexican Americans. *Am.J.Hum.Genet.*64:1127-1140.
33. Stern,M.P., Duggirala,R., Mitchell,B.D., Reinhart,L.J., Shivakumar,S., Shipman,P.A., Uresandi,O.C., Benavides,E., Blangero,J., and O'Connell,P. 1996. Evidence for linkage of regions on chromosomes 6 and 11 to plasma glucose concentrations in Mexican Americans. *Genome Res.* 6:724-734.
34. Mitchell,B.D., Kammerer,C.M., Hixson,J.E., Atwood,L.D., Hackleman,S., Blangero,J., Haffner,S.M., Stern,M.P., and MacCluer,J.W. 1995. Evidence for a major gene affecting postchallenge insulin levels in Mexican-Americans. *Diabetes* 44:284-289.
35. Mitchell,B.D., Cole,S.A., Hsueh,W.C., Comuzzie,A.G., Blangero,J., MacCluer,J.W., and Hixson,J.E. 2000. Linkage of serum insulin concentrations to chromosome 3p in Mexican Americans. *Diabetes* 49:513-516.
36. Ehm,M.G., Karnoub,M.C., Sakul,H., Gottschalk,K., Holt,D.C., Weber,J.L. , Vaske,D., Briley,D., Briley,L., Kopf,J. *et al.* 2000. Genomewide search for type 2 diabetes susceptibility genes in four American populations. *Am J Hum Genet.* 66:1871-1881.
37. Mahtani,M.M., Widen,E., Lehto,M., Thomas,J., McCarthy,M., Brayer,J., Bryant,B., Chan,G., Daly,M., Forsblom,C. *et al.* 1996. Mapping of a gene for type 2 diabetes associated with an insulin secretion defect by a genome scan in Finnish families. *Nat.Genet.* 14:90-94.
38. Ghosh,S., Watanabe,R.M., Hauser,E.R., Valle,T., Magnuson,V.L., Erdos,M.R., Langefeld,C.D., Balow,J., Jr., Ally,D.S., Kohtamaki,K. *et al.* 1999. Type 2 diabetes: evidence for linkage on chromosome 20 in 716 Finnish affected sib pairs. *Proc.Natl.Acad.Sci.U.S.A* 96:2198-2203.
39. Elbein,S.C., Bragg,K.L., Hoffman,M.D., Mayorga,R.A., and Leppert,M.F. 1996. Linkage studies of NIDDM with 23 chromosome 11 markers in a sample of whites of northern European descent. *Diabetes* 45:370-375.

40. Ji,L., Malecki,M., Warram,J.H., Yang,Y., Rich,S.S., and Krolewski,A.S. 1997. New susceptibility locus for NIDDM is localized to human chromosome 20q. *Diabetes* 46:876-881.
41. Bektas,A., Suprenant,M.E., Wogan,L.T., Plengvidhya,N., Rich,S.S., Warram,J.H., Krolewski,A.S., and Doria,A. 1999. Evidence of a novel type 2 diabetes locus 50 cM centromeric to *NIDDM2* on chromosome 12q. *Diabetes* 48:2246-2251.
42. Bowden,D.W., Sale,M., Howard,T.D., Qadri,A., Spray,B.J., Rothschild,C.B., Akots,G., Rich,S.S., and Freedman,B.I. 1997. Linkage of genetic markers on human chromosomes 20 and 12 to NIDDM in Caucasian sib pairs with a history of diabetic nephropathy. *Diabetes* 46:882-886.
43. Warden,C.H., Purcell-Huynh,D.A., Dionne,F.T., Gagnon,J., Nadeau,A., Lusis,A.J. *et al.* 1997. Identification of an obesity quantitative trait locus on mouse chromosome 2 and evidence of linkage to body fat and insulin on the human homologous region 20q. *J.Clin.Invest* 100:1240-1247.
44. Zouali,H., Hani,E.H., Philippi,A., Vionnet,N., Beckmann,J.S., Demenais,F., and Froguel,P. 1997. A susceptibility locus for early-onset non-insulin dependent (type 2) diabetes mellitus maps to chromosome 20q, proximal to the phosphoenolpyruvate carboxykinase gene. *Hum.Mol.Genet.* 6:1401-1408.
45. Shaw,J.T., Lovelock,P.K., Kesting,J.B., Cardinal,J., Duffy,D., Wainwright,B., and Cameron,D.P. 1998. Novel susceptibility gene for late-onset NIDDM is localized to human chromosome 12q. *Diabetes* 47:1793-1796.
46. Hegele,R.A., Sun,F., Harris,S.B., Anderson,C., Hanley,A.J., and Zinman,B. 1999. Genome-wide scanning for type 2 diabetes susceptibility in Canadian Oji- Cree, using 190 microsatellite markers. *J.Hum.Genet.* 44:10-14.
47. Hanson,R.L., Ehm,M.G., Pettitt,D.J., Prochazka,M., Thompson,D.B., Timberlake,D., Foroud,T., Kobes,S., Baier,L., Burns,D.K. *et al.* 1998. An autosomal genomic scan for loci linked to type II diabetes mellitus and body-mass index in Pima Indians. *Am.J.Hum.Genet.* 63:1130-1138.
48. Prochazka,M., Lillioja,S., Tait,J.F., Knowler,W.C., Mott,D.M., Spraul,M. , Bennett,P.H., and Bogardus,C. 1993. Linkage of chromosomal markers on 4q with a putative gene determining maximal insulin action in Pima Indians. *Diabetes* 42:514-519.
49. Ghosh,S., Hauser,E.R., Magnuson,V.L., Valle,T., Ally,D.S., Karanjawala,Z.E., Rayman,J.B., Knapp,J.I., Musick,A., Tannenbaum,J. *et al.* 1998. A large sample of finnish diabetic sib-pairs reveals no evidence for a non-insulin-dependent diabetes mellitus susceptibility locus at 2qter. *J.Clin.Invest* 102:704-709.
50. Hani,E.H., Hager,J., Philippi,A., Demenais,F., Froguel,P., and Vionnet,N. 1997. Mapping NIDDM susceptibility loci in French families: studies with markers in the region of NIDDM1 on chromosome 2q. *Diabetes* 46:1225-1226.
51. Vaxillaire,M., Boccio,V., Philippi,A., Vigouroux,C., Terwilliger,J., Passa,P., Beckmann,J.S., Velho,G., Lathrop,G.M., and Froguel,P. 1995. A gene for maturity onset diabetes of the young (MODY) maps to chromosome 12q. *Nat.Genet.* 9:418-423.
52. McCarthy M., Hattersley A., Walker M., Hitman G., Levy J., O'Rahilly S., Lathrop M., Simecek N., Wishart M., Dhillon R. *et al.* 2000. The British Diabetic Association Warren Type 2 Diabetes Sibpair Repository: interim report on a genome-wide scan for linkage in 439 European sibpair families. *Diabetes* 49:A199 (Abstr.)
53. Mitchell,B.D., Cole,S.A., Hsueh,W.C., Comuzzie,A.G., Blangero,J., MacCluer,J.W., and Hixson,J.E. 2000. Linkage of serum insulin concentrations to chromosome 3p in Mexican Americans. *Diabetes* 49:513-516.
54. Yamada,K., Yuan,X., Ishiyama,S., Koyama,K., Ichikawa,F., Koyanagi,A., Koyama,W., and Nonaka,K. 1997. Association between Ala54Thr substitution of the fatty acid-binding protein 2 gene with insulin resistance and intra-abdominal fat thickness in Japanese men. *Diabetologia* 40:706-710.

55. Sipilainen,R., Uusitupa,M., Heikkinen,S., Rissanen,A., and Laakso,M. 1997. Variants in the human intestinal fatty acid binding protein 2 gene in obese subjects. *J.Clin.Endocrinol.Metab* 82:2629-2632.
56. Hayakawa,T., Nagai,Y., Nohara,E., Yamashita,H., Takamura,T., Abe,T., Nomura,G., and Kobayashi,K. 1999. Variation of the fatty acid binding protein 2 gene is not associated with obesity and insulin resistance in Japanese subjects. *Metabolism* 48:655-657.
57. Baier,L.J., Sacchettini,J.C., Knowler,W.C., Eads,J., Paolisso,G., Tataranni,P.A., Mochizuki,H., Bennett,P.H., Bogardus,C., and Prochazka,M. 1995. An amino acid substitution in the human intestinal fatty acid binding protein is associated with increased fatty acid binding, increased fat oxidation, and insulin resistance. *J.Clin.Invest* 95:1281-1287.
58. Baier,L.J., Bogardus,C., and Sacchettini,J.C. 1996. A polymorphism in the human intestinal fatty acid binding protein alters fatty acid transport across Caco-2 cells. *J.Biol.Chem.* 271:10892-10896.
59. Horikawa,Y., Oda,N., Cox,N.J., Li,X., Orho-Melander,M., Hara,M., Hinokio,Y., Lindner,T.H., Mashima,H., Schwarz,P.E.H. *et al.* 2000. Genetic variation in the calpain 10 gene (CAPN10) is associated with type 2 diabetes. *Nat.Genet.* In press.
60. Cox,N.J., Frigge,M., Nicolae,D.L., Concannon,P., Hanis,C.L., Bell,G.I. , and Kong,A. 1999. Loci on chromosomes 2 (NIDDM1) and 15 interact to increase susceptibility to diabetes in Mexican Americans. *Nat.Genet.* 21:213-215.
61. Frayling T.M., Evans,J.C., Ellard,S., Hattersley,A.T., and Study Group - BDA Warren 2 Consortium . 2000. Transmission disequilibrium at the calpain 1-/NIDDM1 gene in UK Caucasian type 2 diabetes parent-offspring trios. *Diabetes* 49:A8 (Abstr.)
62. Garant, M., Kao, W. H. L., Brancati, F. L., Coresh, J., Hanis, C., Boerwinkle, E., and Shuldiner, A. R. SNP43 of calcium-activated neutral protease (CAPN10) is associated with type 2 diabetes in African Americans: the Atherosclerosis Risk in Communities (ARIC) Study. American Diabetes Association 60th Scientific Sessions, San Antonio, TX, June, 2000 (Poster)
63. Ren,Q., Hasstedt,S., Hanis,C., and Elbein,S.C. 2000. Increased transmission of NIDDM1 variant in Caucasian familial type 2 diabetes. *Diabetes* 49:A200 (Abstr.)

INDEX